SUPPORTIVE CARE
IN CANCER THERAPY

SUPPORTIVE CARE
IN CANCER THERAPY

Edited by

DAVID S. ETTINGER, MD
The Sidney Kimmel Comprehensive Cancer Center at Johns Hopkins,
Baltimore, MD, USA

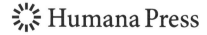 Humana Press

Editor
David S. Ettinger
Department of Oncology
The Sidney Kimmel Comprehensive
  Cancer Center at Johns Hopkins
Baltimore, MD, USA

Series Editor
Beverly A. Teicher
Genzyme Corporation
Framington, MA
USA

ISBN: 978-1-58829-941-3   e-ISBN: 978-1-59745-291-5
DOI: 10.1007/978-1-59745-291-5

Library of Congress Control Number: 2008936258

Printed on acid-free paper

9 8 7 6 5 4 3 2 1

springer.com

Dedication

To my wife Phyllis, whose love, understanding, guidance, and support has made me a better person and physician

Foreword

Patients with cancer, in general, are living longer. Even those with advanced, metastatic disease have shown an increase in the length of their survival. For many, cancer has become a "chronic" disease. This, in part, is due to better therapies, novel treatments, and the multimodality approaches to treating many cancers.

Supportive care of the cancer patient begins with the diagnosis of cancer and terminates with the end of life. The support given to the cancer patient is along a continuum of care whether or not the individual is actively being treated for the malignancy. The supportive care is for symptoms related to the cancer and/or its treatment; physical, psychosocial, and emotional issues associated with the cancer; and, finally, end-of-life decisions. In addition to the cancer patient, supportive care is also provided to family and caregivers of the patient.

As the population ages, cancer has become more prevalent. This book gives special consideration to older patients with cancer because of issues related to their frailty and comorbidities and the effect of these issues on treatment. Reflecting recognition of these needs, there is now an entire discipline called Geriatric Oncology.

In this volume, *Supportive Care in Cancer Therapy*, a part of the "Cancer Drug Discovery and Development" series, the contributors provide an up-to-date, concise review of specific consequences of cancer and its treatment. The chapters will allow the reader to better understand the sequelae associated with all aspects of cancer and how to treat them in order to achieve control of symptoms and provide psychosocial care to improve the quality of life of the cancer patient. In addition, the reader will gain information on the care of the older patient as well as the dying patient.

Chapters 1–6 (1 – Dyspnea, 2 – Skeletal Metastases, 3 – Cancer Pain, 4 – Anorexia and Cachexia, 5 – Fatigue, and 6 – Deep Vein Thrombophlebitis and Clotting Problems) deal with usual consequences of the cancer itself; in addition, the subjects addressed in Chapters 4–6 could also be associated with cancer therapy. Chapter 7 (Depression) is a common problem once the diagnosis of cancer is made. The problems discussed in Chapters 8–13 (8 – Anemia, 9 – Myeloid Growth Factors, 10 – Nausea and Vomiting, 11 – Oral Mucositis, 12 – Constipation and Diarrhea, and 13 – Menopausal Symptoms) for the most part are a consequence of treatment of cancer. Chapter 14, which deals with treating Elderly Patients with Cancer, has great significance as cancer in the older patient becomes more prevalent and older patients are considering the therapeutic options available to them. Chapter 15 (Complementary and Alternative Medicine) discusses therapies that more and more cancer patients want or about which they are seeking information. Chapter 16, the final chapter, deals with End-of-Life Decisions. As many cancers are or become advanced and terminal, this chapter provides the reader with a useful and thoughtful approach to dealing with patients, families, and caregivers when such decisions have to be made.

The contributors to this volume provide the reader with a clearly stated and understandable, practical review of issues relating to supportive care of the cancer patient. It is hoped that this book will assist those individuals whose challenge and privilege it is to care for the cancer patient to better understand all of the consequences of cancer and its treatment as well as how to apply this information to the treatment of their patients.

Baltimore, MD   *David S. Ettinger, MD*

Acknowledgement

To my administrative assistant, Angela Liggins, for all the hours she has spent making this book a reality and for the many years we have worked together as a team.

Contents

Contributors

YESNE ALICI-EVCIMEN • *Department of Psychiatry and Behavioral Sciences, Memorial Sloan-Kettering Cancer Center, New York, NY, USA*

LODOVICO BALDUCCI • *Department of Interdisciplinary Oncology, University of South Florida College of Medicine, and H. Lee Moffitt Cancer Center & Research Institute, Tampa, FL, USA*

ADITYA BARDIA • *Department of Internal Medicine, Mayo Clinic Cancer Center, Rochester, MN, USA*

DEBRA L. BARTON • *Department of Medical Oncology, Mayo Clinic Cancer Center, Rochester, MN, USA*

AL B. BENSON III • *Division of Hematology/Oncology, Robert H. Lurie Comprehensive Cancer Center of Northwestern University, Chicago, IL, USA*

BARRIE CASSILETH • *Integrative Medicine Service, Memorial Sloan-Kettering Cancer Center, New York, NY, USA*

SYDNEY MORSS DY • *Health Policy and Management, Johns Hopkins Bloomberg School of Public Health, Baltimore, MD, USA*

DAVID S. ETTINGER • *Department of Oncology, The Sidney Kimmel Comprehensive Cancer, Center at Johns Hopkins, Baltimore, MD, USA*

MICHAEL J. FISCH • *Community Clinical Oncology Program Research Base, M.D. Anderson Cancer Center, University of Texas, Houston, TX, USA*

STUART A. GROSSMAN • *Department of Oncology, The Sidney Kimmel Comprehensive Cancer, Center at Johns Hopkins, Baltimore, MD, USA*

JYOTHIRMAI GUBILI • *Integrative Medicine Service, Memorial Sloan-Kettering Cancer Center, New York, NY, USA*

JAMES F. HOLLAND • *Department of Medicine, Mount Sinai School of Medicine, New York, NY, USA*

JIMMIE C. HOLLAND • *Department of Psychiatry and Behavioral Sciences, Memorial Sloan-Kettering Center, New York, NY, USA*

JOHN KOSTEVA • *Department of Medicine, Fox Chase Cancer Center, Philadelphia, PA, USA*

COREY LANGER • *Department of Medicine, Fox Chase Cancer Center, Philadelphia, PA, USA*

TARA LIN • *Dept of Pediatrics, Division of Hematology/Oncology, David Geffen School of Medicine at UCLA, Los Angeles, CA, USA*

CHARLES LOPRINZI • *Department of Medical Oncology, Mayo Clinic Cancer Center, Rochester, MN, USA*

SUZANNE NESBIT • *Center for Cancer Pain Research, The Sidney Kimmel Comprehensive Cancer Center at Johns Hopkins, Baltimore, MD, USA*

TAKAO OHNUMA • *Department of Medicine, Mount Sinai School of Medicine, New York, NY, USA*

GEORGE M. RODGERS • *Division of Hematology, University of Utah Health Sciences Center, Salt Lake City, UT, USA*

STEPHEN SONIS • *Department of Oral Medicine, Brigham and Women's Hospital, Dana Farber Cancer Institute, Harvard School of Dental Medicine, Boston, MA, USA*

REGINA STEIN • *Division of Hematology/Oncology, Robert H. Lurie Comprehensive Cancer Center of Northwestern University, Chicago, IL, USA*

MICHAEL B. STREIFF • *Department of Oncology, Sidney Kimmel Comprehensive Cancer Center at Johns Hopkins, Baltimore, MD, USA*

JAY R. THOMAS • *San Diego Hospice & Palliative Care, University of California, San Diego School of Medicine, San Diego, CA, USA*

NATHANIAL TREISTER • *Department of Oral Medicine, Brigham and Women's Hospital, Dana Farber Cancer Institute, Harvard School of Dental Medicine, Boston, MA, USA*

1 Management of Dyspnea

Jay R. Thomas

ABSTRACT

Unfortunately, dyspnea is a common symptom in supportive care and the source of much suffering. As we understand more about the pathophysiology of dyspnea, we can better assess it, reverse its root causes when possible, and symptomatically treat it when reversal is not possible. This chapter focuses predominantly on the symptomatic relief of dyspnea. Because all interventions have benefits and burdens, any particular intervention must be assessed in the context of a patient's goals of care. Although invasive and pharmacologic interventions can be useful in many patients, because dyspnea is a subjective phenomenon, psychosocial/spiritual support is needed in all patients.

Key Words: Dyspnea; Cancer; Opioids; Supportive care; Palliative care; Management.

DEFINITION/EPIDEMIOLOGY

Dyspnea, most simply defined as an uncomfortable sensation or awareness of breathing, can be a very distressing symptom for many cancer patients and, concomitantly, for their caretakers. Because of the subjective nature of this perceived difficult breathing, there are no objective measures of dyspnea. It is not the respiratory rate, oxygen saturation, or pO_2 that defines dyspnea. Moreover, due to its subjective nature, psychological, social, and spiritual/existential issues can amplify the suffering a person experiences. As in the palliation of "total" pain or "total" suffering, optimal dyspnea

From: *Cancer and Drug Discovery Development: Supportive Care in Cancer Therapy*
DOI: 10.1007/978-1-59745-291-5_1, Edited by: D. S. Ettinger © Humana Press, Totowa, NJ

management requires understanding the patient as a whole person in addition to understanding the relevant physiology.

Dyspnea is a common complaint of patients with both cancer and non-cancer diagnoses. Seventy-one percent of terminally ill patients, in a representative sample population of 988 Americans being cared for in their homes, exhibited shortness of breath *(1)*. Among cancer patients, dyspnea prevalence ranges from 21 to 90%, depending on the severity of the underlying cancer and proximity to death *(2–4)*. While dyspnea may be expected in cases with primary or metastatic involvement of the lung, it is also a common complaint of patients with no direct lung involvement. Twenty-four percent of cancer patients in one study complained of dyspnea for which no cardiopulmonary pathology was determined *(4)*. Additionally, preexisting cardiopulmonary problems, such as chronic obstructive pulmonary disease (COPD) and congestive heart failure (CHF), common causes of chronic progressive dyspnea, are present in many patients diagnosed with cancer.

PATHOPHYSIOLOGY OF DYSPNEA

To better understand dyspnea, familiarity with the regulation of normal respiration is required. The respiratory center in the medulla and pons coordinates the activity of the diaphragm, the intercostal muscles, and accessory muscles of respiration (See Fig. 1). Although incompletely understood, the brain appears to receive and integrate the following information in the control of respiration:

1. Chemoreceptor detection of oxygen and carbon dioxide levels
2. The physical effort of breathing
3. Neuromechanical dissociation *(5, 6)*

Chemoreception

Oxygen and carbon dioxide levels are monitored by central and peripheral chemoreceptors. Detection of hypercapnia is the job of medullary chemoreceptors while carotid and aortic body chemoreceptors predominantly sense hypoxemia. Independent of increased respiratory effort, signals from these chemoreceptors can lead to dyspnea *(7, 8)*. Hypoxemia plays a much less significant role in dyspnea than is commonly assumed. Peripheral chemoreceptors require relatively severe levels of hypoxemia for activation *(9)*. Additionally, hypoxemia triggers a compensatory increase in ventilation that drives down the carbon dioxide level, partially negating the effect of the hypoxemia.

Effort of Breathing

Lung expansion and contractile force information is transmitted by peripheral mechanoreceptors in muscles, tendons, and joints. A feeling of dyspnea can be triggered by the increased effort required for breathing against increased resistance (e.g., COPD), or breathing with weakened muscles (e.g., neuromuscular disease or cachexia). This increased work of ventilation is relayed by mechanoreceptors to the central nervous system. Furthermore, dyspnea is enhanced by the efferent signals from the central nervous system that activate the breathing apparatus. There is evidence that these efferent signals are also delivered concurrently to the cortex where they presumably enhance the perception of breathlessness.

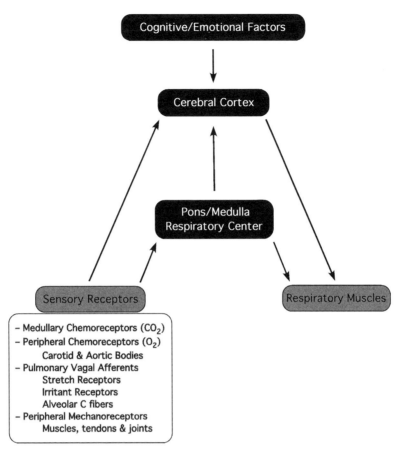

Fig. 1. Respiratory System Afferent and Efferent Signalling

Pulmonary vagal afferents are also involved in respiratory regulation: *(1)* pulmonary stretch receptors are activated by lung inflation, *(2)* pulmonary irritant receptors are triggered by specific chemicals, airflow, and smooth muscle tone, and *(3)* alveolar C fibers respond to pulmonary interstitial and capillary pressure.

Pulmonary afferents may also transmit information directly to the cerebral cortex. The possible role of vagal afferents is elucidated by an experiment comparing dyspnea induced by bronchoconstriction to dyspnea induced by an external increase in breathing load *(10)*. In both cases, the work of breathing was similar but bronchoconstriction induced greater dyspnea. Inhaled lidocaine blocked dyspnea from bronchoconstriction; however, dyspnea from external resistance was not relieved. This result implicates pulmonary afferent involvement in some causes of dyspnea.

Neuromechanical Dissociation

Lastly, the theory of neuromechanical dissociation describes dyspnea as occurring when there is a discrepancy between the brain's expectations for respiration and the sensory feedback it receives *(11)*. One study artificially limited the inspiratory flow rate of subjects, resulting in dyspnea even though there was no change in respiratory work or chemical status *(12)*.

Clinical Causes of Cancer-Related Dyspnea

Potentially there are multiple, independent, and synergistic mechanisms that can trigger dyspnea. Dudgeon and Lertzman *(13)* performed a prospective analysis of 100 advanced cancer patients with dyspnea in an attempt to better understand its causes. They found that 49% had lung cancer; 65% had lung or pleural involvement; 40% were hypoxemic with O_2 saturation < 90%; 12% had $Pa_{CO2} \geq 45$ mmHg; 52% had a component of bronchospasm; 29% had evidence of cardiac ischemia, CHF, or atrial fibrillation; and 20% were anemic with a hemoglobin concentration less than 10 g%. Pulmonary function tests revealed that 5% had an obstructive pattern, 41% had a restrictive pattern, and 47% had mixed obstructive/restrictive pattern. The median maximum inspiratory pressure (MIP) was −16 cm H_2O (normal $\geq$ −50 cm H_2O), indicating that respiratory muscle weakness was significant. None of their patients had received chemotherapy that can cause pulmonary disease but 40% had radiation therapy that included at least a portion of the lungs. Not surprisingly, the average tally of potential causes of dyspnea per patient was five. Although this study is small, limiting its ability to be generalized, it implies that the cause of dyspnea is often multifactorial in cancer patients.

This multifactorial nature is an important consideration in the consideration of potential interventions. While a particular intervention may reduce one contributor to dyspnea, the overall clinical impact depends on the remaining causative factors. As an illustration, a thoracentesis may not necessarily bring relief from dyspnea despite the presence of an identifiable pleural effusion; other sources may be more significant in a particular patient. Therefore, the invasiveness of potential interventions must be weighed against the patient's goals of care and the likelihood of benefit.

The Language of Dyspnea

Given the multiple potential etiologies for dyspnea, there may qualitatively be different types of dyspnea. Based on patient questionnaires, there appear to be different descriptors of dyspnea that may relate to the mechanistic trigger. For example, the bronchospasm of asthma is often characterized as "tightness" whereas hypercapnia is often described as "air hunger" *(7, 14, 15)*. Further study will determine the reliability of this descriptive/mechanistic relationship and its potential use in treatment selection.

Cortical Involvement in the Perception of Dyspnea

To explore the link between cortical activity and perception of dyspnea, researchers are using the functional brain imaging techniques – positron emission tomography (PET) and functional magnetic resonance imaging (fMRI) *(16–21)*. The anterior insula, part of the limbic system, is implicated in all studies to date. Neural connections between the medullary respiratory center and the cortex, including the anterior insula, have been identified in animal studies *(22)*. Neural signals from the respiratory center may simultaneously activate respiratory muscles and targets in the anterior insula, leading to conscious perceptions of breathing. It is of note that the perception of pain, hunger, and thirst also map to the anterior insula *(23–29)* . This leads to speculation on the nature of the perception of unpleasant sensations, suggesting there may be a common final pathway.

DYSPNEA ASSESSMENT AND IDENTIFICATION OF ETIOLOGIES

As in all medical conditions, the history and physical examination are key elements to diagnosis and treatment. The only accurate measure of dyspnea is patient self-report. Validated scales such as a visual analog scale *(30)* or the Borg scale *(31)* are clinically useful to quantify dyspnea and assess palliation. Objective measures such as respiratory rate or arterial blood gas levels may suggest dyspnea and identify potential etiologies, but they are not direct measures. For example, a well-palliated, alert patient with multiple potential causes of dyspnea may report no sense of dyspnea despite being hypoxic, tachypneic, and "looking dyspneic." Therefore it is important for healthcare providers not to treat the look or sounds, but to carefully assess a patient's perceptions. Especially as advanced illness progresses and death approaches, common breathing patterns are encountered, such as Cheynes-Stokes breathing and the breathing sounds associated with terminal secretions (colloquially referred to as the "death rattle"). Loved ones often interpret these patterns as dyspnea and suffering for the patient. However, despite these appearances, there may be no dyspnea or suffering if the patient has been well palliated or is comatose. Educating loved ones to these facts may be a vital intervention. Moreover, since dyspnea is subjective, cognitive and emotional factors may exacerbate it. Thus, the history should also include an assessment of a patient's psychosocial and spiritual stressors. Understanding the meaning the dyspnea has for the patient or how it affects quality of life may be important in treating dyspnea and strengthening the therapeutic alliance.

To identify underlying etiologies for dyspnea, critical diagnostic clues may be obtained from previous medical history, smoking history, occupational history, and knowledge of prior radiation or chemotherapy treatments. Simple studies such as pulse oximetry, complete blood count, and chest X-ray, in conjunction with physical examination, are generally sufficient to clarify the pertinent pathophysiology. Additional studies may be warranted if the possible benefits of further investigation exceed the burdens. These may include arterial blood gas determinations, pulmonary function tests, CAT scans, echocardiograms, or ventilation-perfusion scans.

This thorough evaluation may allow us to identify and treat the underlying causes of dyspnea. Common causes for dyspnea associated with both malignant and nonmalignant processes are listed in Table 1. Description of evidence-based interventions to reverse these etiologies is beyond the scope of this chapter.

Overall, the approach to treatment of dyspnea in supportive care is largely determined by the individual patient's goals of care. Tests and procedures to reverse sources of dyspnea may be justified if they have a reasonable probability of promoting palliation, enhancing quality of life, and if within the parameters of these goals. For example, if a patient has a malignant effusion and obtains relief from a therapeutic thoracentesis, it may be appropriate to proceed to pleurodesis. However, if dyspnea does not improve with a trial thoracentesis, it may be better to palliate the patient through other means,

Table 1
Causes of Dyspnea

Directly related to cancer	Indirectly related to cancer
Primary/metastatic parenchymal lung involvement	Pneumonia
Airway obstruction (intrinsic or extrinsic tumor)	Cachexia
Carcinomatous lymphangitis	Anemia
Pleural tumor	Electrolyte abnormalities
Malignant pleural effusion	Pulmonary embolus
Malignant pericardial effusion	Paraneoplastic syndromes
Superior vena cava syndrome	Ascites
Tumor microemboli	Unrelated to cancer
Phrenic nerve paralysis	Chronic obstructive pulmonary disease
Atelectasis	Asthma
Tracheal esophageal fistula	Congestive heart failure
Chest wall invasion (carcinoma en cuirasse)	Cardiac ischemia
Pathologic chest wall fractures	Arrhythmias
Related to cancer therapy	Pulmonary vascular disease
Surgery (postlobectomy/pneumonectomy)	Obesity
Radiation pneumonitis	Neuromuscular disorders
Chemotherapy-induced pulmonary fibrosis	Aspiration
Chemotherapy-induced cardiomyopathy	Anxiety
	Pneumothorax
	Interstitial lung disease
	Psychosocial/spiritual pain

rather than subjecting them to a painful procedure such as pleurodesis that requires hospitalization and time away from other important life pursuits. Thus, the burdens and benefits of every intervention must be carefully individualized and weighed. Even when the decision has been made to attempt to reverse an underlying cause, every effort should be made to palliate dyspnea while waiting for etiologies to be reversed. Unfortunately, many times, the causes of dyspnea are not reversible or their reversal may not be able to restore a patient to what they define as quality of life. In these circumstances, workup and treatment of potential etiologies may not be appropriate. The primary objective may be symptomatic relief of dyspnea.

SYMPTOMATIC MANAGEMENT OF DYSPNEA

Oxygen

Some practitioners use oxygen as a first-line treatment for dyspnea independent of the etiology. Frequently, patients report improved dyspnea with oxygen even though they are not hypoxemic or when they remain hypoxemic despite oxygen. The placebo effect may be a partial explanation for this observation, potentially due to the medical symbolism inherent in the use of oxygen. Another explanation derives from studies demonstrating that stimulation of the trigeminal nerve (V2 branch) dampens dyspnea *(32–34)*. In experimental subjects with induced dyspnea, cool, moving air directed at the cheek or nasal mucosa is shown to relieve dyspnea and/or decrease ventilatory response to provocation. This result is consistent with the clinical observation that a fan blowing air across a patient's face may improve dyspnea.

In patients suffering from both hypoxemia and dyspnea, the use of oxygen to treat both conditions is reasonable. If dyspnea is unrelieved, continuation of oxygen administration may not necessarily be indicated just to treat the oxygen levels. The decision to use oxygen must be made on an individual basis. In COPD patients with hypoxemia, mortality may decrease with oxygen treatment, but quality of life is not significantly affected. Use of oxygen is not universally recommended for dyspnea unless the benefits outweigh the burdens. Oxygen is costly, explosive, restricts mobility, affects self-image, and may cause CO_2 retention in some patients. As an alternative, and independent of dyspnea etiology, a fan that provides cool, moving air across the trigeminal nerve distribution may provide some relief.

Anxiolytics

Anxiety often accompanies dyspnea, and benzodiazepines are frequently prescribed to alleviate this symptom complex. In general, however, the data do not support the use of benzodiazepines alone as a first line therapy for dyspnea.

Moderate doses of diazepam improved dyspnea in a placebo-controlled single-blind study of COPD patients, but the sample size was only four *(35)*. Subsequently, double-blind studies on both healthy subjects and COPD patients, using diazepam or alprazolam, found them no more effective than placebo *(36, 37, 38)*. Anxiety was correlated with dyspnea by Dudgeon and Lertzman *(13)*, but in their multivariate model, anxiety accounted for only 10% of the variance of dyspnea.

Opioid use, as detailed below, may reduce or remove the perception of dyspnea, and therefore relieve anxiety for many patients. Despite appropriate opioid dosing, some patients may nevertheless continue to suffer from anxiety, possibly due to an underlying anxiety disorder. For such cases, it is both safe and reasonable to coadminister benzodiazepines and opioids. There is no danger of respiratory depression if dosing guidelines are carefully followed. According to a recent single-blind study, midazolam 5 mg SC synergizes with opioids, enhancing the palliation of severe dyspnea in patients with advanced cancer *(39)*.

Studies have also focused on other psychoactive agents. Conflicting results were obtained in two studies using buspirone, a nonbenzodiazepine, hence no recommendations can be made *(40, 41)*. Chlorpromazine, a major tranquilizer, was studied in a small randomized, double-blind trial in healthy volunteers at a dosage of 25 mg orally *(42)*. Dyspnea was significantly reduced compared to placebo without an increase in sedation. Larger studies will be needed to clarify the role of chlorpromazine in the symptomatic treatment of dyspnea. It would be a rational choice for use in dyspneic patients also suffering from psychosis or delirium.

Opioids

The recommended first line therapy for the symptomatic relief of dyspnea is opioids. Though the mechanism of action is not well understood, opioid use is supported by empirical observation and emerging knowledge of the opioid system. Both the central and peripheral nervous systems are known to have mu receptors, the most clinically relevant opioid receptor. Functional brain imaging techniques mentioned previously have implicated the anterior insula region in the perception of dyspnea. Analogously, the same region of the brain appears to be involved in the perception of pain and other suffering. Thus, opioid action may alleviate dyspnea and pain via similar mechanisms altering perception of noxious stimuli. The lungs are also known to contain opioid receptors, notably concentrated in the alveoli, although their role in dyspnea remains controversial *(43)*.

What is known of the involvement of endogenous opioids in the control of dyspnea? In one experiment, opioid-naïve normal volunteers were exerted to the point of dyspnea *(44)*. A systemically acting opioid antagonist, naloxone, was administered intravenously, resulting in an exacerbation of dyspnea. This effect of opioid antagonism implies that dyspnea is normally diminished by endogenous opioids.

Moreover, multiple studies in multiple clinical populations support the safety and effectiveness of opioids in the control of dyspnea.

Bruera et al. demonstrated opioid relief of dyspnea, without a decrease in oxygen saturation or respiratory rate, in a placebo-controlled crossover study in cancer patients *(45)*. Patients were using opioids for pain with tolerable pain control at baseline, but were dyspneic at rest. Increasing the opioid dose was effective in the relief of dyspnea even within a background of chronic opioid use for pain. Furthermore, as little as 5 mg of subcutaneous morphine sulfate was effective in controlling dyspnea in patients that were opioid-naïve at baseline *(46)*. Consistent with morphine's half-life and kinetics of pain relief, the opioid-mediated control of dyspnea persisted for 4 h. In cancer patients, a 25% increase in the baseline opioid pain dose also provided relief of dyspnea for up to 4 h, as shown by Allard et al. *(47)*.

As stated previously, cancer patients often have comorbid conditions that predispose to dyspnea such as CHF and COPD. The use of opioids to relieve dyspnea in opioid-naïve CHF patients has been investigated in three small randomized, double-blind placebo-controlled studies. New York Heart Association (NYHA) class II or III patients with an average ejection fraction of 21.3%, despite a proper medical regimen, were studied by Chua et al. *(48)*. Patients receiving a single oral dose of dihydrocodeine (1 mg/kg) had better exercise tolerance with less dyspnea compared to placebo 1 h after dosing. Williams et al. looked at bolus dosing with intravenous diamorphine (1 or 2 mg) versus placebo just before exercise *(49)*. Diamorphine yielded a significant improvement in aerobic exercise capacity in CHF patients with an average ejection fraction of 35.5%, without suppressing respirations. Stable NYHA class III or IV patients on appropriate medical regimens were treated by Johnson et al. with either placebo or morphine, 5 mg orally four times daily over 4 days, using a cross-over study design *(50)*. Morphine, at steady state, significantly reduced breathlessness on a visual analogue scale without depression of respiration. Chronic opioid treatment was beneficial to several patients who remained on opioids after conclusion of the study.

Opioids have also been used effectively in COPD patients for treatment of dyspnea. Opioid-naïve COPD patients in one study, having an average FEV_1 (forced expiratory volume in one second) of 0.99 L, $Pa_{CO2} < 46$ mmHg, and $Pa_{O2} > 55$ mmHg, were given a single dose of oral morphine (0.8 mg/kg) prior to exercise *(51)*. The typical starting dose of 2.5–5 mg oral morphine for a COPD patient is several fold smaller than this 0.8 mg/kg dosing, for which a 70-kg patient would receive 56 mg of morphine. Despite the large dose, respiration was not suppressed in a life-threatening way, although there was an increase in Pa_{CO2} and decrease in Pa_{O2}. Both exercise tolerance and dyspnea were improved. Another study group was comprised primarily of COPD patients (88%) who were dyspneic at rest despite maximal medical therapy *(52)*. In this randomized, double-blind, placebo-controlled crossover trial, opioid-naïve patients received either placebo or 20 mg of sustained release morphine per day over 4 days. Abernathy et al. show that at steady state, morphine significantly decreased visual analogue scores for dyspnea compared to placebo controls, also without respiratory suppression.

Due to the small sample size in most studies of opioid treatment of dyspnea, generalizability can be questioned. A systematic meta-analysis of previously published studies has been performed by Jennings et al. to address this problem *(53)*. This review assesses the efficacy of opioids in treating dyspnea from any cause, including in the analysis only double-blind, randomized, placebo-controlled studies. Nine studies using parenteral or oral opioids (1 for cancer, 1 for CHF, and 7 for COPD), and 9 studies using nebulized opioids (1 for cancer, 7 for COPD, and 1 for interstitial lung disease) were examined. The meta-analysis demonstrated a statistically significant improvement in dyspnea. The COPD studies alone were analyzed as a subgroup, and they also demonstrated the efficacy of opioids for dyspnea relief. In all studies, opioids caused no deaths; however, common opioid side effects such as nausea, lethargy, and constipation were present. Tolerance typically develops to these side effects, with the exception of constipation, but they are predictable and should be treated proactively when chronic opioids are prescribed. Patients should be monitored for severe adverse events; however, the half-life of short-acting opioids ensures that any adverse event is equally short-lived. In the rare circumstances where adverse events are severe, we also have highly effective specific antagonists as antidotes to quickly reverse any deleterious effects.

Overall, a rational approach to the control of chronic dyspnea might therefore include both a sustained release opioid for baseline control and an immediate release opioid for breakthrough dyspnea, comparable to chronic pain regimens. For an opioid-naïve patient, a reasonable starting dose might be 2.5–5-mg oral morphine equivalent. Maximal clinical response will be evident after waiting for the appropriate amount of time to reach maximal serum concentrations (T_{max}). For hydrophilic opioids, such as morphine, oxycodone, or hydromorphone, oral T_{max} is ~1 h, subcutaneous T_{max} is ~30 min, and IV T_{max} is ~6 min. If dyspnea is not tolerable at this time to C_{max}, the dose can rationally and safely be repeated. In fact, if dyspnea still remains mild to moderate, the dose could be titrated up to 25–50%. If the dyspnea remains moderate to severe, the dose could be titrated up to 50–100%. In this manner, many patients can be acutely titrated to a tolerable level of dyspnea. Twenty-four-hour opioid requirements can then be tallied and converted to a long-acting opioid regimen. To treat breakthrough dyspnea, analogously to breakthrough pain, 5–15% of the 24-h opioid dose can be provided orally every hour (the oral T_{max}) as needed.

Nebulized Opioids

In contrast to the efficacy of systemically acting opioids, a subgroup analysis in the previously cited meta-analysis of studies using nebulized opioids failed to demonstrate any significant benefit despite known lung opioid receptors and anecdotal reports that nebulized opioids improve dyspnea. Opioid antagonists that act exclusively peripherally may help to elucidate the role of opioid receptors outside the central nervous system (CNS), particularly in the lung. Certain antagonists are unable to cross the blood–brain barrier, making it possible to block lung opioid receptors without affecting those in the CNS. In this manner, it will be possible to determine the contribution, if any, of the lung opioid receptors. Two such peripheral antagonists, methylnaltrexone and alvimopan, are currently undergoing clinical trials for opioid-induced constipation. Anecdotally, the author has treated several patients on opioids at least partially for dyspnea, who had opioid-induced constipation. When treated with subcutaneous methylnaltrexone, successful laxation occurred, implying successful antagonism at gastrointestinal mu receptors; however, there was no observed worsening of dyspnea. Presumably, lung mu receptors should have been antagonized as well and the lack of any effect raises the possibility that lung mu receptors play little if any role in the palliation of dyspnea. However, definitive conclusions await formal controlled trials.

Lidocaine

Inhaled lidocaine has been shown to decrease dyspnea that is experimentally induced by bronchoconstriction, as previously cited *(10)*. Lidocaine did not, however, prove more effective than saline placebo in small studies of patients with interstitial lung disease *(54)* and cancer *(55)*. It is possible that only certain subsets of dyspnea are responsive to inhaled lidocaine, but larger studies would be required to discover a clinical role for lidocaine in dyspnea treatment.

Furosemide

Nebulized furosemide has been noted in case reports to relieve severe dyspnea in cancer patients *(56, 57)*. In rat studies, nebulized furosemide increased the activity of pulmonary stretch receptors *(58)*. Manning et al. showed that increased activity of these stretch receptors can diminish dyspnea in humans *(59)*. Nebulized furosemide (40 mg) was partially effective in relieving dyspnea in human clinical trials where dyspnea was experimentally induced *(60, 61)*. Although diuresis was not noted in the case studies, Moosavi et al. observed clinically significant diuresis in their experimental setting. Although more studies in patients with dyspnea are needed, there is mounting evidence that nebulized furosemide may be an effective adjunct to the treatment of dyspnea.

NONPHARMACOLOGIC THERAPIES

Cognitive/Behavioral Interventions

Dyspnea occurs, not in a void, but in the context of a whole person. The philosophy behind supportive and palliative care is that optimal treatment of symptoms, including dyspnea, requires an understanding of the psychological, social, and spiritual/existential milieu of the individual. Resolution of psycho/social issues and problems may enhance the relief of physical symptoms. Assisting patients and families with education, practical care issues, interpersonal relationships, coping with fears, redefining meaning and hope, and attaining a self-defined sense of peace despite illness, are all part of palliation. Addressing the many facets of life, and death, requires the expertise of an interdisciplinary team. Clinical studies are beginning to support this concept.

One multicenter, randomized, controlled trial evaluated the effectiveness of nurse-run clinics for lung cancer patients with dyspnea *(62)*. This approach is similar to that used in pulmonary rehabilitation clinics for COPD patients, which have also been shown to improve quality of life and function *(63)*. Interventions consisted of instruction in breathing control, activity pacing, relaxation techniques, and support for psychosocial issues. Patients randomized to the intervention had better dyspnea scores, performance status, and emotional states than controls.

Integrative Therapies

Integrative therapies, formerly known as complementary or alternative medicine, have been widely used for the treatment of many different conditions. Pan et al. have performed a systematic review of integrative therapies for several symptoms including dyspnea *(64)*. Both acupuncture *(65)* and acupressure *(66)*, in single-blind randomized controlled trials of COPD patients, significantly relieved dyspnea compared to sham interventions. Whether acupuncture or other integrative therapies will attain significant roles in the control of dyspnea depends on the outcome of more comprehensive future studies.

Noninvasive Positive Pressure Ventilation (NIPPV)

NIPPV has been used in cases of respiratory failure due to neuromuscular disease *(67–69)*, COPD *(70)*, and cancer *(71)*. In certain stages of a chronic condition such as amyotrophic lateral sclerosis, and in some acute, reversible clinical situations such as a COPD exacerbation, or pneumonia in a cancer patient, there may be some advantage to the use of NIPPV. Patients may be restored to a better quality of life or enabled to achieve short-term goals. This benefit must be carefully weighed against the burdens of the intervention for each individual. The role NIPPV will play in supportive care remains to be determined.

REFRACTORY DYSPNEA

Unfortunately, some patients may have dyspnea that is refractory to all interventions. In these rare cases, in end-of-life care, palliative sedation is an ethical and legal option with the patient's or surrogate's informed consent. In these cases, sedation is titrated to reduce consciousness to the point that suffering is no longer perceived. An international multicenter survey found that of the cases of sedation on inpatient palliative care services, dyspnea was the precipitating cause ranging from 25 to 53% of the time *(72)*. The principle of double effect is often used to support the use of palliative sedation for refractory suffering. This principle states that if the primary intent of an action is to reduce suffering, even if as an unintended secondary consequence death is hastened, that action remains ethical. Sykes and Thorns argue that in practice the principle of double effect rarely needs to be invoked *(73)*. In their study, they looked at the use of sedation in the last week of life on an inpatient palliative care service. They found that sedation was not correlated with shorter survival and therefore was not hastening death.

SUMMARY

Dyspnea is a subjective phenomenon that can only be quantified through patient self-report. The physiologic triggers for dyspnea include chemical signals (hypoxemia and hypercapnia), the work of breathing, and neuromechanical dissociation. A patient's goals of care dictate the workup and treatment of dyspnea. Sometimes reversible causes can be identified and treated. While waiting for resolution of causes, if causes are irreversible, or attempts to reverse causes are not consistent with a patient's goals, symptomatic relief of dyspnea may be the focus of care. Opioids are the first line therapy for the symptomatic relief of dyspnea. When prescribed appropriately, they are safe and effective for palliating dyspnea. Other pharmacologic agents (e.g., anxiolytics), nonpharmacologic interventions (e.g., a fan blowing air over the trigeminal nerve distribution), and oxygen (in cases of hypoxemia) may also be important adjuncts to opioids. However, optimal control of dyspnea requires an understanding of the patient as a whole person, and all sources of suffering including psychosocial/spiritual issues must be addressed. Occasionally, sedation is required to relieve the suffering from dyspnea. If relief of suffering is the primary intent, sedation is ethical and legal. Moreover, there is evidence that sedation does not in fact hasten death in the majority of cases.

REFERENCES

1. Emanuel EJ, Fairclough DL, Slutsman J, Emanuel LL. Understanding economic and other burdens of terminal illness: the experience of patients and their caregivers. Ann Intern Med 2000;132(6):451–9.
2. Muers MF, Round CE. Palliation of symptoms in non-small cell lung cancer: a study by the Yorkshire Regional Cancer Organisation Thoracic Group. Thorax 1993;48(4):339–43.
3. Higginson I, McCarthy M. Measuring symptoms in terminal cancer: are pain and dyspnoea controlled? J R Soc Med 1989;82(5):264–7.
4. Reuben DB, Mor V. Dyspnea in terminally ill cancer patients. Chest 1986;89(2):234–6.
5. Manning HL, Schwartzstein RM. Pathophysiology of dyspnea. N Engl J Med 1995;333(23):1547–53.
6. Dyspnea. Mechanisms, assessment, and management: a consensus statement. American Thoracic Society. Am J Respir Crit Care Med 1999;159(1):321–40.
7. Banzett RB, Lansing RW, Reid MB, Adams L, Brown R. 'Air hunger' arising from increased PCO2 in mechanically ventilated quadriplegics. Respir Physiol 1989;76(1):53–67.
8. Lane R, Cockcroft A, Adams L, Guz A. Arterial oxygen saturation and breathlessness in patients with chronic obstructive airways disease. Clin Sci (Lond) 1987;72(6):693–8.
9. Eyzaguirre C, Zapata P. Perspectives in carotid body research. J Appl Physiol 1984;57(4):931–57.
10. Taguchi O, Kikuchi Y, Hida W, et al. Effects of bronchoconstriction and external resistive loading on the sensation of dyspnea. J Appl Physiol 1991;71(6):2183–90.
11. O'Donnell DE, Webb KA. Exertional breathlessness in patients with chronic airflow limitation. The role of lung hyperinflation. Am Rev Respir Dis 1993;148(5):1351–7.
12. Manning HL, Molinary EJ, Leiter JC. Effect of inspiratory flow rate on respiratory sensation and pattern of breathing. Am J Respir Crit Care Med 1995;151(3 Pt 1):751–7.
13. Dudgeon DJ, Lertzman M. Dyspnea in the advanced cancer patient. J Pain Symptom Manage 1998;16(4):212–19.
14. Simon PM, Schwartzstein RM, Weiss JW, Fencl V, Teghtsoonian M, Weinberger SE. Distinguishable types of dyspnea in patients with shortness of breath. Am Rev Respir Dis 1990;142(5):1009–14.
15. Binks AP, Moosavi SH, Banzett RB, Schwartzstein RM. "Tightness" sensation of asthma does not arise from the work of breathing. Am J Respir Crit Care Med 2002;165(1):78–82.

16. Evans KC, Banzett RB, Adams L, McKay L, Frackowiak RS, Corfield DR. BOLD fMRI identifies limbic, paralimbic, and cerebellar activation during air hunger. J Neurophysiol 2002;88(3):1500–11.
17. Banzett RB, Mulnier HE, Murphy K, Rosen SD, Wise RJ, Adams L. Breathlessness in humans activates insular cortex. Neuroreport 2000;11(10):2117–20.
18. Brannan S, Liotti M, Egan G, et al. Neuroimaging of cerebral activations and deactivations associated with hypercapnia and hunger for air. Proc Natl Acad Sci U S A 2001;98(4):2029–34.
19. Liotti M, Brannan S, Egan G, et al. Brain responses associated with consciousness of breathlessness (air hunger). Proc Natl Acad Sci U S A 2001;98(4):2035–40.
20. Parsons LM, Egan G, Liotti M, et al. Neuroimaging evidence implicating cerebellum in the experience of hypercapnia and hunger for air. Proc Natl Acad Sci U S A 2001;98(4):2041–6.
21. Peiffer C, Poline JB, Thivard L, Aubier M, Samson Y. Neural substrates for the perception of acutely induced dyspnea. Am J Respir Crit Care Med 2001;163(4):951–7.
22. Gaytan SP, Pasaro R. Connections of the rostral ventral respiratory neuronal cell group: an anterograde and retrograde tracing study in the rat. Brain Res Bull 1998;47(6):625–42.
23. Baciu MV, Bonaz BL, Papillon E, et al. Central processing of rectal pain: a functional MR imaging study. AJNR Am J Neuroradiol 1999;20(10):1920–4.
24. Binkofski F, Schnitzler A, Enck P, et al. Somatic and limbic cortex activation in esophageal distention: a functional magnetic resonance imaging study. Ann Neurol 1998;44(5):811–15.
25. Derbyshire SW, Jones AK, Gyulai F, Clark S, Townsend D, Firestone LL. Pain processing during three levels of noxious stimulation produces differential patterns of central activity. Pain 1997;73(3):431–45.
26. Iadarola MJ, Berman KF, Zeffiro TA, et al. Neural activation during acute capsaicin-evoked pain and allodynia assessed with PET. Brain 1998;121(Pt 5):931–47.
27. Peyron R, Garcia-Larrea L, Gregoire MC, et al. Haemodynamic brain responses to acute pain in humans: sensory and attentional networks. Brain 1999;122(Pt 9):1765–80.
28. Denton D, Shade R, Zamarippa F, et al. Correlation of regional cerebral blood flow and change of plasma sodium concentration during genesis and satiation of thirst. Proc Natl Acad Sci U S A 1999;96(5):2532–7.
29. Tataranni PA, Gautier JF, Chen K, et al. Neuroanatomical correlates of hunger and satiation in humans using positron emission tomography. Proc Natl Acad Sci U S A 1999;96(8):4569–74.
30. Adams L, Chronos N, Lane R, Guz A. The measurement of breathlessness induced in normal subjects: validity of two scaling techniques. Clin Sci (Lond) 1985;69(1):7–16.
31. Borg GA. Psychophysical bases of perceived exertion. Med Sci Sports Exerc 1982;14(5):377–81.
32. Schwartzstein RM, Lahive K, Pope A, Weinberger SE, Weiss JW. Cold facial stimulation reduces breathlessness induced in normal subjects. Am Rev Respir Dis 1987;136(1):58–61.
33. Liss HP, Grant BJ. The effect of nasal flow on breathlessness in patients with chronic obstructive pulmonary disease. Am Rev Respir Dis 1988;137(6):1285–8.
34. Burgess KR, Whitelaw WA. Effects of nasal cold receptors on pattern of breathing. J Appl Physiol 1988;64(1):371–6.
35. Mitchell-Heggs P, Murphy K, Minty K, et al. Diazepam in the treatment of dyspnoea in the 'Pink Puffer' syndrome. Q J Med 1980;49(193):9–20.
36. Stark RD, Gambles SA, Lewis JA. Methods to assess breathlessness in healthy subjects: a critical evaluation and application to analyse the acute effects of diazepam and promethazine on breathlessness induced by exercise or by exposure to raised levels of carbon dioxide. Clin Sci (Lond) 1981;61(4):429–39.
37. Woodcock AA, Gross ER, Geddes DM. Drug treatment of breathlessness: contrasting effects of diazepam and promethazine in pink puffers. Br Med J (Clin Res Ed) 1981;283(6287):343–6.
38. Man GC, Hsu K, Sproule BJ. Effect of alprazolam on exercise and dyspnea in patients with chronic obstructive pulmonary disease. Chest 1986;90(6):832–6.
39. Navigante AH, Cerchietti LC, Castro MA, Lutteral MA, Cabalar ME. Midazolam as adjunct therapy to morphine in the alleviation of severe dyspnea perception in patients with advanced cancer. J Pain Symptom Manage 2006;31(1):38–47.
40. Argyropoulou P, Patakas D, Koukou A, Vasiliadis P, Georgopoulos D. Buspirone effect on breathlessness and exercise performance in patients with chronic obstructive pulmonary disease. Respiration 1993;60(4):216–20.
41. Singh NP, Despars JA, Stansbury DW, Avalos K, Light RW. Effects of buspirone on anxiety levels and exercise tolerance in patients with chronic airflow obstruction and mild anxiety. Chest 1993;103(3):800–4.
42. O'Neill PA, Morton PB, Stark RD. Chlorpromazine – a specific effect on breathlessness? Br J Clin Pharmacol 1985;19(6):793–7.
43. Zebraski SE, Kochenash SM, Raffa RB. Lung opioid receptors: pharmacology and possible target for nebulized morphine in dyspnea. Life Sci 2000;66(23):2221–31.
44. Akiyama Y, Nishimura M, Kobayashi S, et al. Effects of naloxone on the sensation of dyspnea during acute respiratory stress in normal adults. J Appl Physiol 1993;74(2):590–5.

45. Bruera E, MacEachern T, Ripamonti C, Hanson J. Subcutaneous morphine for dyspnea in cancer patients. Ann Intern Med 1993;119(9):906–7.
46. Mazzocato C, Buclin T, Rapin CH. The effects of morphine on dyspnea and ventilatory function in elderly patients with advanced cancer: a randomized double-blind controlled trial. Ann Oncol 1999;10(12): 1511–14.
47. Allard P, Lamontagne C, Bernard P, Tremblay C. How effective are supplementary doses of opioids for dyspnea in terminally ill cancer patients? A randomized continuous sequential clinical trial. J Pain Symptom Manage 1999;17(4):256–65.
48. Chua TP, Harrington D, Ponikowski P, Webb-Peploe K, Poole-Wilson PA, Coats AJ. Effects of dihydrocodeine on chemosensitivity and exercise tolerance in patients with chronic heart failure. J Am Coll Cardiol 1997;29(1):147–52.
49. Williams SG, Wright DJ, Marshall P, et al. Safety and potential benefits of low dose diamorphine during exercise in patients with chronic heart failure. Heart 2003;89(9):1085–6.
50. Johnson MJ, McDonagh TA, Harkness A, McKay SE, Dargie HJ. Morphine for the relief of breathlessness in patients with chronic heart failure – a pilot study. Eur J Heart Fail 2002;4(6):753–6.
51. Light RW, Muro JR, Sato RI, Stansbury DW, Fischer CE, Brown SE. Effects of oral morphine on breathlessness and exercise tolerance in patients with chronic obstructive pulmonary disease. Am Rev Respir Dis 1989;139(1):126–33.
52. Abernethy AP, Currow DC, Frith P, Fazekas BS, McHugh A, Bui C. Randomised, double blind, placebo-controlled crossover trial of sustained release morphine for the management of refractory dyspnoea. BMJ 2003;327(7414):523–8.
53. Jennings AL, Davies AN, Higgins JP, Gibbs JS, Broadley KE. A systematic review of the use of opioids in the management of dyspnoea. Thorax 2002;57(11):939–44.
54. Winning AJ, Hamilton RD, Guz A. Ventilation and breathlessness on maximal exercise in patients with interstitial lung disease after local anaesthetic aerosol inhalation. Clin Sci (Lond) 1988;74(3):275–81.
55. Wilcock A, Corcoran R, Tattersfield AE. Safety and efficacy of nebulized lignocaine in patients with cancer and breathlessness. Palliat Med 1994;8(1):35–8.
56. Stone P, Kurowska A, Tookman A. Nebulized frusemide for dyspnoea. Palliat Med 1994;8(3):258.
57. Shimoyama N, Shimoyama M. Nebulized furosemide as a novel treatment for dyspnea in terminal cancer patients. J Pain Symptom Manage 2002;23(1):73–6.
58. Sudo T, Hayashi F, Nishino T. Responses of tracheobronchial receptors to inhaled furosemide in anesthetized rats. Am J Respir Crit Care Med 2000;162(3 Pt 1):971–5.
59. Manning HL, Shea SA, Schwartzstein RM, Lansing RW, Brown R, Banzett RB. Reduced tidal volume increases 'air hunger' at fixed PCO2 in ventilated quadriplegics. Respir Physiol 1992;90(1):19–30.
60. Nishino T, Ide T, Sudo T, Sato J. Inhaled furosemide greatly alleviates the sensation of experimentally induced dyspnea. Am J Respir Crit Care Med 2000;161(6):1963–7.
61. Moosavi SH, Binks AP, Lansing RW, Topulos GP, Banzett RB, Schwartzstein RM. Effect of inhaled furosemide on air hunger induced in healthy humans. Respir Physiol Neurobiol 2007;156(1):1–8.
62. Bredin M, Corner J, Krishnasamy M, Plant H, Bailey C, A'Hern R. Multicentre randomised controlled trial of nursing intervention for breathlessness in patients with lung cancer. BMJ 1999;318(7188):901–4.
63. Pulmonary rehabilitation-1999. American Thoracic Society. Am J Respir Crit Care Med 1999;159(5 Pt 1):1666–82.
64. Pan CX, Morrison RS, Ness J, Fugh-Berman A, Leipzig RM. Complementary and alternative medicine in the management of pain, dyspnea, and nausea and vomiting near the end of life. A systematic review. J Pain Symptom Manage 2000;20(5):374–87.
65. Jobst K, Chen JH, McPherson K, et al. Controlled trial of acupuncture for disabling breathlessness. Lancet 1986;2(8521–2):1416–19.
66. Maa SH, Gauthier D, Turner M. Acupressure as an adjunct to a pulmonary rehabilitation program. J Cardiopulm Rehabil 1997;17(4):268–76.
67. Voltz R, Borasio GD. Palliative therapy in the terminal stage of neurological disease. J Neurol 1997;244 (Suppl 4):S2–10.
68. Borasio GD, Voltz R. Palliative care in amyotrophic lateral sclerosis. J Neurol 1997;244(Suppl 4):S11–17.
69. Polkey MI, Lyall RA, Davidson AC, Leigh PN, Moxham J. Ethical and clinical issues in the use of home non-invasive mechanical ventilation for the palliation of breathlessness in motor neurone disease. Thorax 1999;54(4):367–71.
70. Lightowler JV, Wedzicha JA, Elliott MW, Ram FS. Non-invasive positive pressure ventilation to treat respiratory failure resulting from exacerbations of chronic obstructive pulmonary disease: Cochrane systematic review and meta-analysis. BMJ 2003;326(7382):185.

71. Nava S, Cuomo AM. Acute respiratory failure in the cancer patient: the role of non-invasive mechanical ventilation. Crit Rev Oncol Hematol 2004;51(2):91–103.
72. Fainsinger RL, Waller A, Bercovici M, et al. A multicentre international study of sedation for uncontrolled symptoms in terminally ill patients. Palliat Med 2000;14(4):257–65.
73. Sykes N, Thorns A. Sedative use in the last week of life and the implications for end-of-life decision making. Arch Intern Med 2003;163(3):341–4.

2 Skeletal Metastases: Optimal Management Today

John Kosteva and Corey Langer

CONTENTS

INTRODUCTION
PATHOPHYSIOLOGY OF SKELETAL METASTASES
PRESENTATION AND COMPLICATIONS OF SKELETAL METASTASES
ECONOMIC IMPACT OF SKELETAL METASTASES
IMAGING OF SKELETAL METASTASES
TREATMENT OF SKELETAL METASTASES
CONCLUSIONS
REFERENCES

ABSTRACT

The skeletal system is a frequent site of metastatic involvement in patients with advanced malignancy, especially in those with breast and prostate cancer, lung cancer, and myeloma. Skeletal metastases involve an imbalance between the osteoclastic and osteoblastic activity of normal bone remodeling. Skeletal metastases may result in various complications, also known as skeletal-related events, including pain, pathologic fractures, hypercalcemia, and nerve or spinal cord compression. The consequences of skeletal metastases and their treatment may have a substantial impact on health care economics. Skeletal metastases can be detected by a variety of radiographic and nuclear imaging modalities. In the modern era, PET imaging may ultimately supplant bone scan as a diagnostic approach. Treatment for skeletal metastases includes rest and analgesics, bisphosphonates, radiation, radionuclides, and surgery. In addition, standard systemic approaches for the underlying cancer may help palliate osseous involvement.

Key Words: Bone metastases; Skeletal metastases; Bisphosphonates; Skeletal-related event; Zoledronic acid; Pamidronate; Radiotherapy; Radionuclides; Economic; Imaging.

From: *Cancer and Drug Discovery Development: Supportive Care in Cancer Therapy*
DOI: 10.1007/978-1-59745-291-5_2, Edited by: D. S. Ettinger © Humana Press, Totowa, NJ

INTRODUCTION

The skeleton represents one of the most frequent sites of metastatic involvement in advanced cancer, which frequently results in significant morbidity in these patients. Skeletal metastases have been most frequently described in multiple myeloma, with an incidence of 95–100% among patients with advanced disease. Among patients with metastatic solid tumors, breast and prostate cancers have been noted to have the highest incidence of skeletal metastases in patients with metastatic disease (65–75%) followed by thyroid (60%), lung (30–40%), and renal cancers (20–25%) *(1)*. It has been estimated that 350,000 people with skeletal metastases die each year in the United States *(2)*. Once the diagnosis of skeletal metastases is made, survival is typically reduced; for example, only 20% of patients with skeletal metastases from breast cancer are alive at five years *(3)*. Data from a Radiation Therapy Oncology Group (RTOG) trial showed that the median survival in patients with a solitary skeletal metastasis was 36 weeks while median survival in patients with multiple skeletal metastases was 24 weeks *(4)*. Patients experiencing skeletal-related events (SREs) from their metastatic disease often have a poor prognosis. The adverse events associated with skeletal metastases such as pathologic fractures, pain, and neurologic complications can result in significant morbidity and generally have a negative impact on patients' quality of life.

PATHOPHYSIOLOGY OF SKELETAL METASTASES

Skeletal metastases are predominantly distributed in the axial skeleton, which suggests that the slow blood flow at these sites may contribute to this pattern of metastasis (Table 1). Batson first described the high-flow, low-pressure, valveless plexus of veins that connects the visceral organs to the spine and pelvis known as the vertebral-venous plexus *(5)*. This network of slow-flowing vessels facilitates the movement of tumor cells from distant organs to the skeleton. Blood flow also tends to be high in areas of red bone marrow, which may contribute to metastases at these sites *(6)*. A "seed and soil" hypothesis has been postulated in describing the predilection of tumor cells for bone. Bone serves as a repository for immobilized growth factors including platelet-derived growth factors, transforming growth factor β, insulin-like growth factors I and II, fibroblast growth factors, bone morphogenetic proteins, and calcium, which may help promote tumor growth *(7)*.

Normal bone remodeling is coordinated by the activity of osteoclasts and osteoblasts. Bone resorption is typically mediated by osteoclasts, which are multinucleated giant cells derived from granulocyte-macrophage precursors. The formation of osteoclasts is induced by the production of both macrophage colony-stimulating factors and receptor activator of nuclear factor-κB (RANK) ligand (RANKL) by stromal cells and osteoblasts *(8, 9)*. Osteoblasts may produce interleukin-6, interleukin-1, and prostaglandin which can also induce the formation of osteoclasts. When RANKL binds the RANK receptor on osteoclast precursors, it stimulates the formation of osteoclasts via signaling through the nuclear factor-κB and Jun N-terminal kinase pathways. Osteoclasts resorb bone by secreting proteases that dissolve the matrix and producing acid that releases bone mineral into the extracellular space *(10)*. Bone formation is mediated by osteoblasts that are derived from mesenchymal fibroblast-like cells. A number of different

Table 1
Anatomic distribution of skeletal metastases in patients
with nonsmall-cell lung cancer
(n = 87 patients)

Anatomic site	Percentage of patients with skeletal metastases
Thoracic spine	52
Lumbar spine	46
Ribs	45
Sacrum	26
Iliac	25
Femur	23
Cervical spine	18
Skull	13
Humerus	11
Scapula	8
Sternum	6
Clavicle	6
Shoulder	5
Spine	2
Patella	1
Tibia	1
Diffuse skeleton	1

From *(65)*

factors may influence the proliferation of osteoblasts including parathyroid hormone, prostaglandins, and cytokines as well as growth factors such as platelet-derived growth factor. The bone matrix itself may produce growth factors such as the bone morphogenetic proteins, transforming growth factor-β, insulin-like growth factors, and fibroblast growth factors.

Under normal circumstances, bone remodeling is carefully regulated by a complex interaction of hormones, paracrine growth factors, and cytokines known as coupling. Malignant cells secrete a number of factors that impact skeletal turnover and remodeling. These factors include prostaglandin E, transforming growth factor-α and $-\beta$, epidermal growth factor, tumor necrosis factor, and interleukin-1 *(11)*. These factors increase the elaboration of RANKL, which induces the formation of osteoclasts and bone resorption. Interleukin-1 is a potent stimulator of bone resorption in vitro in squamous carcinoma cells *(12)*. In osteolytic metastases, the destruction of bone is mediated by osteoclasts rather than the tumor cells. Interleukin-6 may block apoptosis in myeloma cells while stimulating osteoclast formation *(13, 14)*. Procathepsin D is another osteoclast-stimulating factor that has been shown to be a breast cancer cell product *(15)*. The active form of this enzyme stimulates bone resorption in vitro and is associated with activation of transforming growth factor. Cell adhesion molecules from the integrin and selectin families of receptors are involved in the adhesion to basement membrane proteins at the target site *(16)*. Tumor cells also release matrix metalloproteinases to break down host tissue and allow invasion *(17)*.

PRESENTATION AND COMPLICATIONS OF SKELETAL METASTASES

Skeletal metastases are frequently associated with significant morbidity, which may include pain, pathologic fractures, hypercalcemia, and spinal cord compression. These complications along with the radiotherapeutic and surgical interventions required to palliate them are called skeletal-related events. The bone pain associated with skeletal metastases typically involves both biological and mechanical components. The biologic component results from the tumor's presence in bone and is mediated by the local release of cytokines and neuropeptides. In addition, the presence of tumor in bone may elevate intraosseous pressure due to mass effect and irritate periosteal nerve endings. Mechanical pain results from the loss of structural integrity of bone at affected sites. This may result from lytic lesions which result in direct bone loss or from blastic lesions which may result in significantly weakened bone by disrupting the normal trabecular framework.

Pathologic fractures are a potential complication that can have catastrophic effects. For patients with already limited life expectancy, pathologic fractures can be especially devastating in reducing both quality of life and functional capacity. One study found the incidence of pathologic fractures of the humerus or femur in 1,800 patients with a variety of solid tumors to be 8% (17). A more recent study of 250 untreated patients with a variety of solid tumors found the incidence of both vertebral and nonvertebral pathologic fractures to be 12%, respectively (18). The probability of developing a fracture increases with the duration of metastatic involvement. Although surgical intervention, particularly in the case of hip fractures, can stabilize these fractures, recovery can be tedious due to comorbidities, limited functional capacity, and the presence of tumor adversely affecting the bone's ability to heal. As a result, in recent years, greater emphasis has been placed on identifying skeletal lesions and preventing fractures before they develop.

Hypercalcemia of malignancy is estimated to occur in 5–10% of all patients with skeletal metastases, and is most commonly associated with squamous cell lung cancer, breast cancer, and renal cell carcinoma (1). Hypercalcemia is believed to be mediated by multiple factors related to bone destruction such as local osteolysis from skeletal metastases and diffuse osteolysis from immobility. In addition, hypercalcemia may result from tumor secretion of parathyroid hormone-related protein, which may result in the clinical equivalent of secondary hyperparathyroidism. Clinical features of hypercalcemia may include nausea, vomiting, dehydration, confusion, stupor, renal failure, and arrhythmias.

Given that the spine is the most common site of skeletal metastases, neurologic abnormalities such as spinal cord compression may develop. Cord compression often results from spinal instability or from local pressure from intradural or extradural masses. Spinal cord compression often presents with back pain, loss of motor or sensory function, loss of autonomic function, or loss of proprioception. Spinal cord compression is considered an oncologic emergency that requires urgent evaluation and treatment with corticosteroids and either radiotherapy or surgical decompression. Once neurologic function is lost, it is rare for function to return.

ECONOMIC IMPACT OF SKELETAL METASTASES

Because of the high costs of treatment and supportive care that may result when patients develop adverse events from skeletal metastases, recent attention has been given to the economic costs of treating skeletal metastases and their complications.

Several studies have investigated the economic impact of treating skeletal morbidity in patients with prostate cancer, breast cancer, multiple myeloma, and lung cancer. Groot et al. reviewed the economic consequences associated with skeletal metastases in 28 patients with prostate cancer *(19)*. Over 24 months, the authors noted a total of 61 skeletal-related events (SREs) in these patients. On average, approximately 53% of the costs of all medical care received in these patients resulted directly from the cost of treatment of SREs. A study by Delea et al. retrospectively reviewed the impact of SREs in 617 patients with breast cancer *(20)*. Based on survival time from diagnosis of skel-etal metastases and a calculated propensity score based on the patients' baseline char-acteristics, patients with SREs were matched with patients without SREs resulting in 201 matched pairs of patients. Mean follow-up was 13.8 months in the group with SREs and 11.0 months in the group without SREs. In the SRE group, costs of treatment of SREs were \$13,940 (95% CI, \$11,240–\$16,856) per patient. Total medical care costs were \$48,173 (95% CI, \$19,068–\$77,684) greater in the group with SREs ($p = 0.001$). An additional study by Delea et al. conducted a retrospective review of 835 patients with multiple myeloma *(21)*. Three-hundred fifty-two (42%) of these patients devel-oped at least one SRE. Expected lifetime cost of SRE-related care was \$10,247 per patient (95% CI, \$7,921–\$12,573) over a mean follow-up of approximately 18 months. Of the expected costs, 64% were incurred during inpatient hospitalization and 74% in the immediate 6 months after the first SRE claim. A more recently published study retrospectively evaluated 534 patients with lung cancer and skeletal metastases. Two-hundred ninety-five (55%) patients had at least one SRE with the requirement of radio-therapy (68%) and fracture (35%) was noted to be the most common event. Median survival after the first-identified SRE was 4.1 months (95% CI, 3.6–5.5 months). The estimated lifetime SRE-related cost per patient was \$11,979 (95% CI, \$10,193–\$13,766) with radiotherapy accounting for the largest portion of the cost *(22)*. Collectively, these studies demonstrate the high cost of treatment of SREs and their significant impact on health care economics.

IMAGING OF SKELETAL METASTASES

Plain Film Radiography

Plain film radiography is a convenient and inexpensive method for monitoring skel-etal metastases. It is useful in assessing the structural integrity of bone and the risk of impending pathologic fracture. Given the relative cost and convenience in obtaining plain radiographs, they are often the first imaging study used to evaluate bone pain. Plain films are also useful in confirming larger lesions noted on PET or bone scintigra-phy. Plain film radiography is frequently used in surgical planning and to determine response to treatment following surgical stabilization or radiotherapy. Plain film radiog-raphy is often the preferred imaging test for multiple myeloma which often features "cold" lesions on bone scintigraphy. However, plain film radiographs often have limited sensitivity in that approximately 30–50% of bone mineral must be lost before skeletal lesions can be detected.

Skeletal lesions may have either an osteolytic, osteoblastic, or mixed pattern on plain film radiography. Osteolytic lesions result when bone destruction predominates, while osteoblastic lesions result when bone formation predominates. Prostate cancer tends to have a more blastic appearance while lung, thyroid, and renal carcinoma lesions have a more lytic appearance. Breast carcinoma lesions tend to have a more mixed appearance. In patients who undergo radiation for lytic disease, osteoblastic changes will often emerge over time, frequently at the edges of the lesion.

Bone Scintigraphy

Technetium diphosphonate bone scans are valuable studies in detecting occult skeletal lesions. These studies involve the incorporation of tagged diphosphonate into hydroxyapatite during bone mineralization. Historically, bone scintigraphy has been the modality of choice for detecting occult skeletal lesions with sensitivity rates of 72–90% (23–26). Bone scintigraphy can generate nonspecific findings, however, due to increased tracer uptake from a variety of inflammatory or traumatic conditions. These changes are often confused with metastases. Another drawback of bone scintigraphy is that it shows relatively poor anatomic detail compared to other imaging modalities. In addition, lesions such as multiple myeloma that do not involve new bone formation may appear "cold" or "negative" on these studies.

Magnetic Resonance Imaging

Magnetic resonance imaging (MRI) is an additional imaging modality which is useful for detecting skeletal metastases. MRI is a highly sensitive technique for evaluating the bone marrow and early sites of skeletal metastases. The sensitivity of MRI is based on the water content of various tissues; the high water content of skeletal metastases can present a sharp contrast to that of normal bone marrow. Specificity of MRI may be limited in some cases of inflammation or infection which may appear similar to skeletal metastases. The relatively higher cost and impracticality of performing extensive MRI imaging of multiple skeletal sites at the same time in routine clinical practice has resulted in MRI being used mostly for confirmation of lesions at specific symptomatic sites. Recently, however, full-body MRI has been studied as a screening tool for the detection of skeletal metastases and has been shown to be equal to or slightly more sensitive than bone scintigraphy (27). MRI is especially valuable in imaging lesions in the spine as it may be useful in differentiating pathologic compression fractures from osteoporotic compression fractures. In addition, MRI is the preferred modality for evaluating lesions which may be associated with neurologic impairment or epidural extension in the case of vertebral lesions with cord compression or other forms of nerve impingement.

Computed Tomography

Computed tomography (CT) is not a primary method for imaging skeletal metastases, although lesions may be detected on routine CT scans used for evaluating intra-thoracic or intra-abdominal sites of disease. CT is more useful in determining the extent of cortical destruction or soft tissue involvement compared to plain film radiography. CT is often used in the role of surgical planning to assess bone instability due to cortical destruction. CT is also frequently used as a guide or map for biopsies of skeletal lesions. In addition, CT with bone windows may enable assessment in patients in whom pacemakers or vital surgical clips preclude the use of MRI.

Positron Emission Tomography

Positron emission tomography (PET) is an imaging modality that is emerging as a primary method for screening for skeletal metastases. PET scanning employs a radionuclide, fluorine-18, which is bound to a D-glucose analogue yielding [^{18}F]-fluorodeoxyglucose (FDG). FDG is taken up as a glucose analogue in metabolically active cells. Because tumor cells are more metabolically active than normal cells, they usually have a higher rate of glucose uptake, and therefore more FDG uptake, than normal cells. A standard uptake ratio is then used to measure the positron activity in the region of FDG uptake to determine the likelihood that the lesion is malignant.

As with other imaging modalities, PET may have some limitations. FDG physiologically accumulates in the brain and urinary tract. Hence, FDG-PET is relatively useless in assessing for CNS metastases. FDG uptake may also occur in the normal esophagus, stomach, small intestine, large intestine, and thyroid *(28)*. In addition, contracting skeletal muscle, lymph nodes, healing bone, and sites of infection may have physiologically increased FDG uptake. As with bone scintigraphy, degenerative and inflammatory joint disease may demonstrate increased FDG uptake, although at a lower rate. Unlike standard bone scans, PET does not routinely image bones below the pelvis or midfemurs; hence, lesions at these sites may be missed.

Several studies have compared PET to bone scintigraphy for the detection of skeletal metastases. One prospective study evaluated 110 patients with nonsmall cell lung cancer undergoing both PET and bone scintigraphy. Both forms of imaging were noted to have a sensitivity of 90% in the detection of skeletal metastases. Compared to bone scintigraphy, however, PET was determined to have superior specificity (98% vs. 61%), positive predictive value (90% vs. 35%), and negative predictive value (98% vs. 96%) (25).

Another prospective evaluation of 90 patients with nonsmall cell lung cancer undergoing both PET and bone scintigraphy demonstrated greater accuracy with PET. PET correctly staged 98% of patients while bone scintigraphy correctly staged 87% of patients. Compared to bone scintigraphy, PET demonstrated superior sensitivity (92% vs. 50%), specificity (99% vs. 92%), positive predictive value (92% vs. 50%), and negative predictive value (99% vs. 92%) (29).

TREATMENT OF SKELETAL METASTASES

The treatment of skeletal metastases may involve several different modalities, including medical therapy, radiation therapy, and surgery; therefore, the treatment often involves a multidisciplinary approach. Treatment is often aimed at palliation of symptoms such as improving pain control and function while maintaining skeletal integrity. Widespread disease often necessitates systemic therapy such as chemotherapy, hormonal therapy, bisphosphonates, or radionuclides, while localized problems are often managed with radiotherapy or surgery.

Chemotherapy and Hormonal Therapy

Chemotherapeutic agents often have limited utility in the treatment of many types of skeletal metastases. Small cell lung cancer, Hodgkin's and non-Hodgkin's lymphoma, testicular cancer, and small round blue cell tumors have been noted to be very sensitive to traditional chemotherapeutic agents while breast carcinoma, ovarian carcinoma, and germ cell cancers are moderately sensitive *(30)*.

Endocrine therapy has shown some utility in the treatment of skeletal metastases in prostate and breast cancer. Surgical or chemical castration has been shown to be effective in the management of skeletal metastases. For patients with prostate cancer, combined endocrine therapy with antiandrogens and luteinizing hormone-releasing hormone to create a total androgen blockade has shown utility, in some cases quite durable *(3)*. One study investigating oral dexamethasone for hormone-refractory prostate demonstrated reduced pain in 61% of patients and improved bone scan intensity in 19% of patients *(31)*. For the treatment of skeletal metastases in breast cancer, antiestrogen therapy was noted to result in significant tumor shrinkage in 30–65% of patients *(32)*. A large multicenter study examined the use of multiple hormonal manipulations, including megestrol acetate, tamoxifen, aminoglutethimide, dexamethasone, hydrocortisone, and fluoxymesterone, and showed a partial response in 21% and stable disease in 32% of patients *(33)*.

Bisphosphonates

In recent years, bisphosphonates have become a focus in the medical management of skeletal metastases. Bisphosphonates are stable chemical analogues of naturally occurring inorganic pyrophosphates. Bisphosphonates contain a P–C–P central structure instead of the P–O–P structure of the natural pyrophosphates which makes bisphosphonates resistant to phosphatase activity and more easily allows their binding to mineralized bone matrix. Bisphosphonates accumulate in sites of active bone formation making the sites more resistant to dissolution by osteoclasts reducing their survival and modulating the signaling from osteoblasts to osteoclasts. Once deposited, bisphosphonates are internalized by osteoclasts which results in the loss of ability of osteoclasts to resorb bone and promote apoptosis. Bisphosphonates are believed to inhibit osteoclast activity by interrupting the mevalonate metabolic pathway. Bisphosphonates also inhibit both the maturation of osteoclast precursor cells and bone-resorbing cytokine release from adjacent macrophages *(34)*. Bisphosphonates have also shown some antiangiogenesis activity that may impair tumor growth *(35)*.

Different generations of bisphosphonates have been shown to have various potencies and effects with regard to their inhibition of bone resorption. First-generation bisphosphonates such as clodronate and etidronate, which more closely resemble pyrophosphate, act as analogues of ATP and inhibit ATP-dependent intracellular enzymes. Later generation bisphosphonates, the aminobisphosphonates, which contain nitrogen, such as pamidronate, ibandronate, and zoledronate, interrupt the mevalonate metabolic pathway and disrupt the functioning of regulatory proteins *(36)*. These aminobisphosphonates have much less effect on in vivo mineralization and are more widely preferred for treatment of metastatic and metabolic bone diseases.

Typically, bisphosphonates are not metabolized in humans as 50–60% of each dose is rapidly absorbed by bone and later slowly excreted by the kidneys. The remaining 40–50% is rapidly excreted by the kidneys. Bisphosphonates generally have poor oral bioavailability and must be taken on an empty stomach to minimize binding to dietary calcium. The most common toxicities of oral bisphosphonates include gastrointestinal side effects such as nausea, vomiting, indigestion, and diarrhea. The aminobisphosphonates which are given intravenously may be associated with acute-phase reactions as well as renal function impairment.

Beginning in 2003, reports of osteonecrosis of the jaw (ONJ) associated with bisphosphonate use have been reported in the medical literature. ONJ is believed to result from the inability of hypodynamic and hypovascular bone to meet the increased demand for repair and remodeling owing to physiological stress, iatrogenic trauma, and infection. As bisphosphonates are taken up by osteoclasts, they result in a reduction in the rate of formation of new bone and decrease blood flow to these sites. ONJ has been primarily associated with the newer-generation, more potent aminobisphosphonates. A web-based survey of 1,203 respondents (904 patients with multiple myeloma, 299 with breast cancer) was conducted to try to determine the incidence of ONJ *(37)*. Seventy-five patients reported signs and symptoms consistent with ONJ while 77 reported suspicious findings for early ONJ. A higher incidence of ONJ was noted in patients receiving zoledronate compared to pamidronate (10% vs. 4%; $p = 0.002$). Underlying dental problems were noted in 81% of patients with multiple myeloma and 69% of patients with breast cancer who developed ONJ. As this was a web-based survey relying on the self-reporting of patients who were not necessarily evaluated by dental professionals, it is believed that the true incidence of ONJ was very likely overestimated in these patients.

A prospective review of 252 patients with multiple myeloma, prostate cancer, breast cancer, and other solid tumors, receiving either pamidronate, zoledronate, or ibandronate, attempted to better estimate the true incidence of ONJ *(38)*. A total of 17 patients (6.7%) were diagnosed with ONJ. There was noted to be a nonsignificant association with a greater proportion of patients treated with zoledronate who developed ONJ. Prolonged exposure to bisphosphonates was strongly associated with the development of ONJ as the median time on bisphosphonates was 39.3 months for patients with ONJ compared to 19 months for patients without ONJ ($p = 0.001$). Because of the association with longer exposure to bisphosphonates, some groups have recommended that treatment may either be discontinued after 2 years or that the frequency of treatment be reduced *(39)*.

Bisphosphonates have been shown to be effective for treatment of pain associated with skeletal metastases. A review by the Cochrane Pain, Palliative Care, and Supportive Care Group evaluated data from 30 studies involving a total of 3,682 patients with skeletal metastases from breast cancer, prostate cancer, multiple myeloma, and other solid tumors. This study noted a significant benefit favoring the use of bisphosphonates with regard to pain control over 12 weeks with an odds ratio of 2.37 (95% CI, 1.61–3.5) *(40)*.

Several large randomized studies have shown that bisphosphonates may reduce the incidence of skeletal-related events (SREs) in patients with skeletal metastases due to breast cancer. A double-blind, multicenter, parallel group study of 382 women with lytic bone lesions from metastatic breast cancer receiving treatment with pamidronate versus placebo showed a significant reduction in the incidence of skeletal complications (43% vs. 56%; $p = 0.008$) in patients receiving bisphosphonates. In addition, there was a significant reduction in skeletal complications such as vertebral or nonvertebral pathologic fractures, need for radiation or surgery, and hypercalcemia in patients receiving pamidronate. Pamidronate was also shown to increase the median time to development of first skeletal complications from 7.0 months to 13.9 months ($p < 0.001$) *(41, 42)*.

A randomized, double-blind study of 372 women with breast cancer with at least one lytic lesion undergoing hormonal therapy compared patients receiving pamidronate for 24 monthly cycles to patients receiving placebo. Following completion of treatment, there was noted to be a significant difference between the two groups in the proportion of patients with skeletal complications. Fifty-six percent of patients receiving pamidronate developed skeletal complications compared to 67% receiving placebo ($p = 0.027$) *(43)*. Another randomized, double-blind, placebo-controlled trial of 751 women with metastatic breast cancer with osteolytic metastases showed a significant difference in the skeletal morbidity rate as well as the incidence of skeletal complications between the two groups. For the group receiving pamidronate, the skeletal morbidity rate was 2.4% with a 51% incidence of skeletal complications. For the placebo group, these numbers were 3.7% and 64%, respectively ($P < 0.001$ and $p < 0.001$). The median time to first skeletal complication was 12.7 months for patients receiving pamidronate and 7 months for patients receiving placebo ($P < 0.001$). Pain control was also significantly improved among the patients receiving bisphosphonates *(44)*.

A randomized, double-blind trial evaluated the use of pamidronate in 392 patients with skeletal metastases from multiple myeloma. There was noted to be a significantly lower rate of SREs as well as significantly decreased mean number of SREs per year (1.3 vs. 2.2) favoring the use of pamidronate *(45)*.

Zoledronic acid has also been evaluated in a randomized, double-blind study investigating 773 patients with osteolytic, osteoblastic, or mixed skeletal metastases from nonsmall cell lung cancer, small cell lung cancer, renal cell cancer, and other solid tumors. Patients were randomized to receive either zoledronic acid 4 mg, zoledronic acid 8 mg (later adjusted to 4 mg due to concern for renal toxicity at higher dosage), or placebo. The proportion of patients receiving zoledronic acid 4 mg and 8 mg/4 mg experiencing SREs such as radiation to bone, vertebral or nonvertebral pathologic fracture, surgery to bone, spinal cord compression, or hypercalcemia was significantly lower compared to placebo (38%, 35%, and 47%, respectively). Zoledronic acid also significantly delayed the time to first SRE compared to placebo. Median times to first SRE were 230 days and 219 days for the 4-mg and 8-mg/4-mg groups, respectively, and 163 days for the group receiving placebo *(18)*.

Radiation

Local radiation is often used in the control of pain and localized disease. It may also be used in the postoperative setting to limit disease progression following surgical fixation of impending pathologic fractures. Local radiation is effective in obtaining pain relief with 80–90% percent of patients reporting at least partial relief and 50–85% reporting complete relief *(4, 46)*. The full extent of pain relief may not develop until 3–4 weeks after completion of treatment. Local radiotherapy is generally well tolerated with commonly seen acute toxicities including fatigue, skin erythema, nausea, esophagitis, and myelosuppression. Late side effects are relatively uncommon but may include the possibility of further weakening the bone with increased risk of future fractures, although the majority of these events are due to metastatic progression.

Multiple dosing and fractionation schedules have been utilized in the treatment of skeletal metastases. Historically, a treatment schedule of 30 Gy in ten fractions has been used based on the findings from a large study conducted by the Radiation Therapy Oncology Group (RTOG) in the 1970s and 1980s *(4)*. There is some belief that frequent low-dose treatments may allow for a greater total radiation dose with a decrease in late toxicity and more durable symptomatic palliation. More recently, in part due to concerns regarding greater cost effectiveness and patient convenience, single fraction radiation has been investigated as a treatment option for skeletal metastases. Three recent large randomized trials have shown comparable efficacy of single fraction treatment to multiple fraction treatment with regard to palliation of pain. A Dutch multicenter trial assigned 1,171 patients with painful skeletal metastases to either 8 Gy in a single dose or 24 Gy in six fractions. Both the palliative benefit and treatment-related toxicity were similar in the two groups although re-treatment was required in significantly more patients (25% vs. 7%) in the single fraction group *(47, 48)*. A second trial by the Bone Pain Trial Working Party randomized 765 patients to 8 Gy as a single fraction, 20 Gy in five fractions, or 30 Gy in ten fractions. There were no significant differences in any pain end points among the three groups. Patients in the single fraction group were twice as likely to require reirradiation although the majority could be successfully re-treated with a single fraction (49). A third study by the RTOG randomly assigned 949 patients to receive either 8 Gy in a single fraction or 30 Gy in ten fractions. There were no significant differences in the rates for complete and partial pain relief, the use of narcotics, or the incidence of subsequent pathologic fractures. Patients receiving a single fraction were twice as likely to require re-treatment (18% vs. 9%) *(50)*. These studies have demonstrated that single fraction radiotherapy is a cost-effective and more convenient treatment option that is just as effective as multiple fractions of radiotherapy.

Radiotherapy is often utilized in patients undergoing surgical fixation of fractures and in patients with spinal metastases. For patients undergoing surgical fixation of impending and pathologic fractures or decompression and stabilization of the spine, postoperative radiotherapy is often used to treat the entire surgical area. Evidence shows that patients receiving postoperative radiotherapy are less likely to develop loosening of prostheses or hardware requiring revision surgery (3% vs. 15%) *(51)*. For patients who do not have indications for surgical therapy for spinal metastases (spinal instability, structural canal compromise, circumferential epidural tumor, occult primary tumor, and radioresistant tumors), radiotherapy is the first line of treatment.

Because patients frequently develop skeletal metastases at multiple sites, hemibody irradiation (HBI), which involves the treatment of either the upper half body or lower half body, has been investigated. The advantages of this treatment include treating multiple lesions simultaneously and possibly preventing disease progression at asymptomatic sites. Although this form of treatment may provide similar pain relief as focal irradiation, and often in a rapid manner, there may be significant morbidity associated with treatment, and the long-term benefits are small. Many patients often require re-treatment following HBI. As a result, HBI is not used frequently in clinical practice and has been largely replaced by systemic radionuclides.

Radionuclides

Systemic radionuclides have been used in the treatment of skeletal metastases by localizing selectively to skeletal metastases and delivering ionizing radiation in a focal manner. The advantages of this type of treatment include the ability to treat all skeletal sites simultaneously and minimizing the dose delivered to normal soft tissue. Systemic radionuclide treatment is indicated in the presence of widespread painful bony metastases or if there is a contraindication to further external beam radiation such as when normal tissue tolerance has been reached. Because the most common side effect of this treatment is myelosuppression, with counts dropping as much as 20–50% after receiving treatment, patients undergoing chemotherapy should not receive concurrent treatment with systemic radionuclides.

Strontium-89 (^{89}Sr) is the most widely studied radionuclide. ^{89}Sr tends to be more effective for osteoblastic lesions that better allow for effective radionuclide delivery to the bone compared to osteolytic lesions. Several randomized controlled studies have compared ^{89}Sr with either placebo or local external beam radiation. The Trans-Canada study was a phase III study of 126 patients with hormone-refractory, metastatic prostate cancer comparing ^{89}Sr with placebo after the completion of local external beam radiation. Although there was no difference in overall survival, there was noted to be improved pain control, longer time to re-treatment with radiotherapy, and improved quality of life in patients on the treatment arm *(52)*. An additional study of 284 prostate cancer patients with painful skeletal metastases assigned patients to receive either external beam radiation or ^{89}Sr. Overall pain relief and survival was similar in the two groups; however, patients receiving ^{89}Sr were less likely to report new painful sites and were less likely to require reirradiation *(53)*.

Samarium-153 (^{153}Sm) and rhenium-188 (^{188}Re) are two additional lesser-studied agents that have been shown to have some activity in the treatment of skeletal metastases. ^{153}Sm has a shorter physical half-life and higher dose rate than ^{89}Sr. Two prospective, randomized phase III trials have shown significantly improved pain relief compared to placebo in patients with skeletal metastases *(54, 55)*. ^{188}Re has also been shown to be effective in relieving pain due to skeletal metastases from prostate cancer *(56)*.

Surgery

The presence of metastatic lesions can significantly alter the bone's strength and structural properties. Lytic lesions result in the loss of mineral and organic structures of the bone which could diminish its strength. Blastic lesions may disrupt the normal trabecular framework which can alter the bone's structural properties *(57)*. Tumor presence may also adversely affect the bone's ability to heal itself in the case of pathologic fractures. Because surgical treatment of impending pathologic fractures is often associated with less morbidity than pathologic fractures that have already developed, several studies have attempted to develop criteria to predict the likelihood of developing a pathologic fracture at a metastatic site. Although there has been some variation with regard to correlation of risk factors with the likelihood of developing pathologic fractures, several characteristics have been noted to be associated with an increased risk of developing fracture. These factors include pure lytic lesions, subtrochanteric lesions, cortical involvement of tumor, increasing pain, and failure of radiotherapy *(58, 59)*. More sophisticated predictive tools based on computed tomography of sites at risk of fracture are currently under evaluation.

The goals of surgical treatment of pathologic fractures generally involve restoring function and relieving pain. Surgical management should focus on restoring bone strength to allow for immediate weight bearing. Prosthetic replacement and internal fixation are often done to improve healing as conservatively managed pathologic fractures often heal poorly making arthroplasty and internal fixation the most reliable methods of treating pathologic fractures. The choice of surgical procedure depends on the location, number, and size of metastases, as well as the type of primary tumor. Occasionally, external fixation or brace immobilization may be used in patients who are not surgical candidates or in patients who have extensive disease that is not amenable to internal fixation.

Surgical intervention is a valuable treatment option in lesions involving the spine, which is the most common site of skeletal metastases. Surgical intervention may be used to decompress neural elements in the case of cord compression or restore mechanical stability. Both vertebroplasty which involves injection of bone cement into a collapsed vertebrae and kyphoplasty which involves the introduction of inflatable bone tamps into the vertebral body have been shown to reduce pain and improve overall functioning in patients with osteolytic spinal metastases *(60)*.

Biochemical Markers for Bone Turnover

Because of the high morbidity associated with skeletal complications, recent research efforts have focused on identifying biochemical markers for bone turnover, such as *n*-telopeptide of type 1 collagen (NTX), that may help to identify patients at high risk for skeletal complications. Other efforts have focused on identifying biochemical markers, such as bone sialoprotein (BSP) that may help predict the development of skeletal metastases in patients who do not yet have clinical skeletal lesions.

NTX is a marker for bone resorption that has been correlated with an increased number of skeletal-related events (SREs). One study involved monthly measurements of NTX in 121 patients with skeletal metastases. Patients with NTX levels greater than 100-nmol/mmol creatinine were found to be many times more likely to experience SREs than patients with levels less than 100-nmol/mmol creatinine *(61)*. A subsequent larger study again showed that elevated levels of NTX were highly predictive of SREs, progression in bone, and death in both the absence and presence of bisphosphonate treatment. Similar relationships were seen with bone alkaline phosphatase, a bone formation marker, although NTX was more predictive *(62, 63)*.

BSP is another protein implicated in the process of bone resorption that is highly expressed in lung, thyroid, breast, and prostate cancers. One case-control retrospective study of patients with resected nonsmall cell lung cancer evaluating a broad panel of biochemical markers associated with metastatic tumors demonstrated that BSP was strongly associated with bone dissemination *(64)*. The results of this study and others evaluating the role of biochemical markers may have future implications in investigating the treatment of patients without known skeletal metastases with agents such as bisphosphonates in order to prevent skeletal lesions.

CONCLUSIONS

Skeletal metastases remain a common, potentially devastating complication of malignancy. The skeleton is one of the most frequent sites of metastases of several tumor types with the spine, ribs, pelvis, and long bones being the most common sites of involvement. Emerging techniques in imaging skeletal metastases provide an improved ability to detect these lesions. The onset of SREs, such as pathologic fractures or hyper-calcemia, is associated with compromised prognosis and substantial decrements in quality of life. In addition, the costs of treatment of SREs can have a substantial impact on healthcare economics. The treatment of skeletal metastases often involves a multi-disciplinary approach involving medical management, radiotherapy, and surgery. Treatment must be individualized based on primary site, extent of involvement, and degree of pain and functional compromise. In addition to narcotic analgesics, radiation, and surgery, bisphosphonates have emerged as a fundamental component of treatment as they have been shown to be effective in reducing pain associated with skeletal metas-tases. In addition, they have been shown to delay the onset and reduce the rates of development of skeletal metastases in a variety of tumor types. Other treatment options such as radionuclides have recently been noted to be effective in the treatment of diffuse skeletal metastases. The management of patients with skeletal metastases remains an evolving field of cancer research.

REFERENCES

1. Coleman RE. Skeletal complications of malignancy. *Cancer* 1997; 80:1588–1594.
2. Mundy GR. Metastasis to bone: causes, consequences and therapeutic opportunities. *Nat Rev Cancer* 2002; 2:584–593.
3. Coleman RE. Metastatic bone disease: clinical features, pathophysiology and treatment strategies. *Cancer Treat Rev* 2001; 27:165–176.
4. Tong D, Gillick L, Hendrickson FR. The palliation of symptomatic osseous metastases: final results of the study by Radiation Therapy Oncology Group. *Cancer* 1982; 50:893–899.
5. Batson O. The function of the vertebral veins and their role in the spread of metastases. *Ann Surg* 1940; 112:138.
6. Kahn D, Weiner GJ, Ben-Haim S, et al. Positron emission tomographic measurement of bone marrow blood flow to the pelvis and lumbar vertebrae in young normal adults. *Blood* 1994; 83:958–963.
7. Hauschka PV, Mavrakos AE, Iafrati MD, et al. Growth factors in bone matrix: isolation of multiple types by affinity chromatography on heparin-sepharose. *J Biol Chem* 1986; 261:12665–12674.
8. Kodama H, Nose M, Niida S, et al. Essential role of macrophage colony-stimulating factor in the osteoclast differentiation supported by stromal cells. *J Exp Med* 1991; 173:1291–1294.
9. Lacey DL, Timms E, Tan HL, et al. Osteoprotegerin ligand is a cytokine that regulates osteoclast differentia-tion and activation. *Cell* 1998; 93:165–176.
10. Blair HC, Teitelbaum SL, Ghiselli R, et al. Osteoclastic bone resorption by a polarized vacuolar proton pump. *Science* 1989; 245:855–857.
11. Mundy GR. Mechanisms of bone metastases. *Cancer* 1997; 80:1546.
12. Sato K, Fujii Y, Kasano K, et al. Production of interleukin-1 alpha and a parathyroid hormone-like factor by a squamous cell carcinoma of the esophagus derived from a patient with hypercalcemia. *J Clin Endocrinol Metab* 1988; 67:592.
13. Cheung WC, Van Ness B. Distinct IL-6 signal transduction leads to growth arrest and death in B cells or growth promotion and cell survival in myeloma cells. *Leukemia* 2002; 16:1182–1188.
14. Kurihara N, Bertolini D, Suda T, et al. IL-6 stimulates osteoclast-like multinucleated cell formation in long term human marrow cultures by inducing IL-1 release. *J Immunol* 1990; 144:4226–4230.
15. Wo Z, Bonewald LF, Oreffo ROC, et al. The potential role of procathepsin D secreted by breast cancer cells in bone resorption. *Calcium Regulation and Bone Metabolism*. Amsterdam, Elsevier. 1990; 304.
16. Meyer T, Hart I. Mechanism of tumour metastasis. *Eur J Cancer* 1998; 34:214.
17. Higinbotham N, Marcove R. Management of pathologic fractures. *J Trauma* 1965; 5:792.
18. Rosen L, Gordon D, Tchekmedyian S, et al. Zoledronic acid versus placebo in the treatment of skeletal metas-tases in patients with lung cancer and other solid tumors: a phase III, double-blind, randomized trial. The Zoledronic Acid Lung Cancer and Other Solid Tumors Study Group. *J Clin Oncol* 2003; 21:3150–3157.
19. Groot MT, Boeken Kruger CG, Pelger RC, et al. Costs of prostate cancer metastatic to the bone in the Netherlands. *Eur Urol* 2003; 43:226–232.

20. Delea T, McKiernan J, Brandman J, et al. Retrospective study of the effect of skeletal complications on total medical care costs in patients with bone metastases of breast cancer seen in typical clinical practice. *J Support Oncol* 2006; 4:341–347.

21. Delea T, McKiernan J, Liss M, et al. Cost of skeletal complications in patients with multiple myeloma [Abstract]. IX International Multiple Myeloma Workshop; Salamanca, Spain; May 23–27, 2003.

22. Delea T, Langer C, McKiernan J, et al. The cost of treatment of skeletal-related events in patients with bone metastases from lung cancer. *Oncology* 2004; 67(5–6):390–396.

23. Eustace S, Tello R, DeCarvalho V, et al. A comparison of whole-body turboSTIR MR imaging in planar 99mTc-methylene diphosphonate scintigraphy in the examination of patients with suspected skeletal metastases. *AJR Am J Roentgenol* 1997; 169:1655.

24. Galasko C. The detection of skeletal metastases from mammary cancer by gamma camera scintigraphy. *Br J Surg* 1969; 56:757–764.

25. Bury T, Barreto A, Daenan F, et al. Fluorine-18 deoxyglucose positron emission tomography for the detection of bone metastases in patients with non-small cell lung cancer. *Eur J Nucl Med* 1998; 25:1244–1247.

26. Gayed I, Vu T, Johnson M, et al. Comparison of bone and 2-deoxy-2-[18F]fluoro-D-glucose positron emission tomography in the evaluation of bony metastases in lung cancer. *Mol Imaging Biol* 2003; 5:26–31.

27. Lauenstein T, Freudenberg L, Goehde S, et al. Whole-body MRI using a rolling table platform for the detection of bone metastases. *Eur Radiol* 2002; 12:2091.

28. Shreve PD, Anzai Y, Wahl RL. Pitfalls in oncologic diagnosis with FDG PET imaging: physiologic and benign variants. *Radiographics* 1999; 19:61–77.

29. Marom E, McAdams HP, Erasmus J, et al. Staging non-small cell lung cancer with whole-body PET. Radiology 1999; 212:803–809.

30. Savage P, Ward W. Medical management of metastatic skeletal disease. *Orthop Clin North Am* 2000; 31:545–555.

31. Nishimura K, Nonomura N, Yasunaga Y, et al. Low doses of oral dexamethasone for hormone-refractory prostate carcinoma. *Cancer* 2000; 89:2570.

32. Harvey H. Issues concerning the role of chemotherapy and hormonal therapy of bone metastases from breast carcinoma. *Cancer* 1997; 80:1646.

33. Lipton A, Theriault R, Leff R, et al. Long-term reduction of skeletal complications in breast cancer patients with osteolytic bone metastases receiving hormone therapy, by monthly 90 mg pamidronate (Aredia) infusions. *Proc Am Soc Clin Oncol* 1997;16:A531.

34. Rogers MJ, Watts DJ, Russell RGG. Overview of bisphosphonates. *Cancer* 1997; 80(Suppl 8):1652–1660.

35. Vincenzi B, Santini D, Dicuonzo G, et al. Zoledronic acid-related angiogenesis modifications and survival in advanced breast cancer patients. *J Interferon Cytokine Res* 2005; 25:144–151.

36. Luckman SP, Hughes DE, Coxon FP, et al. Nitrogen-containing bisphosphonates inhibit the mevalonate pathway and prevent post-translational phenylation of GTP-binding proteins including Ras. *J Bone Miner Res* 1998; 13:581–589.

37. Durie BG, Katz M, Crowley J. Osteonecrosis of the jaw and bisphosphonates. *N Engl J Med* 2005; 353:99–102.

38. Bamias A, Kastritis E, Bamia C, et al. Osteonecrosis of the jaw in cancer after treatment with bisphosphonates: incidence and risk factors. *J Clin Oncol* 2005; 23:8580–8587.

39. Lacy MQ, Dispenzieri A, Gertz A, et al. Mayo clinic consensus statement for the use of bisphosphonates in multiple myeloma. *Mayo Clin Proc* 2006; 81:1047–1053.

40. Wong R, Witten PJ. Bisphosphonates for the relief of pain secondary to bone metastases. *Cochrane Database Syst Rev* 2003; 2:CD002068.

41. Hortobagyi GN, Theriault RL, Porter L, et al. Efficacy of pamidronate in reducing skeletal complications in patients with breast cancer and lytic bone metastases. *N Engl J Med* 1996; 335:1785–1791.

42. Hortobagyi GN, Theriault RL, Lipton A, et al. Long-term prevention of skeletal complications of metastatic breast cancer with pamidronate. *J Clin Oncol* 1998; 16:2038–2044.

43. Theriault RL,Lipton A, Hortobagyi GN, et al. Pamidronate reduces skeletal morbidity in women with advanced breast cancer and lytic bone lesions: a randomized, placebo-controlled trial. *J Clin Oncol* 1999; 17:846–854.

44. Lipton A, Theriault RL, Hortobagyi GN, et al. Pamidronate prevents skeletal complications and is effective palliative treatment in women with breast carcinoma and osteolytic bone metastases: long term follow-up of two randomized, placebo-controlled trials. *Cancer* 2000; 88:1082–1090.

45. Berenson JR, Lichtemstein A, Porter L, et al. Long-term pamidronate treatment of advanced multiple myeloma patients reduces skeletal events. *J Clin Oncol* 1998; 16:593–602.

46. Vargha ZO, Glickasman AS, Boland J. Single-dose radiation therapy in the palliation of metastatic disease. Radiology 1969; 93:1181–1184.

47. Steenland E, Leer JW, van Houwelingen H, et al. The effect of a single fraction compared to multiple fractions on painful bone metastases: a global analysis of the Dutch Bone Metastasis Study. *Radiother Oncol* 1999; 52:101.

48. Van der Linden YM, Lok JJ, Steenland E, et al. Single fraction radiotherapy is efficacious: a further analysis of the Dutch Bone Metastasis Study controlling for the influence of retreatment. *Int J Radiat Oncol Biol Phys* 2004; 59:528.

49. Bone Pain Trial Working Party. 8 Gy single fraction radiotherapy for the treatment of metastatic skeletal pain: randomized comparison with a multifraction schedule over 12 months of patient follow-up. *Radiother Oncol* 1999; 52:111.

50. Hartsell WF, Scott CB, Bruner DW, et al. Randomized trial of short- versus long-course radiotherapy for palliation of painful bone metastases. *J Natl Cancer Inst* 2005; 97:798.

51. Townsend P, Rosenthal H, Smalley S, et al. Impact of postoperative radiation therapy and other perioperative factors on outcome after orthopedic stabilization of impending or pathologic fractures due to metastatic disease. *J Clin Oncol* 1994; 12:2345.

52. Porter A, McEwan AJ, Powe J, et al. Results of a randomized phase-III trial to evaluate the efficacy of strontium-89 adjuvant to local field external beam irradiation in the management of endocrine resistant metastatic prostate cancer. *Int J Radiat Oncol Biol Phys* 1993; 25:805–813.

53. Quilty PM, Kirk D, Bolger JJ, et al. A comparison of the palliative effects of strontium-89 and external beam radiotherapy in metastatic prostate cancer. *Radiother Oncol* 1994; 31:33–40.

54. Serafini AN, Houston SJ, Resche I, et al. Palliation of pain associated with metastatic bone cancer using samarium-153 lexidronam: a double-blind placebo-controlled clinical trial. *J Clin Oncol* 1998; 16:1574–1581.

55. Sartor O, Reid RH, Hoskin PJ, et al. Samarium-153-lexidronam complex for treatment of painful bone metastases in hormone-refractory prostate cancer. *Urology* 2004; 63:940–945.

56. Palmedo H, Manka-Waluch A, Albers P, et al. Repeated bone-targeted therapy for hormone refractory prostate carcinoma: randomized phase II trial with the new, high-energy radiopharmaceutical rhenium-188 hydroxyethylidenediphosphate. *J Clin Oncol* 2003; 21:2869.

57. Hipp J, Rosenberg A, Hayes W. Mechanical properties of trabecular bone within and adjacent to osseous metastases. *J Bone Miner Res* 1992; 7:1165.

58. Murray J, Bruels M, Landberg R. Irradiation of polymethylmethacrylate. In vitro gamma radiation effect. *J Bone Joint Surg Am* 1974; 56:311.

59. Zickel R, Mourandian W. Intramedullary fixation of pathological fractures and lesions of the subtrochanteric region of the femur. *J Bone Joint Surg Am* 1976; 58:1061.

60. Jang JS, Lee SH. Efficacy of percutaneous vertebroplasty combined with radiotherapy in osteolytic metastatic spinal tumors. *J Neurosurg Spine* 2005; 2:243.

61. Brown JE, Thomson C, Ellis S, et al. Bone resorption predicts for skeletal complications in metastatic bone disease. *Br J Cancer* 2003; 89:2031–2037.

62. Brown JE, Cook RJ, Major P, et al. Bone turnover markers as predictors of skeletal complications in prostate cancer, lung cancer, and other solid tumors. *J Natl Cancer Inst* 2005; 97:59–69.

63. Coleman RE, Major P, Lipton A, et al. The predictive value of bone resorption and formation markers in cancer patients with bone metastases receiving the bisphosphonate zoledronic acid. *J Clin Oncol* 2005; 23:4925–4935.

64. Papotti M, Kalebic T, Volante M, et al. Bone sialoprotein is predictive of bone metastases in resectable non-small-cell lung cancer: a retrospective case-control study. *J Clin Oncol* 2006; 24:4818–4824.

65. Kosteva J, Langer C. Incidence and distribution of skeletal metastases in NSCLC in the era of PET. *Lung Cancer* 2004; 46(Suppl 1):S45.

3 Cancer Pain

Stuart A. Grossman and Suzanne A. Nesbit

ABSTRACT

Cancer pain remains undertreated. Pain occurs in over three-quarters of cancer patients and remains one of the most feared aspects of this illness despite the excellent therapies that are available. Cancer pain commonly results from tumor compressing or invading soft tissue, bone, or nerves or from diagnostic or therapeutic endeavors. Optimal pain management involves determining pain intensity, evaluating the etiology of the pain, implementing a carefully considered therapeutic plan, and repeatedly assessing pain relief following therapeutic interventions. The vast majority of cancer pain can be well controlled with therapies readily available to most physicians. These include nonopioid analgesics, opioid analgesics, adjuvant medications, antineoplastic therapies, nonpharmacologic approaches, and neurostimulatory techniques. Regional anesthetic or neurosurgical approaches should be considered in selected patients with persistent pain or unrelieved toxicities from opioids. Nerve blocks can be extremely useful in selected patients with pancreatic cancer pain and thoracic pain in a dermatomal distribution. Referral to an experienced multidisciplinary pain team may be required in situations which are known to pose special challenges in pain management. These may include patients with unrelieved pain, neuropathic pain, episodic or incident pain, impaired cognitive or communication capabilities, or a history of substance abuse. The special challenges associated with the appropriate management of cancer pain include the subjective nature of pain, the complex multisystem involvement in patients with advanced malignancies, and the ever-changing clinical situation in this patient population.

From: Cancer and Drug Discovery Development: Supportive Care in Cancer Therapy
DOI: 10.1007/978-1-59745-291-5_3, Edited by: D. S. Ettinger © Humana Press, Totowa, NJ

Key Words: Cancer; Pain; Opioid; Assessment; Treatment.

OVERVIEW

Pain is one of the most common and feared symptoms associated with cancer. It occurs in one-quarter to one-half of patients with newly diagnosed malignancies, one-third of those undergoing treatment, and in over three-quarters with advanced disease *(1–3)*. Unrelieved pain directly affects patients' activities and their quality of life. The importance of this symptom and the availability of excellent analgesic therapies require health care providers to be adept at evaluating and treating cancer pain *(4)*.

Ninety percent of pain in cancer patients results from the tumor or its evaluation or therapy while less than 10% is due to unrelated illnesses *(4, 5)*. In 70% of patients, pain develops from tumor invading or compressing soft tissue, bone, or neural structures. The remainder results from diagnostic and therapeutic procedures such as venipunctures, bone marrow aspirations, lumbar punctures, and surgery *(6)*. Nerve injuries are common after mastectomy, thoracotomy, radical neck dissection, and limb amputation *(7)*. Chemotherapy and radiation can result in painful phlebitis, mucositis, cystitis, peripheral neuropathy, dermatitis, enteritis, or proctitis. Painful infections, such as pneumonias, urinary tract infections, wound infections, candida esophagitis, and herpes zoster, are not uncommon in this patient population. In addition, many of these patients also develop painful complications related to other medications, such as osteonecrosis secondary to bisphosphonates.

Although available treatment approaches should result in excellent pain control in the vast majority of patients, studies have routinely demonstrated that cancer pain remains grossly undertreated throughout the world *(8)*. In many developing countries, the unavailability of oral opioids is a major contributing factor *(9, 10)*. However, even in the United States where a wide assortment of opioid analgesics and routes of administration are available, cancer pain is undertreated *(11–13)*. Efforts to improve pain therapy led to the creation of cancer pain initiatives in many states, the development of cancer pain guidelines and algorithms by professional societies, and hospital accreditation requirements by the Joint Commission on Accreditation of Healthcare Organizations *(14–19)*. Inadequate treatment of patients with cancer pain occurs for many reasons (Table 1).

Table 1
Patient and health care provider barriers to providing optimal analgesia

Patient barriers	*Health care providers barriers*
• Failure to adequately communicate pain intensity to health care provider	• Unaware of magnitude of pain in patients
• Concern about addiction, tolerance, side effects	• Concern about addiction, tolerance, side effects
	• Serial quantitative measures of pain intensity poorly documented
	• Inadequate training on pain assessment and management
	• Subjective complaint

As pain is entirely subjective and can only be felt and quantified by the patient, health care providers must rely on patients to inform them of their pain experience. However, patients often do not emphasize pain issues as they (1) expect cancer to be painful, (2) may be concerned about opioid addiction, tolerance, side effects, or (3) do not want to divert physician attention from treating the tumor *(20)*. The underreporting of pain is further complicated by the observation that patients with chronic, severe pain may not "look" or "act" uncomfortable. The net result is that health care providers often do not appreciate the amount of pain their patients are experiencing *(21)*. This problem is further magnified in patient populations where there are additional communication challenges, such as with children, the elderly, those unable to talk, those with significant language or cultural barriers, or individuals with a history of drug abuse *(22–25)*.

Another barrier to the provision of adequate analgesia relates to the lack of training and emphasis on cancer pain management in medical professionals. Determining the etiology of the pain is critical as some pain diagnoses are associated with a unique therapeutic approach or sense of urgency *(26–28)*. For example, providing only opioids to a patient with metastatic cancer and back pain could be a serious error in a patient with an impending epidural cord compression. Similarly, without a basic understanding of opioid equivalencies serious dosing errors can occur when converting from one opioid or route of administration to another.

EVALUATION OF CANCER PAIN

A comprehensive assessment of cancer pain should provide sufficient information to *(1)* estimate the severity of pain, *(2)* form a clinical impression regarding the etiology of the pain, *(3)* determine the need for further diagnostic studies, and *(4)* formulate therapeutic recommendations that take into account the patient's overall medical and psychosocial status. As with any serious medical condition, this requires a detailed history, physical examination, and review of available records, laboratory data, and imaging studies. Special challenges associated with the assessment of cancer pain include the entirely subjective nature of pain, the complex multisystem involvement in patients with advanced malignancies, and the ever-changing clinical situation in this patient population.

A detailed history is the cornerstone of a thorough pain assessment. This may be complex as 75% of patients with advanced cancer have several painful sites and nearly one-third have four or more separate pain problems *(29, 30)*. Each should be identified and characterized with pertinent information on its intensity, location, radiation, how and when it began, how it has changed over time, and what makes it better or worse. Additional information should be collected on the quality of each pain, its temporal pattern, its association with neurologic or vasomotor abnormalities, how it interferes with the patient's life, and successes and failures of current and prior therapies. Many instruments have been developed to aid in pain assessment and serially follow the results of therapy *(31–33)*. Each instrument has shortcomings, but several have been validated in patients with cancer pain and incorporated into clinical practice. Most contain a variant of the unidimensional visual analogue scale (VAS) and a schematic representation of the body for the patient to indicate where their pain is located. The McGill Pain Questionnaire is comprehensive, but too awkward and time-consuming for most oncology patients in a clinical setting *(34, 35)*. The Wisconsin Brief Pain Inventory, which can be completed in 15 min, provides information on the characteristics, severity, and location of the pain, its interference with normal life functions, and the efficacy of prior therapy. The Memorial Pain Assessment Card can be completed in about 1 min and features scales for the measurement of pain intensity and pain relief *(36)*. It is also designed to provide insight into global suffering or psychological distress. The Hopkins Pain Rating Instrument is a validated plastic version of the VAS that simplifies repeated pain intensity measurements *(37, 38)*. A thorough oncologic history is critical as most pain in this patient population is related to the malignancy or cancer treatment. The histology, presentation, stage, sites of involvement, and natural history as well as surgery, radiation, chemotherapy, and hormonal treatments help shape a therapeutic approach. In addition, it is important to note if the malignancy is responding to therapy, stable, or progressing. A general medical history is also helpful as pain treatments can affect coexisting medical problems, exacerbate constitutional symptoms, interact with other medications, or be contraindicated because of allergies. For example, a patient with painful bone metastases and severe peptic ulcer disease would not be an ideal candidate for potent nonsteroidal anti-inflammatory agents. Opioids may be problematic in patients with severe benign prostatic hypertrophy or severe obstructive pulmonary disease. Likewise, knowledge that a patient tolerates food or fluids poorly by mouth, has an indwelling venous access device, or admits to substance abuse may influence decisions about the best way to control his pain. The patient's age, functional status, social support, education, residence, health insurance, finances, and goals for therapy may also figure prominently in planning therapy.

The history, physical examination, and review of other available data should provide sufficient information to formulate a differential diagnosis for each of the patient's distinct pains and to make recommendations regarding the work-up and therapy for each. Somatic, visceral, neuropathic, and sympathetically maintained pain may be approached differently. Prompt institution of therapy reassures patients that their pain will receive immediate attention, ensures patient comfort for diagnostic studies, and can provide information on the accuracy of the pain assessment. Excellent relief suggests an accurate diagnosis while suboptimal control may prompt a new treatment approach or a search for a different etiology to the pain. In this patient population, the status of the underlying malignancy, antineoplastic therapy, and the overall treatment goals will change during the course of the illness. As a result, the etiology and intensity of each new or worsening pain must be reassessed. The toxicities of the analgesics should also be periodically evaluated as they can substantially affect quality of life.

PHARMACOLOGIC MANAGEMENT

Nearly 85% of patients with cancer pain can be well controlled with conventional oral medications *(39, 40)*. More aggressive or invasive therapies should provide pain relief to an additional 10% of patients, leaving only a small fraction of cancer patients with inadequate relief. Pharmacologic approaches are the most commonly used treatments for cancer pain as they are effective, safe, and relatively inexpensive *(40–46)*. These are classified as nonopioids, opioids, and adjuvant analgesics. The site of action of the nonopioids is primarily in the peripheral nervous system. These agents are not associated with physical dependence, tolerance, or addiction, and have a maximum dose associated with analgesia. Many are available in combination with a weak opioid and can be useful in patients with somatic pain from bone metastasis, inflammation or mechanical compression of tendons, muscles, pleura, and peritoneum, and nonobstructive visceral pain (47, 48). As some of these agents can affect platelet and renal function or act as antipyretics, they should be administered thoughtfully to patients receiving chemotherapy. Sustained high doses of acetaminophen can cause renal and hepatic damage especially when combined with alcohol or other agents that cause liver damage or induce hepatic microsomes.

The opioids have their primary effect centrally where they interfere with pain perception. They can be classified into three groups: (1) morphine-like opioid agonists which bind competitively with mu and kappa receptors (codeine, fentanyl, hydromorphone, morphine, oxycodone, and methadone); (2) opioid antagonists which have no agonist receptor activity (naloxone); and (3) mixed agonists–antagonists (pentazocine and butorphanol) or partial agonists (buprenorphine). The mixed agonist–antagonist drugs have limited utility in cancer pain because of their side effect profile and propensity to induce opioid withdrawal in patients who have received opioid agonists. The vast majority of patients can be managed with oral opioids. These are best given "around the clock" to keep pain under control. Although tolerance to these agents occurs, tumor progression is the most common reason for increasing opioid requirements. Tolerance can be easily overcome by raising opioid doses. Addiction is rare in cancer patients taking opioids for pain relief. Most opioid side effects can be managed with appropriate interventions (49). Constipation should be anticipated and treated prophylactically. Proper opioid prescribing is critical to patients with cancer, who often require high doses of opioids for long periods of time. Important tenets of opioid prescribing are provided in Table 2.

Although most patients can be managed with oral opioids, alternate routes of analgesic administration are sometimes needed. Subcutaneous, intravenous, transdermal, transmucosal, or intraspinal opioids can be delivered by intermittent bolus, continuous infusion, or a combination of both as is frequently employed with patient-controlled analgesia. The costs associated with these routes of opioid administration must be carefully considered. In addition, care must be taken to avoid transforming home into a complex health care setting. Subcutaneous opioids administered through a subcutaneous needle on a fixed schedule are effective and less expensive than continuous intravenous or subcutaneous infusions (50). Transdermal fentanyl patches are beneficial in some patients. This delivery system does not eliminate the need for additional analgesics for breakthrough pain. Furthermore, the slow onset of action and the uncertainties associated in conversion from other opioids have led many to reserve transdermal fentanyl for patients with stable opioid requirements who do not have significant incident pain (51). Oral transmucosal fentanyl can be effective in patients with incident or breakthrough pain where rapid onset and short duration of action are desired. This route of delivery is expensive and the optimal dose is found through titration as it cannot be predicted from the total daily dose of administered opioids (52).

Intraspinal opioids can be delivered into the epidural space through a tunneled external catheter or to the subarachnoid space using a totally implanted pump (53).

Table 2
Important principles of opioid prescribing

- Order opioids on a scheduled "around-the-clock" basis to optimize relief
- Order a prn opioid to treat breakthrough or incident pain. For example, if a patient is taking morphine elixir 100 mg po every 4 h, order an additional 25–50 mg of oral morphine elixir every 2 h as needed for pain
- Initiate a prophylactic bowel regimen at the same time opioids are prescribed
- Treat opioid-induced nausea and vomiting aggressively. Patients often become tolerant to this side effect several days after beginning opioids
- Consider converting to sustained release opioid preparations once baseline opioid requirements are determined
- Teach the patient and family about the purpose and benefits of opioids to allay their fears about side effects and addiction. This will improve compliance
- Assess pain relief frequently during the opioid titration period. Titrate doses based on the patient's report of pain and the amount of prn opioid required for patient comfort
- Maximize the dose of one opioid before changing to another agent or route. Changes should be made primarily because of toxicities
- Refer to equi-analgesic tables or opioid conversion software when initiating or changing a patient's analgesic regimen (NCCN guidelines or Hopkins Opioid Conversion Software) *(80, 81)*
- Avoid chronic administration of IM or rectal opioids and the use of meperidine that has a neurotoxic metabolite
- Exercise caution when using methadone that has a long pharmacologic half-life and difficult equianalgesic conversions to and from other opioids *(82)*

As the total daily dose of intraspinal opioid is one-tenth to one-hundredth of parenteral opioid, it is associated with fewer systemic toxicities. Chronic epidural or intrathecal opioids are invasive, expensive, and frequently ineffective in patients requiring high doses of systemic opioids. Tolerance, pruritus, urinary retention, and nausea and vomiting occur in up to 20% of patients receiving spinal opioids. Respiratory depression is unusual. The addition of low doses of anesthetic agents or clonidine to intrathecal and epidural opioids may add considerably to pain relief. Intraspinal opioids are generally used after documentation of the failure of maximal doses of systemic opioids although recent studies suggest that they may be beneficial earlier in patients with cancer pain *(54)*.

Agents that are used primarily for conditions other than pain have been found to be useful "adjuvant" analgesics in specific circumstances *(55)*. Antidepressants and anticonvulsants may be effective in neuropathic pain. Psychostimulants can decrease opioid-induced sedation. Glucocorticoids are effective anti-inflammatory agents and are also used to reduce pain associated with brain edema and epidural metastases. Muscle relaxants, anxiolytic, antispasmodic, and neuroleptic agents are also employed for specific indications. Bisphosphonates reduce the incidence of skeletal complications particularly in patients with myeloma and breast cancer *(56–58)*. Caution must be exercised in the use of adjuvant drugs with sedative properties, as the dose of opioids should not be compromised by the toxicities of these secondary agents.

Therapy directed against the tumor itself can provide pain relief if it reduces the size of lesions invading or compressing normal tissues. Radiation therapy is the treatment of choice for most patients with local pain from tumor progression. It is frequently administered to patients with symptomatic bone, brain, epidural, and plexus metastases. Systemic radiopharmaceuticals such as strontium 89, samarium-153-EDTMP are also used for the treatment of pain from bone metastases (59, 60). Chemotherapy can provide substantial pain relief in malignancies that respond to this therapeutic modality. Surgery can be effective in relieving pain from intestinal obstruction, pathologic fractures, and obstructive hydrocephalus.

NONPHARMACOLOGIC, REGIONAL ANALGESIC, AND SURGICAL APPROACHES

Neurostimulatory techniques, such as transcutaneous electrical nerve stimulation (TENS), are safe, noninvasive, relatively inexpensive, and easily added to other analgesic approaches (61). TENS may provide short-term benefits in cancer patients and a 2–4-week trial will often determine its clinical utility. Nonpharmacologic approaches such as progressive muscle relaxation, massage, heat or cold, guided imagery, biofeedback, hypnosis, and acupuncture (62) are useful adjuncts to pain management. Although psychotherapy is indicated for an associated depression, unrelieved pain may result in depression that is best treated with analgesic therapies (63).

While most cancer pain can be well controlled using the approaches outlined above, some pain remains refractory and some patients experience adverse effects from opioids despite aggressive therapy with psychostimulants, antiemetics, and laxatives. Adding adjuvant medications, changing to another opioid, or using continuous intravenous or subcutaneous infusions to reduce "peak" levels may be helpful. However, in selected patients, regional analgesia or neuroablative procedures may allow the doses of systemically administered opioids agents to be reduced substantially. These invasive approaches should be considered if (1) significant pain persists at doses of analgesics causing dose-limiting side effects, (2) excessive toxicities result from opioid analgesics, or (3) if a careful assessment suggests that a low-risk procedure is likely to result in excellent analgesia.

Regional pain relief can be achieved with long-acting local anesthetics (such as bupivacaine) which provide pain relief for 3–12 h, neurolytic agents (alcohol or phenol) which produce analgesia for weeks to months, or opioids injected into the epidural or subarachnoid space (64). Diagnostic blocks with local anesthetics are usually performed prior to neurolysis. This permits the anesthesiologist to determine the response to local therapy and the patient to decide if the "numbness" that replaces the pain is tolerable. If the pain can be relieved temporarily with local anesthetics, alcohol or phenol can be injected into the subarachnoid or epidural space to destroy nociceptive fibers in the dorsal rootlets simulating a surgical rhizotomy. Injections of these neurolytic agents can augment pain relief for months and can be repeated if the pain recurs. Neurolytic blocks may be particularly useful in the thoracic region where they are associated with few motor complications. In the cervical and lumbar regions, nearly 20% of patients develop motor and/or sphincter dysfunction that may be permanent. In patients with preexisting lower extremity paralysis, colostomy, or nephrostomy tubes where loss of motor or sphincter function may be less critical, lumbar neurolysis may be worthwhile. Other potential side effects of these procedures include hypotension, toxic reactions from accidental intravenous or subarachnoid administration, or pneumothorax following needle placement. Neurolysis is usually restricted to patients with a limited life expectancy as it can produce a painful neuritis that becomes clinically apparent months following the procedure.

Celiac plexus neurolysis is an outpatient procedure associated with few risks that alleviates pain originating in the pancreas, stomach, gallbladder, or other upper abdominal viscera in most patients. This procedure has been shown to decrease opioid requirements and improve pain control (65–67). Although pain may recur months after a celiac block, subsequent blocks are often associated with excellent pain relief. Less commonly used neurolytic procedures include intercostal blocks (chest wall or rib pain), neuroaxial blocks (pain in 2–3 dermatomes), Gasserian ganglion neurolysis (pain in the anterior two-thirds of the head), and brachial plexus blocks (for patients with preexisting limb paralysis). Neuroablative procedures are rarely performed on cancer patients because of the success of more conservative approaches and the risks associated with these surgical approaches. The most commonly performed procedures are radiofrequency ablation and the open unilateral anterolateral cordotomy, percutaneous cordotomy, and commissural myelotomy. Cordotomies are usually performed through a T2 or T3 laminectomy and produce analgesia in the lower part of the body in about 80% of patients. A 5–10% mortality rate and significant morbidity in an additional 15% of patients is reported with this procedure. Hemiparesis, urinary retention, sexual impotence, unmasking pain on the opposite side of the body, and late sensory abnormalities are not infrequent. Bilateral cordotomies are associated with higher complication rates. Percutaneous cordotomy is safer. These procedures are associated with a recurrence of pain within three months in 50% of patients. A commissural myelotomy can be considered in selected patients with bilateral pelvic and perineal pain. This involves surgical division of the crossing fibers of the spinal cord. Although it may result in pain relief with sphincter sparing, few neurosurgeons have expertise with this procedure.

CHALLENGING PAIN PROBLEMS

Patients with impaired cognitive or communicative skills, episodic or incident pain, neuropathic pain, or a history of substance abuse pose special challenges (68). Referral to an experienced multidisciplinary cancer pain team may be helpful if initial attempts to control pain in patients with these problems are not successful.

Patients with Impaired Cognitive or Communicative Function

Problems conveying pain intensity are greatly magnified in patients who cannot communicate with their health care providers or who are cognitively impaired. These deficits complicate the assessment of pain intensity as well as determining the etiology of the pain and the effect of therapeutic efforts. These are not uncommon issues for health care providers caring for cancer patients. Some are unable to speak the language of the health care provider while others may be intubated or have neurologic deficits such as an expressive aphasia. Children and the elderly have special difficulty communicating pain intensity and patients with severe cognitive deficits present obvious challenges in assessing this entirely subjective symptom *(69, 70)*. Delirious patients with cancer are often restless, moaning, and unable to convey the intensity, nature, or even location of their pain. These patients require a review of correctable factors contributing to the delirium. Neurologic events, infections, trauma, bladder distension, fecal impaction, hypoxia, or metabolic abnormalities are common. The patient's drug regimen should be simplified and agents with anticholinergic properties should be discontinued. If the patient is on an opioid, reducing the dose, switching agents, or using a continuous infusion or sustained release preparation to avoid wide fluctuations in drug levels may result in improvement.

Patients with Episodic or Incident Pain

Many patients with cancer experience transient and clinically significant pain that occurs over baseline pain that is well controlled by analgesics *(71–73)*. This can occur at the end of an opioid dosing interval suggesting that the baseline analgesic dose may need to be increased or the interval between dosing should be shortened. Episodic pain associated with voluntary or involuntary movements poses a more difficult therapeutic problem. Examples of these "incident pains" are seen in patients with pelvic or vertebral body metastases or pathologic fractures, who have severe pain with walking or sitting. Patients with rib metastases may experience stabbing chest pain with movement or coughing and patients with esophageal, rectal, or bladder lesions may have severe discomfort with swallowing, defecation, or urination, respectively. Involuntary precipitants can include bowel or ureteral distension. In a recent study, nearly three-quarters of incident pain was related to a neoplastic lesion, 20% resulted from anti-neoplastic therapy, and the remainder was unrelated to the tumor or its treatment *(74)*.

Proper management of these patients requires a comprehensive assessment to determine the origin of the pain. Therapy directed at the underlying etiologic factors is most likely to provide pain relief. Relieving a bowel obstruction, repairing or splinting a fracture, treating a local metastatic lesion with radiation therapy, or performing a neurolytic block for a painful rib lesion are likely to provide better long-term relief than opioids. The frequency and severity of incident pain may also be significantly reduced by anti-inflammatory agents or corticosteroids in bone or nerve compression pain and anticonvulsants or tricyclic antidepressants in neuropathic pain. In addition, therapies to reduce the frequency of precipitating events should be employed. These may include antitussives, laxatives, antiperistaltic drugs, or agents that reduce muscle spasms. Physiotherapy may be useful in musculoskeletal complications and the cognitive and psychological approaches can be helpful to patients with these pains. Carefully selected patients may require invasive anesthetic or neurosurgical approaches or epidural anesthetics and opioids for relief of these transient but severe pains.

Many of the approaches listed above may not be effective, possible, or advisable in the context of a patient's illness. In these situations, opioids remain the mainstay of therapy. The baseline dose of opioid can be escalated until pain relief or intolerable side effects occur. While this may produce relief, patients are often excessively sedated during the intervals between the severe pains. Alternatively, patients may take supplemental analgesics, usually short-acting opioids, 30–60 min before a precipitating event is likely to occur. If the pain is unpredictable, the additional medications are taken as soon as the pain begins. Transmucosal fentanyl or parenteral opioids given by patient-controlled analgesia may be useful if the onset of action is too slow by the oral route. The doses of these supplemental opioids must be determined from the patient's baseline opioid requirements. It is common to begin with 5–10% of the total daily opioid dose ordered every 2–3 h as needed.

Neuropathic Pain

Neuropathic pain is often characterized by paroxysms of shock-like pain on top of a burning or constricting sensation. Neuropathic pain in patients with cancer commonly arises from tumor invading or compressing peripheral nerve, nerve plexus, or spinal cord. It can occur as a result of surgery, radiation, or chemotherapy as exemplified by post-mastectomy and post-thoracotomy syndromes, radiation-induced plexopathies, and chemotherapy-induced neuropathies *(75)*. Neuropathic pain may also accompany disorders that are unrelated to the tumor or its treatment, such as diabetes mellitus, nerve entrapment syndromes, and herpes zoster. Providing adequate relief from neuropathic pain is often difficult even for the most experienced physicians. Although this pain may improve on opioids, it appears to respond less well to these agents than nociceptive pain. Optimal therapy of neuropathic pain often relies on opioids used in combination with nonopioid "adjuvant" analgesics. Tricyclic antidepressants have been studied most extensively in this situation and may work through the inhibition of serotonin and norepinephrine. Although the most convincing efficacy data is with amitriptyline, this agent is associated with significant anticholinergic effects and sedation. As a result, desipramine, which has a more favorable toxicity profile, is prescribed more commonly. Serotonin and nonserotonin reuptake inhibitors including duloxetine and venlafaxine have also been helpful in some patients. Anticonvulsants are also helpful in the management of neuropathic pain, particularly if it has lancinating qualities *(76)*. The doses of these agents are similar to those used for the control of seizures. Care must be taken to avoid abrupt withdrawal as this may induce seizures. The most commonly used agents are gabapentin, pregabalin, lamotrigine *(77, 78)*. Anesthetic creams that produce few systemic side effects are also available. Capsaicin, a neurotoxin that selectively destroys nociceptors, is manufactured as a topical preparation and provides relief in some patients. If oral agents and topical creams are ineffective, afferent input can be reduced with TENS *(79)* regional anesthetic techniques such as long-term epidural catheters or intrathecal pumps for the delivery of local anesthetics.

Patients with a History of Substance Abuse

The overall assessment and management of cancer pain are not different in patients with a history of drug abuse. These patients should not be permitted to remain in pain merely because of a history of drug abuse. It is helpful to divide patients with a drug abuse history into three different subgroups. The first may have used drugs inappropriately in the very distant past. The second may have more recent drug exposure but for months or years have done well, perhaps with a steady job and enrollment in a long-term methadone program suggesting that this may be a problem in the past. In these two patient groups, the primary challenge is often to encourage the patient and involved family members that opioids are indicated and needed to control their cancer pain. Those on methadone may require higher than usual doses of opioids because of tolerance to these agents. Many of these patients have difficulty finding physicians who believe their reports of pain and who will provide the high doses of analgesics required. As a result, they may become angry, frustrated, and more persistent in their demands for opioids. This constellation of symptoms is also seen in patients who do not have a history of drug abuse but have severe, untreated pain. Their "appropriate" preoccupation with obtaining analgesics is referred to as "pseudo-addiction" and tends to disappear rapidly when they are provided with appropriate pain medications *(79)*.

The third group is comprised of those actively abusing drugs. These patients are difficult to engage in a therapeutic relationship and frequently have poor social support networks. They require a coordinated plan and a dedicated team as well as frank discussions relating to the proper use of opioid analgesics for pain management. Oral agents are preferred and local therapies to painful sites, such as radiation therapy or nerve blocks, which may limit the need for opioids should be considered. Early referrals to tertiary care centers are often required if the care of these patients does not go smoothly.

REFERENCES

1. Cleeland CS. The impact of pain on patients with cancer. Cancer 1984: 54:2635–2641.
2. Foley KM. The treatment of cancer pain. N Engl J Med 1985: 313:84–95.
3. van den Beuken-van Everdingen, Mde Rijke J, Kessels A, Schouten H, van Kleef M, Patijn J. Prevalence of pain in patients with cancer: a systematic review of the past 40 years. Ann Oncol 2007; 18:1437–1449.
4. Twycross R, Harcourt J, Bergl S. A survey of pain in patients with advanced cancer. J Pain Symptom Manage 1996: 12:273–282.
5. Cleeland CS, Gonin R, Hatfield AK, et al. Pain and its treatment in our patients with metastatic cancer. N Engl J Med 1996: 330:595–596.
6. Portnow J, Lim C, Grossman SA. Assessment of pain caused by invasive procedures in cancer patients. J NCCN 2003: 1:435–439.
7. Cherny NI. Cancer pain: principles of assessment and syndromes, in Berger AM, Portenoy RK, Weissman DE (eds), Principles and Practice of Supportive Oncology, Philadelphia: Lippincott-Raven Publishers, 1998: 3–42.
8. Joranson DE. Availability of opioids for cancer pain: recent trends, assessment of system barriers, New World Health Organization guidelines, and the risk of diversion. J Pain Symptom Manage 1993: 8:353–360.
9. Angarola RT. Availability and regulation of opioid analgesics. Adv Pain Res Ther 1990: 16:513–525.
10. Koshy RC, Rhodes D, Devi S, Grossman SA. Cancer pain management in developing countries: a mosaic of complex issues resulting in inadequate analgesia. Support Care Cancer 1998: 6:430–437.
11. Cleeland CS, Gonin R, Hatfield AK, et al. Pain and its treatment in outpatients with metastatic cancer. N Engl J Med 1994: 330:592–596.
12. Cleeland CS, Pandya KJ, Loehrer P, et al. Pain and treatment of pain in minority patients with cancer. The Eastern Cooperative Oncology Group Minority Outpatient Pain Study. Ann Intern Med 1997: 127:813–816.
13. van Roenn JH, Cleeland CS, Gonin R, et al. Physician attitudes and practice in cancer pain management. A survey from the Eastern Cooperative Oncology Group. Ann Intern Med 1993: 119:121–126.
14. Ad Hoc Committee on Cancer Pain. Cancer pain assessment and treatment curriculum guidelines. J Clin Oncol 1992: 10:1976–1982.
15. American Pain Society Quality of Care Committee: Quality improvement guidelines for the treatment of acute pain and cancer pain. J Am Med Assoc 1995: 274:1874–1880.
16. Spross JA, McGuire DB, Schmitt R. Oncology Nursing Society position paper on cancer pain. Oncol Nurs Forum 1990: 17:595–614 (Part I); 17:751–757 (Part II); 17:825, 944–955 (Part III).
17. Jacox A, Carr DB, Payne R, et al. Management of Cancer Pain: Clinical Practice Guideline No. 9. AHCPR Publication No. 94–0592. Rockville, MD: Agency for Health Care Policy and Research, US Dept of Health and Human Services, Public Health Service, 1994.
18. Grossman SA. Management of Cancer Pain: National Comprehensive Cancer Network Guidelines. Oncology 1999: 13:33–44.

19. Curtiss CP. JCAHO: meeting the standards for pain management. Orthop Nurs 2001: 20:27–30.
20. Ward SE, Goldberg N, Miller-McCauley V, et al. Patient-related barriers to management of cancer pain. Pain 1993: 52:319–324.
21. Grossman SA, Sheidler VR, Swedeen K, et al. Correlation of patient and caregiver ratings of cancer pain. J Pain Sympt Manage 1991: 6:53–57.
22. Schechter NL. Pain in children with cancer. Adv Pain Res Ther 1990: 16:57–72.
23. McGrath PA. Development of the World Health Organization Guidelines on Cancer Pain Relief and Palliative Care in Children. J Pain Symptom Manage 1996: 12:87–92.
24. Cleary JF, Carbone PP. Palliative medicine in the elderly. Cancer 1997: 80:1335–1347.
25. Passik SD, Portenoy RK. Substance abuse issues in palliative care, in Berger AM, Portenoy RK, Weissman DE (eds), Principles and Practice of Supportive Oncology, Philadelphia: Lippincott-Raven Publishers, 1998: 513–529.
26. Mortimer JE, Bartlett NJ. Assessment of knowledge about cancer pain management by physicians in training. J Pain Symptom Manage 1997: 14:21–28.
27. Sheidler VR, McGuire DB, Gilbert MR, et al. Analgesic decision making skills of nurses. Oncol Nurs Forum 1992: 19:1531–1534.
28. Au E, Loprinzi CL, Dhodapkar M, et al: Regular use of a verbal pain scale improves the understanding of oncology inpatient pain intensity. J Clin Oncol 1994: 12:2751–2755.
29. Twycross RG: Relief of pain, in Saunders CM (ed), The Management of Terminal Disease, 1978: Chicago Yearbook Publishers, 1978: 65.
30. Twycross RG. Incidence of pain. Clin Oncol 1984: 3:5.
31. Vallerand AH: Measurement issues in the comprehensive assessment of cancer pain. Semin Oncol Nurs 1997: 13:16–24.
32. Paice JA, Cohen FL. Validity of a verbally administered numeric rating scale to measure cancer pain intensity. Cancer Nurs 1997: 20:88–93.
33. Chibnal JT. Pain assessment in cognitively impaired and unimpaired older adults: a comparison of four scales. Pain 2001: 92:173–186.
34. Melzack R: The McGill pain questionnaire: major properties and scoring methods. Pain 1975: 1:277–299.
35. Graham C, Bond SS, Gerkovich MM, et al. Use of the McGill pain questionnaire in the assessment of cancer pain: replicability and consistency. Pain 1980: 8:377–387.
36. Fishman B, Pasternak S, Wallenstein S, et al. The Memorial pain assessment card: a valid instrument for the evaluation of cancer pain. Cancer 1987: 60:1151–1158.
37. Grossman SA, Sheidler VR, McGuire DB, et al. A comparison of the Hopkins Pain Rating Instrument with standard visual analogue and verbal descriptor scales in patients with cancer pain. J Pain Symptom Manage 1992: 7:196–203.
38. Rhodes DJ, Koshy R, Sheidler VR, Waterfield W, Wu A, Grossman SA. Feasibility of quantitative pain assessment in outpatient oncology practice. J Clin Oncol 2001: 19:501–508.
39. Wiffen PJ, Edwards JE, Barden J, McQuay JH. Oral morphine for cancer pain. Cochrane Database Syst Rev 2003: 4:CD003868.
40. Zech DF, Grond S, Lynch J, et al. Validation of the World Health Organization guidelines for cancer pain relief: a 10-year prospective study. Pain 1995: 63:65–76.
41. Cherny NI, Foley KM. Nonopioid and opioid analgesic pharmacotherapy of cancer pain. Hematol Oncol Clin North Am 1996: 10:79–102.
42. Hanks G, Cherny N. Analgesic therapy, in Doyle D, Hanks G, MacDonald N (eds), Oxford Textbook of Palliative Medicine, Oxford: Oxford Medical Publications, 1998: 331–355.
43. Cancer Pain Relief and Palliative Care. Report of a WHO Expert Committee. Geneva: World Health Organization, 1990 (WHO Technical Report Series, No. 804).
44. Grossman SA, Staats PS. Current management of pain in patients with cancer. Oncology 1994: 8:93–107.
45. Portenoy RK. Pharmacologic management of cancer pain. Seminars in Oncology 1995: 22(2 Suppl 3):112–120.
46. Levy MH. Pharmacologic treatment of cancer pain. N Engl J Med 1996: 335:1124–1132.
47. Eisenberg E, Berkey CS, Carr DB, et al. Efficacy and safety of nonsteroidal antiinflammatory drugs for cancer pain: a meta-analysis. J Clin Oncol 1994: 2:2756–2765.
48. McNicol E, Strassels S, Goudas L, et al. Nonsteroidal anti-inflammatory drugs, alone or combined with opioids, for cancer pain: a systematic review. J Clin Oncol 2004: 22:1975–1992.
49. McNicol E, Horowicz-Mehler N, Fisk RA, et al. Management of opioid side effects in cancer-related and chronic noncancer pain: a systematic review. J Pain 2003: 4:231–256.
50. Crane RA. Intermittent subcutaneous infusion of opioids in hospice home care: an effective, economical, manageable option. Am J Hosp Palliat Care 1994: 11:8–12.
51. Stanley TH. Fentanyl. J Pain Symptom Manage 2005: 29(5 Suppl) S67–S71.

52. Streisand JB, Busch MA, Egan TD, et al. Dose proportionality and pharmacokinetics of oral transmucosal fentanyl citrate. Anesthesiology 1998: 88:305–309.

53. Ballantyne JC, Carwood CM. Comparative efficacy of epidural, subarachnoid, and intracerebroventricular opioids in patients with pain due to cancer. Cochrane Database Syst Rev 2005: 1:CD005178.

54. Smith TJ, Staats PS, Deer T, et al. Randomized clinical trial of an implantable drug delivery system compared with comprehensive medical management for refractory cancer pain: impact on pain, drug-related toxicity, and survival. J Clin Oncol 2002: 20:4040–4049.

55. Lussier D, Huskey AGB, Portenoy RK. Adjuvant analgesics in cancer pain management. Oncologist 2004: 9:571–591.

56. Body JJ, Piccart M, Coleman RE. Use of bisphosphonates in cancer patients. Cancer Treat Rev 1996: 22:265–287.

57. Seaman J, Knight RD. Efficacy of pamidronate in reducing skeletal events in patients with advanced multiple myeloma. N Engl J Med 1996: 334:488–493.

58. Hortobagyi GN, Theriault RL, Lipton A, et al. Long-term prevention of skeletal complications of metastatic breast cancer with pamidronate. J Clin Oncol 1998: 16:2038–2044.

59. Janjan NA. Radiation for bone metastases: conventional techniques and the role of systemic radiopharmaceuticals. Cancer 1997: 80(8 Suppl):1628–1645.

60. Rogers CL, Speiser BL, Ram PC, et al. Efficacy and toxicity of strontium-89 for symptomatic osseous metastases. J lBrachyther Int 1998: 14:133–142.

61. Long DM. Fifteen years of transcutaneous electrical stimulation for pain control. Stereotact Funct Neurosurg 1991: 56:2–19.

62. Cohen AJ, Menter A, Hale L. Acupuncture: role in comprehensive cancer care--a primer for the oncologist and review of the literature. Integr Cancer Ther 2005: 4:131–143.

63. Patrick DL, Ferketich SL, Frame PS, et al. National Institutes of Health State-of-the-Science Conference Statement: Symptom Management in Cancer: Pain, Depression, and Fatigue. J Natl Cancer Inst 2003: 95:1110–1117.

64. Bonica JJ, Ventafridda V,Twycross RG. Section E: Regional Analgesia/Anesthesia in The Management of Pain, 2nd ed. Malvern, Pa: Lea & Febiger; 1990: 1878–2039.

65. Lillemoe KD, Cameron JL, Kaufman HS, et al. Chemical splanchnicectomy in patients with unresectable pancreatic cancer. Ann Surg 1993: 217:447–455.

66. Mercadante S. Celiac Plexus block versus analgesics in pancreatic cancer pain. Pain 1993: 52:187–192.

67. Wong GY, Schroeder DR, Carns PE, et al. Effect of neurolytic celiac plexus block on pain relief, quality of life, and survival in patients with unresectable pancreatic cancer: a randomized controlled trial. JAMA 2004: 291:1092–1099.

68. Hanks G, Portenoy RK, MacDonald N, et al. Difficult pain problems, in Doyle D, Hanks G, MacDonald N (eds), Oxford Textbook of Palliative Medicine (2nd edn), Oxford: Oxford Medical Publications, 1998: 454–477.

69. Balducci L. Management of cancer pain in geriatric patients. J Support Oncol 2003: 1:175–191.

70. Levy MH, Samuel TA. Management of cancer pain. Semin Oncol 2005: 32:179–193.

71. Zeppetella G, Ribeiro MD. Opioids for the management of breakthrough (episodic) pain in cancer patients. Cochrane Database Syst Rev 2006: 25:CD004311.

72. Payne R. Recognition and diagnosis of breakthrough pain. Pain Med 2007: 8(Suppl 1):S3–S7.

73. Svendsen KB, Andersen S, Arnason S, et al. Breakthrough pain in malignant and non-malignant diseases: a review of prevalence, characteristics and mechanisms. Eur J Pain 2005: 9:195–206.

74. Portenoy RK, Hagen NA. Breakthrough pain: definition, prevalence, and characteristics. Pain 1990: 41:273–282.

75. Paice JA. Mechanisms and management of neuropathic pain in cancer. J Support Oncol 2003: 1:107–120.

76. Wiffen P, Collins S, McQuay H, et al. Anticonvulsant drugs for acute and chronic pain. Cochrane Database Syst Rev 2005: 3:CD001133.

77. Moulin DE, Clark AJ, Gilron I, et al. Pharmacological management of chronic neuropathic pain - consensus statement and guidelines from the Canadian Pain Society. Pain Res Manag 2007: 12:13–21.

78. Bosnjak S, Jelic S, Susnjar S, Luki V. Gabapentin for relief of neuropathic pain related to anticancer treatment: a preliminary study. J Chemother 2002: 14:214–219.

79. Weissman DE, Haddox JD. Opioid pseudoaddiction: an iatrogenic syndrome. Pain 1989: 36:363–366.

80. Mercadantc S, Bruera W. Opioid switching: a systemic and critical review. Cancer Treat Rev 2006: 32:304–315.

81. Grossman SA, Nesbit S. Hopkins Opioid Conversion Software for PDA's and web-based use. www.hopweb.org.

82. Ripamonti C, Groff L, Brunelli C, et al. Switching from morphine to oral methadone in treating cancer pain: what is the equianalgesic dose ratio? J Clin Oncol 1998: 16:3216–3221.

4 Anorexia and Cachexia

Takao Ohnuma and James F. Holland

ABSTRACT

Cachexia is a complex syndrome presenting wasting of muscle and adipose tissues, weight loss, anorexia, early satiety, fatigue, anemia, hyperlipidemia, systemic inflammatory responses, and often a hypercatabolic state. Cachexia differs from starvation, where visceral proteins are also depleted. Profound anorexia and early satiety are partly responsible, but metabolic abnormalities are the major cause of cachexia. Mechanisms of cachexia include production of inflammatory cytokines including TNF-α, Interleuken-1 (IL-1), IL-6, and IFN-γ; secretion of tumor byproducts, which include lipolytic factors and proteolysis-inducing factor; hormonal aberration; prostaglandin elevation; possible dysfunction of neuropeptidergic circuits; and metabolic derangement produced by treatment. A variety of agents have been used in attempts to reverse cachexia, including corticosteroids, megestrol acetate and medroxyprogesterone acetate, anabolic steroids, cannabinoids, growth hormones, somatostatin and GHRP-2, insulin-like growth factor 1, metoclopramide and cisapride, hydrazine sulfate, anti-inflammatory agents such as indomethacin and ibuprofen, pentoxifylline and lisofylline, proteasome inhibitors and NF-κB inhibitors, clenbuterol, thalidomide, adenosine triphosphate, 5′-deoxy-5-fluorouridine, proinflammatory-cytokine inhibitors including proinflammatory cytokine antibodies and anti-inflammatory cytokines, eicosapentaenoic acid, enteral and parenteral nutrition, branched-chain amino acids, orexigenic mediators, melatonin and cyproheptidine. Currently, the most commonly used agent is megestrol acetate; however, megestrol-induced weight gain is mainly from water and fat, rather than muscle protein. Side effects include thromboembolic phenomena. In early studies, thalidomide and NF-κB inhibitors appear effective at attenuating loss of

From: *Cancer and Drug Discovery Development: Supportive Care in Cancer Therapy*
DOI: 10.1007/978-1-59745-291-5_4, Edited by: D. S. Ettinger © Humana Press, Totowa, NJ

weight and lean body mass in cancer cachexia. Development of agents that prevent or reverse loss of lean body weight mass is eagerly awaited.

Key Words: Anorexia; Cachexia; Mechanisms; Serotonin; Inflammatory cytokines; Lipid-mobilizing factor; Prostaglandin; Proteolysis-inducing factor; Corticosteroids; Megestrol acetate; NF-κB inhibitors; Thalidomide; Eicosapentaenoic acid.

INTRODUCTION

Cachexia and anorexia are commonly associated with a number of acute and chronic diseases, including cancer, acquired immunodeficiency syndrome, sepsis, chronic heart failure, kidney failure, burn injury, severe trauma, and chronic arthritis *(1)*.

Cachexia is a complex syndrome presenting as wasting of muscle and adipose tissues, weight loss, anorexia, early satiety, fatigue, anemia, hyperlipidemia, systemic inflammatory responses including elevated proinflammatory cytokines and often a hypercatabolic state.

In a study to establish factors influencing survival of cancer patients after diagnosis of terminal cancer of the lung, breast, or gastrointestinal tract, shorter survival was independently associated with a weight loss of greater than 8.1 kg in the previous 6 months *(2)*. In addition to a reduction in survival time, patients had a reduced quality of life. Chronic pain and fatigue were common, and there was a poor tolerance to surgery, chemotherapy, and radiotherapy *(3)*.

Extensive loss of skeletal muscle mass and adipose tissue in cachexia may be contrasted with simple starvation in which fat replaces glucose as the preferred fuel to spare lean body mass *(4–6)*. Cancer cachexia results from altered metabolism rather than just an energy deficit, and it cannot be reversed by forced feeding *(7, 8)*. This article serves as an update of the authors' previous work *(9)*.

ETIOLOGY AND MECHANISMS

The causes of cancer-related cachexia are multifold and can be grouped into three interrelated categories: anorexia and early satiety, mechanical obstruction of the alimentary tract, and metabolic derangement.

Anorexia and Early Satiety

Anorexia in cancer patients can be divided into three categories: disease-related, treatment-related, and emotional distress-related. Anorexia may result from early satiety, nausea, or dysgeusia, a change in taste.

Abnormalities of taste sensation and olfaction for food aromas have been demonstrated in cancer patients *(10, 11)*. Patients displayed a distaste for sweet foods as compared to healthy subjects, which correlated with a loss of taste sensation. Patients experiencing food aversion found the odors of chocolate, pork, roast beef, and chicken significantly less pleasant than controls *(11)*.

Etiologic Factors of Anorexia and Early Satiety

Animal studies and clinical trials have identified many factors as causes of cancer anorexia. Examples are listed in Table 1, which illustrates that cancer anorexia is probably multifactorial. Among these factors, serotonin and cytokines as well as neuropeptidergic circuit dysfunction are worthy of additional comments.

SEROTONIN

Abnormal tumor cell utilization of tryptophan, the precursor of serotonin, with resultant excess-free tryptophan levels in the plasma has been reported in cancer patients *(12)*. Increase in blood tryptophan results in elevated tryptophan levels in the cerebrospinal fluid, which appears to induce increased serotonin synthesis/secretion in the ventromedial hypothalamic (VMH) serotonergic system. A close relationship between elevated plasma-free tryptophan and anorexia was observed in patients with cancer *(13)*. Increases in urinary excretion of 5-hydroxyindoleacetic acid, the main metabolite of serotonin, have been identified after cisplatin treatment in cancer patients *(14)*. As described below, studies of cytokines and neuropeptide circuits have led to identification of CNS serotonin as a major mediator of cancer anorexia *(15)*.

CYTOKINES

Certain cytokines, such as tumor necrosis factor-α (TNF-α) and interleukin-1 (IL-1), have been shown to be mediators of anorexia. While TNF-α induces IL-1, both cytokines appear to be operative in mediating their anorectic effect through the brain as well as directly on the gastrointestinal tract, e.g., decrease in gastric emptying time *(16, 17)*. Peripherally infused IL-1 increased brain tryptophan and serotonin concentrations, whereas intracerebrally infused IL-1 increased neural firing rate and serotonin release in the VMH, suggesting that IL-1 production during tumor growth facilitated tryptophan conversion in the brain.

Using methylcholanthrene-induced tumors in rats, various specific components of the cytokine-induced anorectic reactions were examined in the tumor tissue, the liver, and the brain including IL-1β system components (ligand, signaling receptor, receptor accessory proteins, and receptor antagonist), TNF-α, TGF-β1, and IFN-γ. IL-1β, TNF-α,

Table 1
Possible causes of cancer anorexia

(a) Bombesin, a neuropeptide produced by small-cell lung cancer *(288)*

(b) Certain cytokines, e.g., TNF-a and IL-1 *(13)*

(c) Emetogenic anticancer agents, e.g., cisplatin, nitrogen mustard, doxorubicin *(14)*

(d) Glucagon or glucagon-like peptides *(289)*

(e) Hypercalcemia, a common paraneoplastic syndrome *(290)*

(f) Increases in serum lactate, known to be produced abundantly by tumor *(291)*

(g) Dysfunction of neuropeptidergic circuits in the brain *(27)*

(h) Satietins, proteins isolated from human plasma *(292, 293)*

(i) Increases in serotonin levels in serum and central nervous system (CNS) in cancer patients *(12–15)*

(j) Toxohormone-L, a lipolytic factor purified from ascitic fluid of patients with hepatoma *(96)* and interferon-γ (IFN-γ mRNA were detected in the tumor tissue of anorectic tumor-bearing rats, whereas in brain regions, anorexia was associated with the upregulation of only IL-1β and its receptor mRNA. All other mRNAs remained unchanged in the brain regions examined. This observation suggests that IL-1β and its receptor played a major role in this model of cancer-associated anorexia *(18)*.

While IFN-γ infusion produced anorexia in patients with renal cell cancer, the appearance in mice of anorexia associated with tumor growth was similar whether mice were IFN-γ knockout or intact, suggesting that endogenous IFN-γ plays little role in producing anorexia in the tumor-bearing host *(19, 20)*. Interleukin-6 (IL-6) appears to have no direct anorectic effect *(21, 22)*.

Immunohistochemical image analyses of the time course of various proinflammatory cytokines in the CNS of tumor-bearing mice did not find that upregulation of brain cytokines could explain cancer anorexia *(23)*.

Animal studies showed development of tolerance to injections of TNF-α and IL-1 *(24)*. IL-1 infusion was not anorexigenic in food-deprived rats *(25)*.

Serum levels of circulating TNF-α, IL-1, IL-6, and IFN-γ did not correlate with the anorexia/weight loss syndrome in cancer patients *(26, 27)*. These studies imply that anorexigenic actions of these cytokines are processed by intermediate mediator molecules, such as melanocortins *(28)*. Cytokines not only produce anorectic effects but also exert direct catabolic activity on muscle and adipose tissues. This will be discussed in a separate section below.

Dysregulation of Neuropeptidergic Circuits

Both *insulin*, secreted from the exocrine pancreas, and *leptin*, produced primarily by adipocytes, circulate at levels proportional to body fat content and enter the CNS in proportion to their plasma levels. As weight increases, insulin secretion is increased both at the basal state and in response to meals to compensate for insulin resistance. As obesity progresses, increased insulin secretion promotes insulin delivery to the brain, where it helps to limit further weight gain. Insulin also promotes both fat storage and leptin synthesis by fat cells. Leptin has a more important role than insulin in the CNS control of energy homeostasis. Thus, leptin deficiency causes severe obesity with hyperphagia that persists despite high insulin levels. In contrast, obesity is not induced by insulin deficiency *(29, 30)*.

Several studies have dealt with the role of leptin in cancer-induced anorexia. In cachectic tumor-bearing animals, lower circulating levels of leptin together with decreased adipose tissue leptin mRNA content have been described *(31)*. Similarly, serum leptin levels were reduced in patients with both advanced lung cancer and colon cancer, suggesting that cancer anorexia and cachexia are not solely due to the dysregulation of leptin production *(32, 33)*. Plasma leptin levels showed gender-dependent associations, and significantly lower levels were found among cachectic women but not among cachectic men *(34)*.

Ghrelin, secreted predominantly from the stomach, is the natural ligand for the growth hormone secretagogue receptor (GHS-R) in the pituitary gland. It has profound orexigenic, adipogenic, and somatotrophic properties, thereby increasing food intake and body weight *(35)*. The brain–gut axis is the effector of anabolism, regulating feeding, metabolism, and growth via vagal efferents mediating ghrelin signaling.

Studies of ghrelin and of IL-6 levels in cancer patients provided conflicting data. Ghrelin and IL-6 levels were either increased, equal, or lower in cachectic cancer patients than those in noncachectic groups *(36–39)*.

In a study examining whether ghrelin counteracted tumor-induced anorexia in MCG 101 tumor-bearing mice, ghrelin treatment increased food intake, body weight, and whole body fat in normal controls, whereas tumor-bearing mice showed improved intake and body composition at the high dose of ghrelin only. Exogenous ghrelin normalized the growth hormone secretagogue receptor (GHS-R) expression in the hypothalamus from tumor-bearing mice without alterations in the gastric fundus expression of ghrelin. Tumor growth was not altered by exogenous ghrelin. These results indicated that MCG 101-bearing mice became ghrelin resistant despite upregulation of hypothalamic GHS-R expression. Thus, other factors downstream of the ghrelin-GHS-R system appear to be more important than ghrelin to explain cancer-induced anorexia *(40)*.

Seven cancer patients who reported loss of appetite were subjected to a short-term randomized cross-over clinical trial examining whether ghrelin stimulated appetite in cancer patients with anorexia *(41)*. A marked increase in energy intake was observed with ghrelin infusion compared with saline control, and every patient ate more. The meal appreciation score was greater with ghrelin treatment. No side effects were observed. No long-term effects were studied to examine whether ghrelin improved performance status, maintained lean body mass, or improved overall survival. Further research on high-dose ghrelin is needed to ascertain its role as a therapeutic agent.

Both insulin and leptin interact with several distinct hypothalamic neuropeptide-containing pathways *(42)*. Neuropeptides implicated in the control of energy homeostasis are divided into orexigenic (anabolic) and anorexigenic (catabolic) signaling molecules (Table 2). Peripheral leptin enters into the CNS where leptin receptors exist in the hypothalamus. Leptin interacts with numerous hypothalamic neuropeptidergic effector molecules, which are downstream of the leptin signal. Leptin suppresses hypothalamic orexigenic neuropeptides, which include *neuropeptide Y (NPY), agouti-related protein (AgRP), melanin-concentrating hormone (MCH),* and *orexin.* Leptin also stimulates anorexigenic neuropeptides including α*-melanocytes-stimulating hormone* (α*-MSH), corticotropin-releasing hormone (CRH), cocaine, and amphetamine-related transcript (CART).* The arcuate nucleus transduces leptin signals from the periphery. The leptin receptor is coexpressed with NPY and AgRP in the arcuate nucleus neurons, and is also expressed in pro-opiomelanocortin/CART neurons. NPY/AgRP neurons are inhibited by leptin and activated by a decrease in leptin levels. NPY stimulates food intake and decreases energy expenditure, primarily from a reduction in thermogenesis in brown adipose tissue and by facilitating fat deposition in white adipose tissue, partly through increased insulin activity. Both insulin and leptin have been shown to activate the hypothalamic phosphoinositol-3-kinase pathway *(43)*. From this apparently contradictory observation, possible mechanisms of insulin- and leptin resistance were inferred *(44)*. While synthesis and secretion of leptin appear to be stimulated by cytokines such as IL-1, circulating leptin levels are not elevated in cachectic cancer patients *(45, 46)*.

Dysregulation of the neuropeptidergic circuit controlling food intake, energy expenditure, and thus energy homeostasis may play a role in the development of the cancer anorexia-cachexia syndrome *(47)*. Thus, rats bearing methylcholanthrene-induced

Table 2
Orexigenic (anabolic) and anorexigenic (catabolic) neuropeptides

Orexigenic molecules
Neuropeptide Y (NPY)
Agouti-related protein (AGRP)
Melanin-concentrating hormone (MCH)
Hypocretin 1 and 2 (Orexin A and B)
Galanin
Norepinephrine
Opioids
Anorexigenic molecules
Melanoxyte-stimulating hormone (MSH)
Coricotropin-releasing hormone (CRH)
Thyrotropin-releasing hormone (TRH)
Cocaine- and amphetamnine-regulated transcript (CART)
Urocortin
Glucagon-like peptide 1 (GLP-1)
Oxytocin
Neurotensin
Serotonin

Adapted from Schwartz MW et al. *(29)*

sarcomas were refractory to intrahypothalamic injection of NPY as an orexigen when compared to controls *(48)*. NPY mRNA levels are not always increased in anorectic tumor-bearing rats when compared with pair-fed or control animals *(49)*. Reduced affinity of hypothalamic NPY receptors as well as refractory adenylate cyclase in response to NPY suggested that the postsynaptic NPY-signaling systems were altered in the hypothalamus of tumor-bearing rats *(50, 51)*.

Cytokines produce a more potent effect on feeding and metabolism when injected directly into the CNS rather than peripherally. A central mechanism of action in the production of cachexia has been postulated for many cytokines, including IL-1, IL-6, IL-8, TNF-α, IFN-α, and other chemokines *(42, 52)*.

TNF-α acts peripherally to increase leptin mRNA and centrally upon neural activity of glucose-sensitive neurons within the ventromedial nucleus and the lateral hypothalamic area. Episodic TNF administration has been reported to induce anorexia but does not appear to be able to induce cachexia. Tolerance to the cytokine eventually develops, and food intake and body weight return to normal *(53)*.

IL-1β blocked hypothalamic NPY mRNA levels and decreased NPY-induced feeding, whereas it stimulated CRH in parallel with suppression of food intake *(53, 54)*. Conversely, at different doses NPY blocked and reversed IL-1β-induced anorexia *(55)*. IL-1-induced anorexia is mainly due to development of early satiety and such early satiety has long been linked to enhanced serotonergic activity *(56)*. In addition, TNF-α and IFN-γ were also shown to stimulate CRH expression and/or release *(57)*. Cytokines may play an important role in long-term inhibition of feeding by mimicking the hypothalamic effect of excessive negative feedback signaling from leptin by persistent stimulation of anorexigenic neuropeptides such as CRH or by inhibition of the NPY orexigenic network *(47)*.

In summary, a number of factors have been proposed as putative mediators of cancer anorexia, including hormones (e.g., leptin), neuropeptides (e.g., NPY), cytokines (e.g., IL-1, TNF), and neurotransmitters (e.g., serotonin and dopamine). Rather than representing separate and distinct pathogenic entities, it appears that close interrelationships exist among these factors. Indeed, many studies suggest that different anorexia-related factors converge on a common final pathway as a major target, i.e., hypothalamic monoaminergic neurotransmission and serotonergic activity *(58, 59)*. In patients with cancer, it is likely that cytokines and anorexia are related. Compelling evidence is lacking because cytokines may be released episodically and many of their biologic effects are mediated by paracrine and autocrine mechanisms. Circulating concentrations of cytokines may not reliably reflect their role in determining specific biological responses, including cachexia *(29, 40, 60)*.

Alimentary Tract Dysfunction

Abnormalities in perception of taste and smell have been described in cancer patients. Tumors of the mouth, oropharynx, esophagus, stomach, pancreas, liver, and peritoneum may compromise oral intake from mechanical interference with anatomical structures. Intestinal obstruction is a common complication of cancer. Malabsorption secondary to pancreatic insufficiency due to pancreas carcinoma or secondary to the infiltration of the intestine or mesentery by lymphoma has been described *(61, 62)*.

Direct encroachment of a tumor on the gastrointestinal tract, atrophic changes in the mucosa and muscles of the stomach, a reduction in the duration or activity of digestive enzymes which may lead to delayed gastric emptying, and slowing of peristalsis are all pathogenic mechanisms that may contribute to early satiety *(63, 64)*. Early satiety is common in patients with decreased upper gastrointestinal motility *(65)*.

Major surgery for cancer, particularly on the gastrointestinal tract, may produce abnormalities in taste and difficulties in swallowing, digestion, or absorption that may contribute indirectly to anorexia. Chemotherapy commonly induces abnormal perception of taste, mucositis, and nausea and vomiting. Radiotherapy to the head and neck can induce stomatitis, xerostomia, and alterations in taste and smell. Radiotherapy to the abdomen can induce anorexia, nausea, vomiting, diarrhea, and malabsorption.

Biochemical and Metabolic Derangement
Increased Glucose Utilization and Futile Substrate Cycles

High rates of glucose utilization with production of lactic acid are characteristic features of the neoplastic cell. In mice bearing transplantable colon tumors, glucose utilization by the tumors was second only to that by the brain *(66)*. Hexokinase, which catalyzes the first step of the glycolytic pathway and which is often highly overexpressed in tumor cells, is a major player in this process. Binding of tumor hexokinase to the outer mitochondrial membrane provides the enzyme with preferential access to ATP generated in the mitochondrion and increases the activity and stability of the enzyme *(67)*. The end product of the hexokinase reaction, glucose-6-phosphate, serves not only as a source of ATP via glycolysis but is also a key intermediate in the metabolic processes essential for cell growth and proliferation. Alteration of an isozyme appears closely linked to this process. Thus, the promoter activity of the type II isoform of hexokinase, the dominant form expressed in AS-30 hepatoma cells, was found to be resistant to normal hormonal control *(68)*. The distal region of the promoter was found to display consensus motifs for hypoxia-inducible factor (HIF-1). Subjecting transfected hepatoma cells to hypoxic conditions activated the type II hexokinase promoter almost sevenfold in the presence of glucose *(69)*. The tumor cell was able to maintain glycolysis regardless of the metabolic state of surrounding normal cells.

Lactic acid produced via glucose metabolism may be utilized by other tissues for energy purposes or may be transported to the liver for resynthesis to glucose. The cyclic metabolic pathway, in which glucose is converted to lactic acid by glycolysis in tumor tissue and then reconverted to glucose in the liver, is referred to as the Cori cycle. Conversion of glucose to lactate in cancer cells yields two ATPs, whereas lactate to glucose conversion in the liver requires six ATPs. Thus a systemic energy-losing or futile substrate cycle, involving this interplay of tumor glycolysis and host gluconeogenesis may be an important cause of cancer cachexia *(70)*. Assuming that all lactate produced is recycled to glucose, the cancer cell acts as an energy parasite. It may be calculated, however, that if 85% of lactate passes through the gluconeogenic pathway and 15% is oxidized, the host's handling of tumor-produced lactate would be energy neutral. It has been suggested that the increase in the Cori cycle is insignificant in terms of energy expenditure and that increased glucose catabolism itself is responsible for weight loss and development of cachexia *(71)*.

CYTOKINES

TNF-α, IL-1, IL-6 (and its subfamily members such as ciliary neurotrophic factor (CNTF) and Leukemia Inhibitory Factor (LIF)), and IFN-γ produced by host immune cells and/or tumor cells have all been implicated as mediators of cancer cachexia *(72–74)*. These cytokines are characterized by the induction of anorexia, weight loss, an acute-phase protein response, protein and fat breakdown, rises in levels of cortisol and glucagon and falls in insulin level, insulin resistance, anemia, fever, and elevated energy expenditure in animals. Direct interaction with leptin, neuropeptides, or serotonin as mechanisms of induction of cancer anorexia has been described above.

TNF-α: TNF-α was independently and simultaneously discovered as cachectin because it caused systemic suppression of lipoprotein lipase and development of hypertriglyceridemia, a state frequently seen in cachectic animals *(75)*. One mechanism by which TNF-α induces a net catabolic state in the host is by mediating increased catabolism at the level of specific tissues such as muscle and fat *(76)*. TNF-α increases activities of both phosphofructokinase and fructose bisphosphate phosphatase in myocytes in culture, producing an increased substrate cycling between fructose-6-phosphate and fructose-1,6-bisphosphate. Each of the fructose-6-phosphate/fructose-1,6-bisphosphate cycles loses one ATP. TNF also increased ubiquitin gene expression in isolated rat muscle.

Elevation of serum TNF-α and/or TNF-α-receptor levels has been associated with the clinical status of patients with B-cell chronic lymphocytic leukemia and with endometrial carcinoma and other solid tumors *(77, 78)*. Administration of TNF-α in humans induced anorexia, negative nitrogen balance, and increases in serum triglycerides and in very low-density lipoprotein *(79, 80)*. In contrast, TNF-α was rarely detected in patients with clinical cancer cachexia and administration of recombinant TNF-α did not produce demonstrable cachexia *(26, 27, 81)*. Patients with type I hyperlipidemia caused by an inherited deficiency in lipoprotein-lipase have normal fat stores and are not cachectic. These observations suggest that neither TNF-α nor suppression of lipoprotein-lipase alone can explain loss of adipose tissue and cachexia in cancer patients.

IL-1, The genotype for a diallelic polymorphism of the IL-1β gene was examined in patients with pancreatic cancer *(82)*. The possession of a genotype resulting in increased 1β production was associated with shortened survival and increased serum C-reactive protein (CRP) level. This may reflect the role of IL-1β in inducing an acute-phase protein response and cachexia in cancer.

IL-6: A significant role of IL-6β in cancer anorexia is detailed in the earlier section. Involvement of IL-6 in the development of cancer cachexia has been suggested from a number of animal models. Prevention of muscle atrophy in tumor-bearing mice by anti-IL-6 receptor antibody appears to be mediated by modulation of lysosomal and ATP-ubiquitin-dependent proteolytic pathways *(83)*. The influence of IL-1 on cachexia appears to be mediated through IL-6, and IL-6 seems to act in concert with other cytokines in a final common pathway of cachexia *(84, 85)*.

In patients with lung cancer, increased IL-6 levels were correlated with extensive disease, impaired performance status, enhanced acute-phase response, weight loss, and malnutrition *(86, 87)*.

The exact role of IL-1 and IL-6 in the development of cancer cachexia in humans remains speculative, however. Serum IL-6 concentrations were significantly elevated in tumor-bearing animals but only minimally in patients with cancer *(88)*. IL-1 and IL-6 serum levels were not always measurable *(89)*. IL-6 administration produced no changes in ubiquitin gene expression, and no effect on body weight or food intake, despite being associated with increased acute-phase protein production *(22)*. Likewise, transgenic mice constitutively expressing IL-6 did not develop cachexia *(90, 91)*. It has been suggested that IL-6 is necessary but not sufficient for the induction of cachexia, and that additional factor(s) besides IL-1β control production of IL-6 and other cachexigenic factors *(18)*.

The superfamily of IL-6 includes LIF and CNTF. LIF will be discussed in the section of Tumor Byproducts. The role of CNTF in cancer anorexia/cachexia in humans has not been established.

IFN-γ: IFN-γ may have a bearing on the development of cancer cachexia. Interferon and TNF were shown to have similar catabolic effects on NIH 3T3 cells in vitro *(92)*. Monoclonal antibody against IFN-γ given prior to injection of Lewis lung tumor cells prevented cachexia from developing *(93)*. IFN-γ was found to be increased in 51% of patients with multiple myeloma *(94)*. The levels of IFN-γ had no correlation with clinical parameters, however.

As to the link between inflammatory cytokines and energy expenditure, involvement of the transcriptional coactivator, peroxisome proliferator-activated receptor (PPAR) gamma coactivator-1 (PGC-1) has been suggested. Thus, many cytokines activate PGC-1 through phosphorylation by p38 kinase, resulting in stabilization and activation of PGC-1 protein. Cytokine-induced activation of PGC-1 in cultured muscle cells or muscle tissue in vivo caused increased respiration and expression of genes linked to mitochondrial uncoupling and energy expenditure. These data illustrated a direct thermogenic action of cytokines through PGC-1 *(95)*.

Tumor Byproducts

Various pharmacologically active tumor byproducts have been reported as causal factors of cachexia.

Lipolytic Factors

Three different lipolytic factors have been characterized or purified. First, a lipolytic factor termed *Toxohormone-L* was found in pleural effusions of patients with malignant lymphoma as well as in ascites from patients with ovarian carcinoma and hepatoma *(96)*. It is an acidic protein with a molecular weight of 65–75 kDa. Toxohormone-L elicited fatty acid release in rat adipose tissue in vitro and injections into rats resulted in suppression of food and water intake. Toxohormone-L and related substances were considered responsible for the cancer cachexia syndrome in nude mice bearing human cancer cell lines *(97)*.

Second, *LIF (leukemia inhibitory factor)* was originally isolated from conditioned medium of Krebs II ascites tumor cells. This factor has a differentiation-inducing activity on myeloid leukemia cell lines. In an independent work, the identical material was purified from a conditioned medium of human melanoma cell line SEKI. The substance was found to be an effective lipoprotein-lipase inhibitor *(98)*. Comparisons among nude mice bearing various human melanoma cell lines revealed that the degree of LIF mRNA expression correlated with the development of cachexia *(98)*. LIF caused smaller increases in lipolysis and catabolic effects than those of TNF *(99, 100)*.

Third, British workers purified and characterized what they termed *lipid-mobilizing factor (LMF)* which was derived from MAC16 murine adenocarcinoma and from urine of cancer patients with cachexia *(101, 102)*. LMF, an acidic peptide, lacked triglyceride lipase activity and was different from natural lipolytic hormones, which were all basic. LMF isolated from either the murine tumor or from patients' urine had an apparent MW of 43 kDa and was homologous to the plasma protein Zn-α2-glycoprotein (ZAG) *(101)*. Both caused direct lipolysis in isolated murine adepocytes and caused selective loss of adipose tissue in male mice *(102)*. Both caused stimulation of adenylate cyclase in murine adipocyte plasma membranes in a GTP-dependent process, and release of glycerol from isolated adipocytes. Adenylate cyclase stimulation and thus oxygen consumption in brown adipose tissue (BAT) by LMF is mediated by a β3-adrenergic receptor *(103, 104)*. Brown adipocytes express abundant amounts of β3-adrenergic receptors. An increase in oxygen uptake by interscapular brown adipose tissue suggested that LMF exerted its effect by increases in energy expenditure *(102)*. This increase may be related to changes in expression of uncoupling proteins (UCP) because mice bearing MAC16 tumor showed higher UCP-1 mRNA levels in BAT than did controls *(105)*. Three types of UCPs are known. UCP1 is present only in BAT, UCP2 is expressed ubiquitously, and UCP3 is expressed abundantly and specifically in skeletal muscle in humans and also in BAT of rodents. LMF increased expression of UCP1, 2, and 3 in brown adipose tissue and UCP-2 in liver and skeletal muscle *(106)*. UCPs function as mitochondrial protein carriers that stimulate heat production by dissipating the proton gradient generated during respiration across the inner mitochondrial membrane, thereby uncoupling respiration from ATP synthesis.

In rodents, UCP2 and UCP3 mRNAs were elevated in skeletal muscle during tumor growth; TNF was able to mimic this increase in gene expression *(107)*.

Recent studies showed that ZINC-alpha2-glycoprotein (ZAG) is produced not only by certain tumors, but also by BAT and white adipose tissue *(108)*. Glucocorticoids stimulate lipolysis through an increase in ZAG expression, and they are responsible for the increase in ZAG expression seen in adipose tissue of cachectic mice *(109)*. These findings suggest that increased cortisol levels seen in cachectic cancer patients may lead to an increased lipolysis through ZAG overexpression.

In cancer patients with weight loss, LMF/ZAG levels found in serum and urine were much higher than those in noncancer control patients with comparable weight loss and were proportional to the degree of weight loss *(110)*. Patients who responded to therapy showed a decrease in the plasma levels of LMF/ZAG, which correlated with the levels of response *(111)*.

Proteolysis-Inducing Factor (PIF)

Serum from cachectic mice bearing MAC16 adenocarcinoma as well as urine and plasma from cancer patients with weight loss contained factors that induced proteolysis in skeletal muscles *(6, 112, 113)*. These factors are termed PIF. The PIFs derived from murine and human sources are identical: both are characterized as a sulfated glycoprotein with a molecular weight of 24 kDa, with a unique amino acid sequence. A murine monoclonal antibody can attenuate weight loss induced by human PIF in mice. PIF was readily detected in the urine of cachectic cancer patients, whereas it was absent in the urine of normal subjects and of patients with weight loss due to trauma or sepsis. Weight loss was associated with loss of skeletal muscles, but there was no effect on the heart and an increase in liver weight *(113)*. Protein degradation induced by PIF appears to be mediated through the ubiquitin-proteasome pathway specifically in skeletal muscles *(114)*. Increased muscle proteasome activity was correlated with disease severity in gastric cancer patients *(115)*. Effects of PIF on increased expression of proteasome subunits and the ubiquitin-conjugating enzyme ($E2_{14k}$) were also demonstrated in vitro. The action of PIF on the protein degradation was mediated by the phospholipase A2 catalyzed release of arachidonic acid from membrane phospholipid and its conversion to the lipoxygenase product 15-hydroxyeicosatetraenoic acid *(114)*.

Production of PIF appears to be associated specifically with cancer cachexia and it was not found in the urine of patients undergoing major surgery or in those with burns, multiple injuries, sepsis, or sleeping sickness, even though the rate of weight loss exceeded that found in cancer patients *(116)*. Patients with cancer of the pancreas, lung, colon, breast, rectum, liver, and ovary, in whom the rate of weight loss was greater than or equal to 1 kg/month, showed evidence of PIF excretion in the urine *(117)*. Eighty percent of patients with pancreas cancer excreted PIF in the urine *(116)*.

INVOLVEMENT OF SIGNAL TRANSDUCTION PATHWAY

Research in recent years has elucidated essential functions of the nuclear factor-kappaB (NF-κB) family of transcription factors in skeletal myogenesis and muscle disease. The first hint that NK-κB was relevant in cachexia came from studies showing that

NF-κB by cachectic factors TNF plus IFN-γ caused a block in muscle differentiation by targeting the myogenic transcription factor MyoD in mouse myocytes. Both TNF and IFN-γ signaling were required for NF-κB-dependent downregulation of MyoD, the nuclear transcription factor, and dysfunction of skeletal myofibers. MyoD mRNA was also downregulated by TNF and IFN-γ expression in mouse muscle in vivo (118).

Further study in using myogenic cell cultures, treatment with a combination of TNF-α and IFN-γ resulted in selective and progressive depletion of myosin heavy chain, whereas none of other core myofibrillar proteins, troponin T, tropomyosin α and β, actin or actinin were affected (119). Again, treatment with TNF-α alone or IFN-γ alone had negligible effect on the myosin heavy chain depletion. Depletion of myosin heavy chain of cultured myotubes with TNF-α and IFN-γ was associated with a decrease in MyoD. These results imply that TNF-α and IFN-γ selectively trigger a reduction in the expression of the myosin heavy chain through a MyoD-mediated block in gene transcription. The implantation of cells expressing both TNF-α and IFN-γ into muscles of mice led to a similar, specific reduction in the synthesis of the myosin heavy chain relative to that of other myofibrillar proteins such as actin and tropomyosin. Interestingly, transplantation of C-26 adenocarcinoma, which is known to produce IL-6 rather than TNF-α and IFN-γ resulted in downregulation of myosin heavy chain, but from a different mechanism, via ubiquitin-dependent proteasome-mediated protein degradation. These observations highlight the importance of myosin heavy chain as a target of cachexia, which occurs through different pathways.

In resting conditions, NF-κB is sequestered in the cytoplasm bound to its inhibitor, I-kB. TNF-α, IL-β, and PIF induce degradation of the wild type (but not the mutant) I-κBα. This degradation leads to nuclear accumulation of NF-κB, which mediates proteolytic loss of the myofibrillar protein myosin in myotubes (120). PIF also induces expression of the ubiquitin-proteasome pathway. PIF is able to activate the transcription factor NF-κB and NF-κB-inducible genes in isolated human Kupffer cells and in monocytes, resulting in production of proinflammatory cytokines, TNF-α, IL-8, and IL-6. PIF also activates the transcription factor STAT3 in Kupffer cells. The proinflammatory effect of PIF, mediated via NF-κB and STAT3, may contribute to the inflammatory procachectic process in the liver (121).

It is of note that muscle protein degradation in humans may not necessarily be mediated though the ubiquitin-proteasome pathway. Thus, mRNA levels of the lysosomal protease cathepsin B were shown to be much higher in patients with early stages of lung cancer who had weight loss and muscle wasting (122). In using cDNA microarrays of mouse myoblasts, the nitric oxide (NO) synthase gene was demonstrated to be an important downstream target of NF-κB, suggesting that NO production might be a direct cause of MyoD mRNA degeneration (123).

Other signaling molecules are also identified as relevant in cancer cachexia (124). These molecules include: myostatin, a member of the transforming growth factor-β superfamily that functions as a negative regulator of muscle mass (125), and dystrophin glycoprotein complex that forms a link from the extracellular matrix to the cytoskeleton (126).

HORMONAL ABERRATION

Hormonal aberration may be a contributory factor to cancer cachexia. In a unique endocrine animal tumor model, estrogen was incriminated as the cause of cancer cachexia *(127)*. Abnormally low levels of testosterone or hypogonadism have been described in male patients with advanced cancer; these findings correlated with weight loss and adverse outcome *(128, 129)*. Plasma cortisol values and arterial glucagon levels in patients with malignant tumors were significantly increased, however, compared with patients with benign surgical disorders *(130, 131)*. This finding is in accord with the hypothesis that glucocorticoids are involved in the increased protein catabolism of skeletal muscles and other organs in cachectic cancer patients.

PROSTAGLANDIN ELEVATION

Marked weight loss and wasting of muscle and adipose tissue after tumor transplantation to rats were associated with the presence of circulating TNF-α and high levels of prostaglandin E_2 *(132)*. Indomethacin reduced weight loss and increased survival of mice with transplantable tumors receiving chemotherapy, and ibuprofen, a cyclooxygenase inhibitor, abrogated IL-1-induced anorexia in rats *(133, 134)*. Close interaction of host- and tumor-derived cytokines and prostaglandins in the CNS were suggested by these animal models *(134)*. Recent work, however, showed that prostaglandin E and prostaglandin I receptor levels in the CNS seemed to have little role in cancer anorexia/cachexia. Rather, expression of overall prostaglandin E receptors in the liver, fat, and skeletal muscles appeared to be directly contributory to metabolic alterations in cancer cachexia *(135)*.

TUMOR PARASITISM

Selective parasitism of the host by the tumor in the form of a successful competition for substrates with limited availability may be a cause of cachexia. Some animal studies suggest that translocation of nitrogen from host to tumor constitutes nearly the total nitrogen depletion of the host *(136)*. Tumors are effective nitrogen traps independent of protein intake, despite the wasting of normal host tissue *(137)*. Since cachexia can appear in patients with very small tumors, however, and the total tumor mass in the majority of cancer patients at death rarely exceeds 0.5 kg, it is unlikely that a simple competition of available nitrogen between tumor and host is responsible for the development of cachexia, especially in early stage cancer.

DYSFUNCTION OF THE NEUROPEPTIDERGIC CIRCUIT

Dysfunction of neuropeptidergic circuits as the mechanism of the cancer anorexia-cachexia syndrome has been discussed in the section on anorexia above.

METABOLIC DERANGEMENT PRODUCED BY TREATMENT

Postoperative weight loss results from increased energy expenditure due to the stress response and decreased dietary intake *(138)*. Pancreatic resection can result in pancreatic exocrine and endocrine insufficiency creating major nutritional problems such as steatorrhea and hyperglycemia. Major hepatic resections can cause metabolic abnormalities in the immediate postoperative period. Extensive resection of the small bowel can lead to malabsorption of many nutrients.

A majority of chemotherapeutic agents are toxic, producing a variety of metabolic effects. L-asparaginase and IL-12 exemplify this: profound weight loss and/or hypoalbuminemia are among the common manifestations in patients treated with these compounds *(139–141)*.

TREATMENT OF CANCER ANOREXIA/CACHEXIA

The definitive treatment of cancer cachexia is removal of the causative tumor. Short of achieving this goal, various measures have been undertaken with limited success.

Supportive Care

Patients with anorexia from decreased physical activity, concomitant infection, and toxicities to the alimentary tract from chemotherapy and radiotherapy are managed symptomatically for maintenance of nutritional status and quality of life. Such management includes the use of mouthwash for stomatitis, frequent small volume feedings, antiemetics, antibiotics, transfusions of blood components, and/or oral and parenteral nutritional supplement. Consideration of the patient's food preferences and service of food in a dining room atmosphere may also be important to stimulate appetite. When a patient is unable to consume a regular diet to obtain adequate nutrition, food supplements, both home-made and commercially available, are an effective means of providing additional calories, protein, fat, vitamins, and minerals, although overall consumption may not increase much. In specific instances such as the malabsorption syndrome secondary to pancreas carcinoma, exogenous pancreas extract improves fat and protein absorption.

Frequent nutritional counseling may increase daily energy and protein intake as well as triceps skinfold measurements. However, response rates and overall survival cannot be improved by counseling alone.

Pharmacologic Management

CORTICOSTEROIDS

A number of uncontrolled studies have suggested that corticosteroids can diminish such symptoms as anorexia, asthenia, and pain in patients with cancer. The mechanism of action may include a euphoriant activity, anti-inflammatory action through the inhibition of TNF release and suppression of IL-1β activity, as well as inhibition of prostaglandin metabolism. Significant improvements in appetite and a sense of well-being have been reported in randomized trials with prednisolone, methylprednisolone, or dexamethasone *(142–145)*. Unfortunately, the improvements were not long lasting and upon completion of the studies all nutritional parameters returned to their baseline. There were no differences in mortality rate or in survival.

In a randomized comparison of dexamethasone and megestrol acetate, both drugs caused a similar degree of appetite enhancement and similar changes in nonfluid weight status, but dexamethasone was found to be less favorable *(146)*. Dexamethasone had more corticosteroid-type toxicity and a higher rate of drug discontinuation because of toxicity and/or patient refusal than megestrol acetate.

Although corticosteroids have been postulated to be responsible for muscle wasting and cancer cachexia, studies involving treatment with RU38486, a glucocorticoid receptor antagonist, of experimental animals bearing cachexia-producing tumors suggested that glucocoricoids are not involved in skeletal muscle wasting associated with cancer cachexia. Receptor blockade did not abrogate tumor-induced cachexia *(147, 148)*.

MEGESTROL ACETATE AND MEDROXYPROGESTERONE ACETATE

Megestrol acetate, a progestational agent, is frequently used in the treatment of patients with metastatic breast cancer. It is generally well tolerated, except that it may cause undesirable weight gain. Subsequently, it was shown that megestrol acetate produced weight gain in a variety of cachectic cancer patients. Significant reduction in serum levels of IL-1a and b, IL-2, IL-6, and TNF-α were observed in cancer patients treated with megestrol acetate which may bear on the mechanism of improved appetite and body weight gain *(149)*. It has also been postulated that the effect is, at least in part, mediated by NPY, a potent central appetite stimulant *(150)*.

In a review of 15 randomized clinical trials including more than 2,000 patients, there was a statistically significant advantage for high-dose progestins in regard to improved appetite and gain of body weight *(151)*. Treatment morbidity was low, due to the brief period of the treatment in most of the studies. A meta-analysis of 26 studies confirmed the usefulness of megestrol acetate in promoting gains in appetite and body weight of cancer patients with anorexia-cachexia syndrome *(152)*

Weight gain produced by megestrol acetate was found to be mainly from increased body fat stores rather than accretion of lean tissue *(153, 154)*. It has been argued that the gain of adipose tissue as opposed to lean tissue during treatment with megestrol acetate, although suboptimal, should not be disparaged because depletion of body fat is generally an undesirable outcome of cancer.

The addition of megestrol acetate to chemotherapy for patients with melanoma resulted in higher objective responses and prolonged median survival compared to historical controls with chemotherapy alone *(155)*. Megestrol acetate is contraindicated in pediatric cachectic patients, since a significant proportion of such patients developed adrenal insufficiency *(156)*. Megestrol acetate should also be used with caution in geriatric cancer patients because they are prone to develop deep vein thrombosis because of immobility and increases in serum fibrinogen levels.

Medroxyprogesterone acetate is a more widely used synthetic progestagen. Medroxyprogesterone acetate reduced production of cytokines and serotonin *(157)*. Two placebo-controlled randomized studies have been reported in which increased appetite was described *(158, 159)*. In one study, significant increases in rapid turnover proteins such as serum thyroid binding prealbumin and retinol binding protein were reported *(158)*. In spite of increased appetite, no weight gain was produced in either study.

ANABOLIC STEROIDS

Anabolic androgenic steroids have been used by athletes to promote muscle growth and strength. In MCG sarcoma-bearing mice with progressive cachexia, administration of nandrolone propionate resulted in significant weight gain *(160)*. The weight gain was, however, mainly attributed to water retention, and food intake and survival were not affected. Randomized clinical trials were carried out to test whether supplements of nandrolone decanoate influenced the outcome of chemotherapy in patients with nonsmall cell lung cancer *(161, 162)*. Although the treated group experienced less weight loss, response to chemotherapy and survival were comparable. In a three-arm phase III randomized clinical trial for the treatment of cancer anorexia/cachexia, fluoxymesterone, an anabolic steroid, showed significantly less appetite enhancement and did not have as favorable a toxicity profile as megestrol acetate, a progestational agent, or dexamethasone, a corticosteroid *(146)*.

CANNABINOIDS (DRONABINOL)

While using dronabinol (Delta 9-tetrahydocannabinol, THC) as an antiemetic, it was found that the agent enhanced appetite in healthy individuals and in cancer patients. To study this phenomenon further, an open dose-ranging study was carried out in patients with cancer *(163, 164)*. All patients reported improvement in appetite. Higher doses, 5.0 mg or 7.5 mg/day, were more effective than the low dose of 2.5 mg/day. Patients in all groups nonetheless continued to lose weight although the rate of weight loss decreased with therapy. It is of note that these effects were observed at doses lower than those producing antiemetic effects and without overt psychotropic symptoms.

Recently, a randomized study was carried out to compare dronabinol, megestrol acetate, and the combination for palliating cancer-associated anorexia *(165)*. Megestrol acetate provided superior anorexia palliation among advanced cancer patients compared with dronabinol alone. The combination of megestrol and dronabinol did not appear to confer additional benefit.

GROWTH HORMONE (GH), SOMATOSTATIN, AND GHRH (GHRP-2)

Anabolic properties of GH have been examined in animals. Administration of GH to tumor-bearing rats resulted in increased muscle weight, muscle protein content, and preserved host-body composition *(166)*. GH did not stimulate tumor growth *(167)*. The effect of a combination of insulin, GH, and somatostatin on tumor growth, metastasis, and host metabolism was evaluated in rats bearing MAC-33 mammary tumor *(168)*. The triple therapy supported host anabolism, increased hamstring muscle weight and protein content, and inhibited tumor growth kinetics. The rationale for including somatostatin in the treatment was based on the fact that insulin treatment alone led to limited success in treating cancer cachexia due to insulin-induced hypoglycemia and subsequent glucagon secretion. Somatostatin alone is known to have antitumor activity, however, and the contribution of each component to the observed changes was not clear.

The effect of recombinant human GH and insulin administration on protein kinetics was examined in 28 cancer patients *(169)*. Whole-body protein net balance was higher in patients treated with both GH and insulin than in insulin-only or GH-only controls. Skeletal muscle protein net balance in the GH/insulin group was higher than in no-treatment controls. Recombinant human GH and insulin reduced whole-body and skeletal muscle protein loss in cancer patients. Simultaneous use of these agents during nutritional therapy may benefit cancer patients *(169)*.

In another study, 30 patients undergoing surgery for upper GI tract malignancies were prospectively randomized into one of three nutritional support groups after surgery: standard TPN, TPN plus GH, and TPN, GH, and systemic insulin. Patients who received standard TPN only were in a state of negative skeletal muscle protein net balance. Those who received GH and insulin had improved skeletal muscle protein net balance. Whole-body protein net balance was improved in the GH and the GH and insulin groups compared with the TPN-only group. GH and insulin combined did not improve whole-body net balance more than GH alone. GH administration significantly increased serum IGF-1 and GH levels. Insulin infusion significantly increased serum insulin levels and the insulin/glucagon ratio. Thus, GH and GH plus insulin regimens improved protein kinetic parameters in patients with upper GI tract cancer who were receiving TPN after undergoing surgery. The study was carried out for only 5 days. It is unknown whether the TPN plus GH improved wound healing and shortened hospital stay *(170)*. Whether prolonged use of TPN plus GH would play any role in reversal of cancer cachexia in humans has not been tested.

Daily subcutaneous injections of a more stable synthetic ghrelin receptor agonist GHRP-2 (growth hormone releasing peptide-2) in mice produced dose-dependent increases in food intake and body weight *(171)*. Pre- and post-treatment analysis of body composition indicated increased fat and bone masses but not lean mass. GHRP-2-induced positive energy balance leading to fat gain occurred in the absence of involvement of hypothalamic NPY neurons. Indeed, GHRP-2 administration to healthy volunteers resulted in increased food intake *(172)*. Further studies are needed to ascertain whether ghrelin receptor agonists offer a treatment option for syndromes like anorexia nervosa, cancer cachexia, or AIDS wasting.

As a more recent approach, a myogenic plasmid that expresses GH-releasing hormone (GHRH *(1, 40)*) was tested in dogs for prevention and/or treatment of cancer anorexia and cachexia. Seventeen geriatric and five cancer-afflicted companion dogs were enrolled. Effects of the treatment were documented for at least 180 days post treatment, with ten animals followed for more than one year post treatment. Treated dogs showed increased IGF-1 levels, and increases in scores for weight, activity level, exercise tolerance, and appetite. No adverse effects associated with the GHRH plasmid treatment were found. Most importantly, the overall assessment of the quality of life of the treated animals improved. Hematological parameters such as red blood cell count, hematocrit, and hemoglobin concentrations were increased and maintained within their normal ranges. It was concluded that intramuscular injection of a GHRH-expressing plasmid was both safe and capable of improving the quality of life in animals for an extended period of time in the context of aging and disease *(173)*.

INSULIN-LIKE GROWTH FACTOR-1 (IGF-1)

IGF-1, also known as somatomedin-C, mediates many of the anabolic properties of GH, including stimulation of amino acid uptake and protein synthesis *(174)*. Other studies have shown its important role in muscle cell proliferation and differentiation, as well as inhibition of lipolysis *(174, 175)*. Continuous subcutaneous IGF-1 administration in rat bearing methylcholanthrene-induced sarcoma resulted in host preservation of lean tissue and attenuation of host muscle protein depletion *(176)*. The treatment did not stimulate tumor growth.

Ten subjects with AIDS-associated cachexia received either low- or high-dose iv recombinant IGF-1 daily for 10 days *(177)*. Cumulative nitrogen retention was positive for both dosage groups, but a significant increase in daily nitrogen retention occurred only in the low-dose group. The anabolic response was transient, however. Repeated administration of IGF-1 decreased IGF-binding protein-3 levels, producing lower intrainfusion levels of IGF-1 and limiting its therapeutic efficacy. The basal metabolic rate increased with high-dose IGF-1 and may have contributed to the lack of anabolic effect. The authors concluded that partial growth hormone resistance occurred in AIDS-associated cachexia.

A randomized placebo-controlled 12-week trial of a combination of recombinant human GH (rhGH, Nutropin) and rhIGF-1 was carried out in 142 subjects with HIV wasting *(178)*. At three weeks, the treatment group had a significantly larger weight increase, but this difference was not observed at any later time point. Similarly, fat-free mass, calculated from skinfold measurements, increased transiently in the treatment group at six weeks. No significant differences in isokinetic muscle strength or endurance testing or in quality of life were observed between the groups. The authors concluded that the combination of rhIGF-I and low-dose rhGH had no significant anabolic effect on HIV wasting. IGF-I has not been tested in patients with cancer cachexia.

METOCLOPRAMIDE AND CISAPRIDE

In advanced cancer patients with delayed gastric emptying or gastroparesis, oral administration of a prokinetic agent, metoclopramide, 10 mg orally 4 times daily before meals and at bedtime, was shown to be effective in stimulating appetite and relieving other dyspeptic symptoms associated with anorexia *(179, 180)*. A controlled release preparation appears to be more effective than an immediate release drug due to its control of nausea associated with advanced cancer even without demonstrated abnormalities of the GI tract *(181)*. Patients with head and neck cancer undergoing radiotherapy were randomized to three groups: megestrol acetate, cisapride, and placebo. Megestrol significantly prevented body weight loss and deterioration of appetite, whereas cisapride lacked these clinical benefits *(182)*.

HYDRAZINE SULFATE

Hydrazine sulfate, an inhibitor of the enzyme phosphoenolpyruvate carboxykinase, has been shown to interrupt gluconeogenesis in animals *(183)*. Based on a theory that increased gluconeogenesis and enhanced Cori cycle activity were the central mechanism of tumor-induced cachexia, clinical studies of hydrazine sulfate were carried out in attempts to prevent or reverse cancer-related cachexia and weight loss. Three multicenter group studies were reported in patients with nonsmall cell lung cancer or colorectal cancer *(184–186)*. All three studies failed to show beneficial results in appetite, body weight, quality of life, or survival from hydrazine sulfate.

INDOMETHACIN, IBUPROFEN, AND CELECOXIB

It has been proposed that cell growth may be controlled by the interconversion of different types of prostagladins *(187, 188, 189)*. In animal studies, ability of prostagladin biosynthesis inhibitors to reverse cancer cachexia is not universally positive. In one study, indomethacin, ibuprofen, or aspirin inhibited growth of Walker 256 carcinoma in rats *(190)*. All drug-treated rats partially recovered body weight and food intake compared to a saline-treated group. In another study using the same tumor system, indomethacin and ibuprofen retarded tumor growth and lowered body temperature compared with controls, but these agents had no effect on food intake or body weight of tumor-bearing animals *(191)*. Celecoxib, a COX-2 inhibitor, was reported to rapidly reverse weight loss in two murine models: colon 26, which induced high levels of circulating IL-6, and a human head and neck tumor, 1483 HNSCC xenograft *(192)*.

In clinical trials, indomethacin reduced fever and granulocytosis and was claimed to have improved the well-being of cancer patients *(193, 194)*. In cachectic cancer patients, indomethacin or ibuprofen was reported to decrease resting energy expenditure and

C-reactive protein values, to produce body weight gain and to improve survival *(195–197)*. In a randomized study in patients with advanced gastrointestinal cancer with more than 5% weight loss, megestrol acetate alone resulted in weight loss and deterioration of quality of life, whereas the combination of megestrol/ibuprofen appeared to reverse weight loss and appeared to improve quality of life *(198)*. Impact of erythropoietin was studied in a randomized fashion in unselected weight-losing cancer patients who were treated with indomethacin. The combination resulted in an improvement of hematocrit together with increased serum albumin levels, decreases in C-reactive protein, improved body weight, and greater exercise capacity compared to indomethacin-alone controls *(199, 200)*. Study and control patients did not differ in survival, however. Well-designed randomized clinical studies are needed to assess therapeutic values of prostaglandin inhibitors alone and in combination with other anticachectic agents.

PENTOXIFYLLINE AND LISOFYLLINE

These agents are methylxanthine analogues with anti-inflammatory properties. They were shown to have profound stimulatory effects on vascular endothelial production of the noninflammatory prostaglandins I_2 and E_2, while inhibiting TNF-α synthesis by blocking gene transcription *(201)*. Pentoxifylline, originally used for the treatment of vascular insufficiency because of its hemorheological properties, prevented muscle atrophy and suppressed increased protein breakdown in tumor-bearing rats. Pentoxifylline suppressed the enhanced expression of ubiquitin, the 14-kDa ubiquitin conjugating enzyme E2, and the C2 20S proteasome subunit in muscle from cancer-bearing rats and inhibited the activation of a nonlysosomal, Ca(2+)-independent ubiquitin-proteasome proteolytic pathway *(202)*.

Prophylactic oral administration of pentoxifylline in allograft recipients together with chemotherapy and radiotherapy resulted in significant reduction in the incidence and severity of treatment-related complications: mucositis, hepatic veno-occlusive disease, renal insufficiency, and the incidence of graft versus host disease *(203)*.

In an initial study in cancer patients, pentoxifylline suppressed TNF-α mRNA levels, increased the sense of well-being, improved appetite and improved the ability to perform activities of daily living. Patients who normalized their TNF levels had a weight gain. In a randomized controlled trial in patients with solid tumors, however, pentoxifylline failed to provide improvements in appetite or body weight compared to a placebo group *(204)*. Likewise, for patients with acute myelocytic leukemia or myelodysplastic syndrome once in complete remission with idarubicin/ara – C chemotherapy, lisofylline provided no favorable effects in terms of rates of infection, overall mortality rates, or outcome *(205)*. Lisofylline did not alter the toxicities of high-dose IL-2 and thus did not impact the overall dose intensity in the treatment of advanced renal cancer and malignant melanoma *(206)*.

PROTEASOME INHIBITORS AND NF-κB INHIBITORS

As detailed above, the ubiquitin-proteasome pathway plays an important role in muscle protein catabolism during cancer cachexia and may be a potential therapeutic target for muscle wasting *(207)*. Arginine methylester and alanine methylester, selective inhibitors of ubiquitin ligase E3α, as well as bortezomib, a direct inhibitor of the protease complex, have not been examined in cachectic cancer patients.

Activation of nuclear factor-kappaB (NF-κB) leads to the induction of proteasome expression and protein degradation by PIF. SN50, a synthetic cell permeable peptide NF-κB inhibitor, attenuated the expression of 20S proteasome α-subunits, two subunits of the 19S regulator MSS1 and p42, and the ubiquitin-conjugating enzyme, E2(14k) *(208)*. SN50 also decreased myosin expression in murine myotubes. The potential for curcumin, a natural product from tumeric, and resveratrol, a natural phytoalexin found in red wine, to act as inhibitors of muscle protein degradation in cancer cachexia, because they are inhibitors of NF-κB activation, has been evaluated in vitro and in vivo *(208, 209)*. Both agents completely attenuated total protein degradation in murine myotubes at all concentrations of PIF, and attenuated the PIF-induced increase in expression of the ubiquitin-proteasome proteolytic pathway. However, curcumin was ineffective in preventing weight loss and muscle protein degradation in the animal tumor model, however; whereas resveratrol significantly attenuated weight loss and protein degradation in skeletal muscle, and produced a significant reduction in NF-κB DNA-binding activity *(208, 209)*. The inactivity of curcumin was probably due to low bioavailability. Agents that inhibit nuclear translocation of NF-κB may prove useful for the treatment of muscle wasting in cancer cachexia *(208)*. Administration of dehydroxymethyl-epoxyquinomicin, a NF-κB inhibitor, ameliorated cachexia in tumor-bearing mice *(210)*. It was also shown to inhibit IL-6 production in patients with prostate cancer. Clinical studies are eagerly awaited.

CLENBUTEROL

Clenbuterol is a β2-adrenoceptor agonist. It prevented muscle protein wasting in tumor-bearing animals and increased muscle mass and function in healthy animals *(211–213)*. There was no change in food intake or tumor growth. A combination of naproxen, clenbuterol, insulin, and eicosapentaenoic acid ameliorated cancer cachexia and reduced tumor growth in Walker 256 tumor-bearing rats *(214, 215)*. In a randomized trial, clenbuterol was able to improve muscle strength of patients after knee surgery *(216)*. Its effects on muscle preservation appeared to occur without the need for exercise. Clenbuterol has not yet been studied in patients with cancer cachexia.

THALIDOMIDE

Thalidomide, a drug associated with over 10,000 cases of severe malformation in newborn children, has been revived because of its ability to suppress TNF production in monocytes in vitro and to normalize elevated TNF levels in animals. The drug also possesses antiangiogenic properties. Thalidomide inhibited TNF-α production in patients with leprosy, tuberculosis, AIDS, and cancer *(217–221)*.

In a randomized placebo-controlled trial, 50 patients with advanced pancreatic cancer who had lost at least 10% of their body weight received thalidomide 200 mg daily or placebo for 24 weeks *(221)*. At four weeks, patients who received thalidomide had gained on average 0.37 kg in weight and 1.0 cm^3 in arm muscle mass compared to a loss of 2.21 kg and 4.46 cm^3, respectively, in the placebo group. At eight weeks, patients in the thalidomide group had lost 0.06 kg in weight and 0.5 cm^3 in arm muscle mass compared with a loss of 3.62 kg and 8.4 cm^3, respectively, in the placebo group. Improvements in physical function correlated positively with weight gain. Thalidomide was well tolerated and appeared effective at attenuating loss of weight and lean body mass in patients with cachexia due to advanced pancreatic cancer. Beneficial effects of thalidomide have not been compared with other anticachexia agents such as megestrol acetate. Lenalidomide, a newer analogue of thalidomide, has not been tested in patients with cancer cachexia.

Adenosine Triphosphate (ATP)

Extracellular ATP is involved in the regulation of a variety of biologic processes including neurotransmission, muscle contraction, and hepatic metabolism of glucose, via purinergic receptors. In nonrandomized studies involving patients with different tumor types, ATP infusion appeared to inhibit loss of weight and deterioration of quality of life and performance status.

Patients with nonsmall cell lung cancer, stage IIIB or IV, were randomized to receive either 10 intravenous, 30-hour ATP infusions every 2–weeks, or no ATP (222, 223). In the ATP group, no change in body composition occurred over the 28-week follow-up period, whereas, the control group lost 0.6 kg of fat mass, 0.5 kg of fat-free mass, 1.8% of arm muscle area, and 0.6% of body cell mass/kg body weight per 4 weeks. Appetite remained stable in the ATP group but decreased significantly in the control group, by 568 KJ/d in energy intake. These effects were ascribed to maintenance of energy intake by exogenous ATP.

These reports contrast with a strategy of ATP suppression as a means of cancer therapy. ATP suppression in tumor tissue by means of direct intra-arterial delivery of 3-bromopyruvate, a potent inhibitor of ATP production, to the site of the primary tumor, or by a combination of 6-methylmercaptopurine riboside, a purine de novo synthesis inhibitor, and 6-aminonicotinamide, an inhibitor of glycolysis, which were given concomitantly with N-(phosphonacetyl)-L-aspartic acid (PALA), a pyrimidine synthesis inhibitor was reported to show marked therapeutic enhancement (224, 225). Furthermore, imatinib and other tyrosine kinase inhibitors with major activity in chronic myelocytic leukemia and gastrointestinal sarcomas expressing c-kit do so by blocking the ATP receptor site.

5′-Deoxy-5-Fluorouridine (5′-dFUrd)

The fluorinated pyrimidine nucleoside, 5′-dFUrd, was shown to effectively attenuate the progress of cachexia in mice bearing the murine adenocarcinomas MAC16 or colon 26, as well as in the human uterine cervical carcinoma xenograft, Yumoto. The anticachexia effect of 5′-dFUrd was shown to be independent of its antitumor activity and appears to be at least in part related to its inhibition of proteolysis-inducing factor (PIF), thought to be responsible for the development of cachexia in the murine MAC16 model (226, 227). 5′-dFUrd has not yet been evaluated as an anticachectic agent in humans.

Proinflammatory Cytokine Inhibitors, Proinflammatory Cytokine Antibodies, and Anti-Inflammatory Cytokines

In addition to pentoxifylline and thalidomide, a number of cytokine inhibitors and antibodies have been developed.

Anti-TNF-α antibody, anti-IL-1 antibody, and anti-IL-1 receptor antibody were reported to have attenuated the cachexia produced by either chronic TNF-α administration or implantation of a tumor in experimental animals (228, 229). Administration of TNF-α antibody to tumor-bearing rats decreased protein degradation rates in skeletal muscle, heart, and liver as compared to controls; the antibody was unable to prevent a reduction in body weight, however *(230)*. Decreases in protein degradation in skeletal muscle by TNF-α antibody appear to be due to inhibition of tumor-induced increases in muscle ubiquitin gene expression *(230)*.

Randomized clinical trials using anti-TNF antibody failed to increase survival or reverse the protein catabolism associated with severe sepsis or septic shock compared to those who received standard supportive care and antimicrobial therapy *(231)*. Similarly, clinical trials involving anti-TNF strategies such as etanercept (a dimeric fusion protein consisting of the extracellular ligand-binding portion of the human tumor necrosis factor receptor [TNFR] linked to the Fc portion of human IgG1) or infliximab (monoclonal antibody against TNF-α) in patients with chronic heart failure showed no improvements in clinical outcome as compared to placebo controls *(232)*.

Suramin, an antitrypanosomal polyanion, prevented the binding of IL-6 to its cell surface receptor subunits in vitro and inhibited colon-26-mediated cancer cachexia in mice *(233)*. Treatment of mice bearing AB 22 mesothelioma with anti-IL-6 antibody curtailed the clinical symptoms, as did treatment with recombinant human (rhu) IFN-α *(234)*. Neither anti-IL-6 antibody nor rhuIFN-α had a direct growth-inhibitory effect on the tumor cell line in vitro; however, in vivo rhuIFN-α attenuated both IL-6 mRNA expression in the tumors and serum IL-6 levels, ameliorated the depression of lymphocyte activities, and enhanced the number of tumor-infiltrating lymphocytes and macrophages. A combination therapy of rhuIFN-α and anti-IL-6 antibody may be beneficial in the palliative treatment for patients with malignant mesothelioma *(234)*.

Administration of an anti-IL-6 antibody in patients seropositive for human immunodeficiency virus-1 and suffering from an immunoblastic or a polymorphic large-cell lymphoma resulted in partial remission or stabilization of the disease *(235)*. The neutralizing effect of the anti-IL-6 antibody as measured by C-reactive protein levels in the serum was accompanied by abrogation of B clinical symptoms including fever and cachexia.

Production of anti-inflammatory cytokine IL-12 and type 2 immune responses is markedly decreased in cachectic patients with colorectal and gastric cancer *(236)*. Administration of IL-12 was reported to reduce serum levels of IL-6 in mice bearing colon 26 carcinoma and prevented development of cachexia *(237)*. The IL-12 activity was T-cell-dependent and the anticachexia effect resulted from at least two mechanisms: the downregulation of IL-6 and the upregulation of IFN-α. Similarly, a gene transfer of IL-10, another IL-6 inhibitor, prevented cachexia in an animal model *(238)*. IL-15 treatment partly inhibited skeletal muscle wasting in AH-130-bearing rats by decreasing protein degradation rates to values even lower than those observed in nontumor-bearing animals *(239)*. These alterations in protein breakdown rates were associated with an inhibition of the ATP-ubiquitin-dependent proteolytic pathway. Administration of IL-15 to rats bearing ascites hepatoma resulted in a significant reduction of muscle wasting and reversal of the increased DNA fragmentation observed in skeletal muscle *(240)*. IL-15 decreased apoptosis apparently by affecting TNF-α signaling. Administration of IL-15 decreased the inducible nitric oxide synthase protein levels by 73%, suggesting that nitric oxide formation and muscle apoptosis during tumor growth could be related. IL-12, IL-10, and IL-15 have not been evaluated as anticachectic agents in humans.

EICOSAPENTAENOIC ACID (EPA)

ω-3 polyunsaturated fatty acids are an essential component of the diet and are involved in the synthesis of eicosanoids (prostaglandins, leukotriens, and thromboxanes) and in membrane, receptors and enzyme functions. EPA, an ω-3 polyunsaturated fatty acid found in oily fish such as sardines, salmon, and mackerel, has been shown to possess antitumor as well as anticachexia activities in animal cachexia models *(241, 242)*. EPA-induced inhibition of weight loss was accompanied by increases in total body fat and muscle mass. EPA administration resulted in downregulation of ZAG (see Tumor Byproducts) expression in both white and brown adipose tissue and suppression of well-characterized mediators of cancer-associated wasting, including IL-6, as well as an attenuation of protein degradation by the ubiquitin-proteasome proleolytic pathway mediated by PIF (see Tumor Byproducts) in cachectic mice *(243–245)*. PIF in skeletal muscle releases arachidonic acid, which is rapidly metabolized to prostaglandins E2 and F2a as well as 5-, 12- and 15-hydroxyeicosatetraenoic acids (HETEs). Of all the metabolites, only 15-HETE produces a significant increase in protein degradation. EPA induced inhibition of arachidonic acid release and subsequent decreases in 15-HETE, which serves as a second messenger, abrogate the enhancer effect on the promoter region of the proteasome C3 subunit gene *(246)*. EPA also decreased glucose utilization of skeletal muscle, inhibited lipolysis in adipocytes by preventing prostaglandin synthesis and by a rising cyclic AMP in response to the LMF (see Tumor Byproducts). EPA also inhibited translocation of the nuclear transcription factor NF-κB, by preventing degradation of the inhibitor protein I-κB in the cytosol *(247–249)*.

Early clinical trials of fish oils were encouraging. Patients with pancreas cancer treated with supplements of fish oil capsules (EPA and docosahexaenoic acid) showed body weight gain accompanied by significant reduction in acute-phase protein production and by stabilization of resting energy expenditure *(250)*. While nutritional supplements alone did not attenuate the development of weight loss in cachectic cancer patients, nutritional supplements enriched with EPA produced significant weight gain along with an improvement in appetite and performance status *(251)*. Significant increases of lean body mass were noteworthy among various therapeutic interventions reported. A randomized controlled study was carried out to investigate the effects of dietary EPA plus vitamin E on the immune system and survival of well-nourished and of malnourished cancer patients *(252)*. EPA had a considerable immunomodulating effect by increasing the ratio of T-helper cells to T-suppressor cells in the subgroup of malnourished patients. EPA doubled the survival of patients compared with the placebo arm.

More recent randomized clinical studies, however, cast a serious doubt on any unique benefit of EPA. No significant differences in symptomatic or nutritional parameters were found in 60 patients with advanced cancer and loss of both weight and appetite who were randomized to fish oil capsules or placebo *(253)*. The majority of the patients were not able to swallow more than ten fish oil capsules per day. After 2 weeks of treatment, fish oil did not significantly improve appetite, tiredness, nausea, well-being, caloric intake, nutritional status, or function. In an international multicenter randomized double-blind trial, 200 patients with weight-losing inoperable pancreas cancer were randomized to receive EPA (2.2 gm/day) plus nutritional supplement or the nutritional supplement alone for 8 weeks *(254)*. Enrichment with EPA did not provide advantage over nutritional supplement alone. Both treatment groups equally benefited in arresting weight loss, but no differences were seen in body mass index, lean body mass, quality of life, or survival. In a third trial, 221 patients with cancer-associated wasting were randomized to either EPA supplement alone, megestrol acetate alone, or EPA plus megestrol acetate for a median of 3 months *(255)*. Weight gain of ≥10% was seen in a higher percentage of patients with megestrol acetate than EPA. Overall weight gain, functional assessment of anorexia/cachexia therapy (FAACT), and QOL were essentially identical among the three groups. To meet the criticisms of too short a treatment period in some studies, and of compliance issues of taking large amounts of EPA in randomized trials, a new randomized study comparing placebo versus two doses of EPA, 2 g or 4 g per day for 8 weeks, was undertaken in 518 patients with weight-losing advanced gastrointestinal or lung cancer. There were no statistically significant improvements in survival, weight, or other nutritional variables *(256)*. Thus, available data do not support a value of EPA in the treatment of cancer cachexia in humans.

β-Hydroxy-β-methylbutyrate (HMB)/l-Arginine/l-Glutamine

HMB, a metabolite of the amino acid leucine, interferes with the activation of NF-κB. HMB inhibited PIF-induced protein degradation and attenuated the increased protein degradation during cachexia in tumor-bearing mice. In a randomized study, the effects of HMB were examined during exercise training. Regardless of gender or training status, HMB increased upper body strength and minimized muscle damage when combined with an exercise program *(257)*. In a randomized study of patients with acquired immunodeficiency syndrome (AIDS), supplements containing HMB, arginine, and glutamine were shown to produce weight gain mainly as a lean body mass *(258)*. Immune status was also improved as evidenced by an increase in CD3 and CD8 cells and a decrease in the HIV viral load.

Thirty-two patients with solid tumors who had demonstrated a weight loss of at least 5% were randomly assigned in a double-blind fashion to either an isonitrogenous control mixture of nonessential amino acids or an experimental treatment containing HMB (3 g/d), l-arginine (14 g/d), and l-glutamine (14 g/d) (HMB/Arg/Gln) *(259)*. The primary outcomes measured were the change in body mass and fat-free mass (FFM), which were assessed at up to 6 months. The patients supplemented with HMB/Arg/Gln gained 0.95 ± 0.66 kg of body mass in 4 weeks, whereas control subjects lost 0.26 ± 0.78 kg during the same time period. This gain was the result of a significant increase in fat-free mass (FFM) in the HMB/Arg/Gln-supplemented group (1.12 ± 0.68 kg), whereas the control subjects lost 1.34 ± 0.78 kg of FFM ($P = 0.02$). The effect of HMB/Arg/Gln on FFM increase was maintained over 24 weeks. The exact reason for this improvement was unclear. The increases of FFM were attributed to the observed effects of HMB on slowing the rate of protein breakdown, with improvements in protein synthesis observed with arginine and glutamine. For the last 5 years, no follow-up or confirmatory studies have been published. Whether this combination improved survival or improved tolerance to chemotherapy is unclear. Additional randomized studies are needed to fully assess the benefit of the combination.

Enteral and Parenteral Nutrition

Cancer cachexia is different from simple starvation, in that nutritional support, either enteral or parenteral, has only limited value. For the correction of cancer-related malnutrition, therefore, enteral and parenteral administration of nutrient solutions must be used discreetly. In patients with oro-pharyngeal dysfunction from head and neck neoplasm or esophageal obstruction, blenderized food and liquid supplement can often achieve an adequate level of nutritional repletion. When necessary, percutaneous gastrostomy or jejunostomy offer bypass feeding. For patients who cannot tolerate the use of the gastrointestinal tract because of nausea, vomiting, obstruction, malabsorption, or absence, it may be necessary to begin total parenteral nutrition (TPN, "hyperalimentation").

The needs of nutritional support in cancer patients during tumor progression and the role of TPN in cancer surgery, chemotherapy, and radiotherapy should be considered at several different levels. Benefits of TPN in patients who underwent cancer surgery have been reported to include improved wound healing, a decreased rate of infection, fewer major complications, and a decrease in postoperative mortality. In other studies, however, no advantage of TPN was found; one report described an increase in the rate of major postoperative complications (260). TPN in cancer patients with obstructions of the gastrointestinal tract, gastrointestinal fistulae, evisceration, and intra-abdominal infection appears justified during and after surgery, however, since it constitutes a treatment for starvation, not cancer cachexia (261).

No significant benefit of TPN has been demonstrated in patients undergoing chemotherapy and/or radiotherapy in terms of treatment tolerance, response to chemotherapy or radiotherapy, or in survival (262, 263). Furthermore, other authors have reported that TPN is detrimental. Controversies related to TPN in the treatment of cancer cachexia have been reviewed (264–266).

Recently, in a randomized trial of more than 300 patients with malignant neoplasms who experienced progressive cachexia, indomethacin and epogen, or these drugs plus oral or parenteral nutritional support were compared (267). Patients in the latter group had significant improvements in food intake, energy balance, and overall survival. It is unclear, however, whether improved survival was due to the combined effects of two drugs plus nutritional intervention or nutritional intervention alone. This question is relevant because a large percentage (92.1%) of patients had GI cancer, suggesting that many patients might have had nausea and vomiting, GI obstruction, ascites, diarrhea, or other GI-specific causes of weight loss rather than simply cancer cachexia. Confirmatory studies are needed, specifically accruing patients with non-GI malignancies.

BRANCHED-CHAIN AMINO ACIDS

Branched-chain amino acids (leucine, isoleucine, and valine) are utilized by skeletal muscle but not by the liver. They have been shown to be uniquely effective in regulating nitrogen balance in muscle by reducing protein catabolism and increasing protein synthesis in both injured and tumor-bearing animals. Randomized studies have shown improved nitrogen retention, improved protein utilization, and increased protein and albumin synthesis in patients who received parenteral nutritional support with a high content of branched-chain amino acids (268, 269). In contrast, in another randomized study, the effects of a balanced amino acid solution with or without supplementation of α-ketoisocaproate or a branched-chain amino acid solution were compared in patients with gastrointestinal cancer who underwent surgery (270). The balanced amino acid solution itself with an adequate energy supply had an optimal nitrogen-sparing effect. Branched-chain amino acids or α-ketoisocaproate did not improve nitrogen balance or reduce protein degradation.

Interestingly, the tryptophan (precursor of serotonin) uptake into the brain is competitive with that of branched-chain amino acids *(271)*. A trial to reduce tryptophan uptake by increasing plasma levels of branched-chain amino acids resulted in a decrease in the severity of anorexia in cancer patients *(272)*.

Glutamine Tumor cells are major glutamine consumers both for protein synthesis and for oxidation *(273)*. A glutamine-enriched solution has been used to compensate for the uptake of the amino acid by the tumor to enhance host immune response against tumor growth *(274)*. In patients undergoing bone marrow transplantation for hematological malignancies, glutamine supplementation was found to be beneficial, improving nitrogen balance and diminishing the incidence of clinical infection *(275)*. The role of glutamine supplementation on cancer cachexia has not been reported.

OREXIGENIC AND ANOREXIGENIC MEDIATORS

Insulin Some of the metabolic alterations associated with cancer cachexia include glucose intolerance, increased gluconeogenesis, and Cori cycle activation. These metabolic changes are accompanied by insulin resistance. These observations led to the study of exogenous insulin administration. Animal studies show that insulin administration has improved the food intake, the host preservation of nitrogen, fat, and potassium, and decreased muscle wasting *(276, 277)*. Indeed, daily subcutaneous insulin administration resulted in a marked weight gain in AIDS patients *(278)*. Insulin administration alone has not been evaluated in the treatment of cancer cachexia (see sections "Growth Hormone (GH)," "Somatostatin," and "GHRH (GHRP-2) and Clenbuterol").

Ghrelin, an orexigenic mediator has recently been reported to have a key role in increasing appetite and food intake. The circulating levels of ghrelin have been reported to be increased in patients with chronic heart failure and muscle wasting and in patients with cancer cachexia.

Anticachexic effects of ghrelin have been demonstrated in nude mice bearing human melanoma cells *(279)*. Ghrelin has not been tested in patients with cancer cachexia.

MELATONIN

Melatonin is an indole amine primarily secreted from the pineal gland during the hours of darkness. The functions of melatonin are obscure but it has been claimed to modulate sleep, cardiac rhythms, sexual behavior, the reproductive system, immunologic functions, as well as antioxidative and anti-inflammatory activities. Melatonin has been reported to decrease the level of circulating TNF in patients with advanced cancer, prevent weight loss, and reduce chemotherapy-induced malaise and asthenia as well as thrombocytopenia *(280–283)*.

Based on observations that melatonin amplified IL-2-induced antitumor effects in animals, a randomized study was carried out in patients with metastatic solid tumors comparing a combination of low-dose IL-2 plus melatonin with best supportive care *(284)*. In the treated group, the percentage of patients with improved performance status as well as overall survival was significantly higher than the controls. Another randomized study of chemotherapy with cisplatin and etoposide plus/minus melatonin was carried out in poor-risk patients with advanced nonsmall cell lung cancer *(285)*. There was no significant difference in survival between the two groups, but the melatonin group had less frequent myelosuppression, neuropathy, and cachexia. In a recent

Swedish trial, the effect of fish oil, melatonin, or the combination of the two was investigated in 24 patients with advanced GI cancer. None induced major biochemical changes indicative of a strong anticachectic effect. Nonetheless, the interventions may have produced a weight-stabilizing effect *(286)*. Additional clinical studies appear indicated to define the role of melatonin in the treatment of cancer cachexia.

CYPROHEPTADINE

As has been discussed above, anorexia may be mediated by an increased serotonergic activity in the brain. Cyproheptadine is a serotonin antagonist with antihistaminic properties, usually prescribed for allergies. In several clinical situations, the agent produced appetite stimulation and weight gain. A randomized trial in patients with advanced malignant neoplasms showed that cyproheptadine produced a decrease in nausea and mild enhancement in appetite. The agent did not abate progressive weight loss in these patients, however *(287)*. Additional studies are needed with use of other antiserotogenic drugs.

CONCLUDING REMARK

Patients with cancer cachexia are characterized by the presence of anorexia, early satiety, anemia, weakness, and weight loss accompanied by muscle and adipose tissue loss. Patients with gastric cancer may present weight-loss as an initial and only sign of the disease whereas, in patients with lymphoma, weight loss and cachexia may be simply a terminal event. Cachexia occurs to a variable extent in different types of cancer at different stages, likely from different mechanisms. The multifactorial nature of cachexia precludes a uniform pathophysiological definition. Inability to translate animal studies to humans may lie in this context. These factors have hindered clinical studies not only at biochemical and molecular levels, but also in terms of the introduction of effective therapy. The advent of novel therapeutic targets (e.g., ubiquitin-proteasome pathway and NF-κB) and biological response modifiers (e.g., thalidomide) has opened possibilities for new clinical research in cachexia. Regulatory authorities feel it is important not only to demonstrate efficacy in terms of patients' nutritional status (e.g., lean body mass) but also in terms of functional status (e.g., performance status, tolerance to treatment, and survival).

In spite of extensive research on the mechanisms of cachexia, there has been little success in developing effective agents to treat cancer cachexia. Differences in therapeutic targets among cachectic cancer patients suggest no single agent will be able to treat all kinds of cachexia. There will likely be no all-in-one panacea for cancer cachexia. Combined anticachectic treatments and individualized approaches based on targets in individual patients are today's standard.

Several potentially promising leads beg for well-designed clinical trials. The following agents with suggestive activity in animal experiments or preliminary clinical explorations deserve critical clinical investigation: TPN plus GH or TPN/GH plus insulin, GHRP-2, megestrol plus ibuprofen, resvcratrol, dehydroxymethyl-epoxyquinomicin, clenbuterol, thalidomide/lenalidomide, 5′-doeoxy-5-fluorouridine, IL-12, IL-10, IL-15, HMB/Arg/Gln, ghrelin, and antiserotogenic agents.

Effective prevention or control of cachexia would significantly improve cancer therapy.

REFERENCES

1. Tisdale MJ. Clinical anticachexia treatments. Nutr Clin Pract 2006;2:168–174.

2. Vigano A, Bruera E, Jhangri GS, et al. Clinical survival predictors in patients with advanced cancer. Arch Intern Med 2000;160:861–868.

3. Persson C, Glimelius B. The relevance of weight loss for survival and quality of life in patients with advanced gastrointestinal cancer treated with palliative chemotherapy. Anticancer Res 2002;22:3661–3668.

4. Thomas DR. Distinguishing starvation from cachexia. Clin Geriatr Med 2002;18:883–891.

5. Giordano A, Calvani M, Petillo O, et al. Skeletal muscle metabolism in physiology and in cancer disease. J Cell Biochem 2003;90:170–186.

6. Tisdale MJ. Tumor-host interactions. J Cell Biochem 2004;93:871–877.

7. Nixon DW, Lawson DH, Kutner M, et al. Hyperalimentation of the cancer patient with protein-calorie undernutrition. Cancer Res 1981;41:2038–2045.

8. Brennan MF. Uncomplicated starvation versus cancer cachexia. Cancer Res 1977;37:2359–2364.

9. Ohnuma T. Cancer anorexia and cachexia. In: DW Kufe, RC Bast Jr, WN Hait, WK Hong, RE Pollack, RR Weichselbaum, JF Holland, E Frei III, Eds. Cancer Medicine (7th Edition) B C Decker, Hamilton, Ontario, Canada, 2006, pp. 2037–2054.

10. DeWys WD, Walters K. Abnormalities of taste sensation in cancer patients. Cancer 1975;36:1888–1896.

11. Nielsen SS, Theologides A, Vickers ZM. Influence of food odors on food aversion and preference in patients with cancer. Am J Clin Nutr 1980;33:2253–2261.

12. Krause R, Humphrey C, von Meyenfeldt M, et al. A central mechanism for anorexia in cancer: a hypothesis. Cancer Treat Res 1981;65(Suppl 5):15–21.

13. Cangiano C, Testa U, Muscaritoli M, et al. Cytokines, tryptophan and anorexia in cancer patients before and after surgical tumor ablation. Anticancer Res 1994;14:1451–1455.

14. Cubeddu LX, Hoffmann IS, Fuenmayor NT, Finn AL. Efficacy of ondansetron (GR 38032F) and the role of serotonin in cisplatin-induced nausea and vomiting. New Engl J Med 1990;322:810–816.

15. Laviano A, Meguid MM, Yang ZJ, et al. Cracking the riddle of cancer anorexia. Nutrition 1996;12:706–710.

16. Bodnar RJ, Pasternak GW, Mann PE, et al. Mediation of anorexia by human recombinant tumor necrosis factor through a peripheral action in the rat. Cancer Res 1989;49:6280–6284.

17. Plata-Salaman CR, Oomura Y, Kai Y. Tumor necrosis factor and interleukin-1 beta: suppression of food intake by direct action in the central nervous system. Brain Res 1988;448:106–114.

18. Turrin NP, Ilyin SE, Gayle DA, et al. Interleukin-1beta system in anorectic catabolic tumor-bearing rats. Curr Opin Clin Nutr Metab Care 2004;7:419–426.

19. [No authors listed] Phase II study of recombinant human interferon gamma (S-6810) on renal cell carcinoma. Summary of two collaborative studies. Recombinant Human Interferon Gamma (S-6810) Research Group on Renal Cell Carcinoma. Cancer 1987;60:929–933.

20. Cahlin C, Korner A, Axelsson H, et al. Experimental cancer cachexia: the role of host-derived cytokines interleukin (IL)-6, IL-12, interferon-gamma, and tumor necrosis factor alpha evaluated in gene knockout, tumor-bearing mice on C57 Bl background and eicosanoid-dependent cachexia. Cancer Res 2000;60:5488–5493.

21. Llovera M, Carbo N, Lopez-Soriano J, et al. Different cytokines modulate ubiquitin gene expression in rat skeletal muscle. Cancer Lett 1998;133:83–87.

22. Espat NJ, Auffenberg T, Rosenberg JJ, et al. Ciliary neurotrophic factor is catabolic and shares with IL-6 the capacity to induce an acute phase response. Am J Physiol 1996;271(1 Pt 2):R185–R190.

23. Wang W, Lonnroth C, Svanberg E, et al. Cytokine and cyclooxygenase-2 protein in brain areas of tumor-bearing mice with prostanoid-related anorexia. Cancer Res 2001;61:4707–4715.

24. Otterness IG, Seymour PA, Golden HW, et al. The effects of continuous administration of murine interleukin-1α in the rat. Physiol Behav 1988;43:797–804.

25. Mrosovsky N, Molony LA, Conn CA, et al. Anorexic effects of interleukin 1 in the rat. Am J Physiol 1989;257:R1315–R1321.

26. Maltoni M, Fabbri L, Nanni O, et al. Serum levels of tumour necrosis factor alpha and other cytokines do not correlate with weight loss and anorexia in cancer patients. Support Care Cancer 1997;5:130–135.

27. Jatoi A, Egner J, Loprinzi CL, et al. Investigating the utility of serum cytokine measurements in a multi-institutional cancer anorexia/weight loss trial. Support Care Cancer 2004;12:640–644.

28. Wisse BE, Schwartz MW, Cummings DE. Melanocortin signaling and anorexia in chronic disease states. Ann N Y Acad Sci 2003;994:275–281.

29. Schwartz MW, Woods SC, Porte D Jr, et al. Central nervous system control of food intake. Nature 2000;404:661–671.

30. Porte D Jr, Baskin DG, Schwartz MW. Leptin and insulin action in the central nervous system. Nutr Rev 2002;60(10 Pt 2):S20–S29.

31. Lopez-Soriano J, Carbo N, Tessitore L, et al. Leptin and tumor growth in rats. Int J Cancer 1999;81:726–729.

32. Aleman MR, Santolaria F, Batista N, et al. Leptin role in advanced lung cancer. A mediator of the acute phase response or a marker of the status of nutrition? Cytokine 2002;19:21–26.

33. Arpaci F, Yilmaz MI, Ozet A, et al. Low serum leptin level in colon cancer patients without significant weight loss. Tumori 2002;88:147–149.

34. Wolf I, Sadetzki S, Kanety H, et al. Adiponectin, ghrelin, and leptin in cancer cachexia in breast and colon cancer patients. Cancer 2006;106:966–973.

35. Wu JT, Kral JG. Ghrelin: integrative neuroendocrine peptide in health and disease. Ann Surg 2004;239:464–474.

36. Garcia JM, Garcia-Touza M, Hijazi RA, et al. Active ghrelin levels and active/total ghrelin ratio in cancer-induced cachexia. J Clin Endocrinol Metab 2005;90:2920–2926.

37. Shimizu Y, Nagaya N, Isobe T, et al. Increased plasma ghrelin level in lung cancer cachexia. Clin Cancer Res 2003;9:774–778.

38. Inui A, Meguid MM. Ghrelin and cachexia. Diabetes Obes Metab 2002;4:431.

39. Huang Q, Fan YZ, Ge BJ, Zhu Q, Tu ZY. Circulating ghrelin in patients with gastric or colorectal cancer. Dig Dis Sci 2007;52:803–809.

40. Wang W, Andersson M, Iresjo BM, et al. Effects of ghrelin on anorexia in tumor-bearing mice with eicosanoid-related cachexia. Int J Oncol 2006;28:1393–1400.

41. Neary NM, Small CJ, Wren AM, et al. Ghrelin increases energy intake in cancer patients with impaired appetite: acute, randomized, placebo-controlled trial. J Clin Endocrinol Metab 2004;89:2832–2836.

42. Ramos EJ, Suzuki S, Marks D, et al. Cancer anorexia-cachexia syndrome: cytokines and neuropeptides. Curr Opin Clin Nutr Metab Care 2004;7:427–434.

43. Niswender KD, Morton GJ, Stearns WH, et al. Intracellular signalling. Key enzyme in leptin-induced anorexia. Nature 2001;413:794–795.

44. Niswender KD, Schwartz MW. Insulin and leptin revisited: adiposity signals with overlapping physiological and intracellular signaling capabilities. Front Neuroendocrinol 2003;24:1–10.

45. Plata-Slaman CR. Immunoregulators in the nervous system. Neurosci Biobehav Rev 1991;15:185–215.

46. Chance WT, Sheriff S, Moore J, et al. Reciprocal changes in hypothalamic receptor binding and circulating leptin in anorectic tumor-bearing rats. Brain Res 1998;803:27–33.

47. Inui A. Cancer anorexia-cachexia syndrome: are neuropeptides the key? Cancer Res 1999;59:4495–4501.

48. Chance WT, Bakasubramaniam A, Thompson H, et al. Assessment of feeding response of tumor-bearing rats to hypothalamic injection and infusion of neuropeptide Y. Peptides 1996;17:797–801.

49. Rossi-Fanelli F, Laviano A. Role of brain tryptophan and serotonin in secondary anorexia. Adv Exp Med Biol 2003;527:225–232.

50. Chance WT, Bakasubramaniam A, Fischer JE. Neuropeptide Y and the development of cancer anorexia. Ann Surg 1995;221:579–589.

51. Chance WT, Balasubramaniam A, Borchers M, Fischer JE. Refractory hypothalamic adenylate cyclase in anorectic tumor-bearing rats. Brain Res 1995;691:180–184.

52. Sarraf P, Frederich RC, Turner EM, et al. Multiple cytokines and acute inflammation raise mouse leptin levels: potential role in inflammatory anorexia. J Exp Med 1997;185:171–175.

53. Argiles JM, Moore-Carrasco R, Busquets S, et al. Catabolic mediators as targets for cancer cachexia. Drug Discov Today 2003;8:838–844.

54. Gayle D, Ilyin SE, Plata-Salaman CR. Central nervous system IL-1 beta system and neuropeptide Y mRNAs during IL-1 beta-induced anorexia in rats. Brain Res Bull 1997;44:311–317.

55. Hellerstein MK, Meydani SN, Maydani M, et al. Interleukin-induced anorexia in the rat. J Clin Invest 1989;84:228–235.

56. Sato T, Laviano A, Meguid MM, et al. Involvement of plasma leptin, insulin and free tryptophan in cytokine-induced anorexia. Clin Nutr 2003;22:139–146.

57. Sonti G, Ilyin SE, Plata-Salaman CR. Neuropeptide Y blocks and reverses interleukin-1 beta-induced anorexia in rats. Peptides 1996;17:517–520.

58. Simons JP, Schols AM, Campdfield LA, et al. Plasma concentration of total leptin and human lung cancer-associated cachexia. Clin Sci (Colch) 1997;93:273–277.

59. Wallace AM, Satter N, McMillan DC. Effect of weight loss and the inflammatory response on leptin concentrations in gastrointestinal cancer patients. Clin Cancer Res 1998;4:2977–2979.

60. Laviano A, Russo M, Freda F, Rossi-Fanelli F. Neurochemical mechanisms for cancer anorexia. Nutrition 2002;18:100–105.

61. Perez MM, Newcomer AD, Moertel CG, et al. Assessment of weight loss, food intake, fat metabolism, malabsorption, and treatment of pancreatic insufficiency in pancreatic cancer. Cancer 1983;52:346–352.

62. Ramot B. Malabsorption due to lymphomatous diseases. Ann Rev Med 1971;22:19–24.

63. Armes PJ, Plant HJ, Allbright A, et al. A study to investigate the incidence of early satiety in patients with advanced cancer. Br J Cancer 1992;65:481–484.

64. Willox JC, Corr J, Shaw J, et al. Prednisolone as an appetite stimulant in patients with cancer. Br Med J 1984;288:27.

65. Nelson KA, Walsh TD, Sheehan FG, et al. Assessment of upper gastrointestinal motility in the cancer-associated dyspepsia syndrome (CSDS). J Palliat Care 1993;9:27–31.

66. Mulligan HD, Tisdale MJ. Metabolic substrate utilization by tumour and host tissue in cancer cachexia. Biochem J 1991;277:321–326.

67. Pedersen PL, Mathupala S, Rempel A, et al. Mitochondrial bound type II hexokinase: a key player in the growth and survival of many cancers and an ideal prospect for therapeutic intervention. Biochim Biophys Acta 2002;1555:14–20.

68. Mathupala SP, Rempel A, Pedersen PL. Glucose metabolism in cancer cells: isolation, sequence, and activity of the promotor for type II hexokinase. J Biol Chem 1995;270:16918–16925.

69. Mathupala SP, Rempel A, Pedersen PL. Glucose catabolism in cancer cells: identification and characterization of a marked activation response of the type II hexokinase gene to hypoxic conditions. J Biol Chem 2001;276:43407–43412.

70. Gold J. Cancer cachexia and gluconeogenesis. Ann NY Acad Sci 1974;230:103–110.

71. Lundholm K, Edstrom S, Karlberg I, et al. Glucose turnover, gluconeogenesis from glycerol and estimation of net glucose cycling in cancer patients. Cancer 1982;50:1142–1150.

72. Ramos EJ, Suzuki S, Marks D, et al. Cancer anorexia-cachexia syndrome: cytokines and neuropeptides. Curr Opin Clin Nutr Metab Care 2004;7:427–434.

73. Deans C, Wigmore SJ. Systemic inflammation, cachexia and prognosis in patients with cancer. Curr Opin Clin Nutr Metab Care 2005;8:265–269.

74. Henderson JT, Mullen BJM, Roder JC. Physiological effects of CNTF-induced wasting. Cytokins 1996;8:784–793.

75. Beutler B, Greenwald D, Hulmes JD, et al. Identity of tumour necrosis factor and the macrophage-secreted factor cachectin. Nature (London) 1985;316:552–554.

76. Tisdale MJ. Loss of skeletal muscle in cancer: biochemical mechanisms. Front Biosci 2001;6:D164–D174.

77. Adami F, Guarini A, Pini M, et al. Serum levels of tumor necrosis factor-a in patients with B-cell chronic lymphocytic leukemia. Eur J Cancer 1994;30A:1259–1263.

78. Aderka D, Englemann H, Hornik V, et al. Increased serum levels of soluble receptors for tumor necrosis factor in cancer patients. Cancer Res 1991;15:5602–5607.

79. Sherman ML, Spriggs DR, Arthur KA, et al. Recombinant human tumor necrosis factor administered as a five-day continuous infusion in cancer patients: Phase I toxicity and effects on lipid metabolism. J Clin Oncol 1988;6:344–350.

80. Starnes HF Jr, Warren RS, Jeevanandam M, et al. Tumor necrosis factor and the acute metabolic response to tissue injury in man. J Clin Invest 1988;82:1321–1325.

81. Socher SH, Martinez D, Craig JB, et al. Tumor necrosis factor not detectable in patients with clinical cancer cachexia. J Natl Cancer Inst 1988;80:595–598.

82. Barber MD, Powell JJ, Lynch SF, et al. A polymorphism of the interleukin-1 beta gene influences survival in pancreatic cancer. Br J Cancer 2000;83:1443–1447.

83. Fujita J, Tsujinaka T, Yano M, et al. Anti-interkeukin-6 receptor antibody prevents muscle atrophy in colon-25 adenocarcinoma-bearing mice with modulation of lysosomal and ATP-ubiquitin-dependent proteolytic pathways. Int J Cancer 1996;68:637–643.

84. Oldenburg HS, Rogy MA, Lazarus DD, et al. Cachexia and the acute phase protein response in inflammation are regulated by Interleukin-6. Eur J Immunol l993;23:1889–1894.

85. Strassmann G, Masui Y, Chizzonite R, Fong M. Mechanism of experimental cancer cachexia. Local involvement of IL-1 in colon 26 tumor. J Immunol l993;150:2341–2345.

86. Scott HR, McMillan DC, Crilly A, et al. The relationship between weight loss and interleukin 6 in non-small-cell lung cancer. Br J Cancer 1996;73:1560–1562.

87. Martin F, Santolaria F, Batista N, et al. Cytokine levels (IL-6 and IFN-gamma), acute phase response and nutritional status as prognostic factors in lung cancer. Cytokine 1999;11:80–86.

88. Jablons DM, McIntosh JK, Mule JJ, et al. Induction of interferon b2/interleukin-6 (IL-6) by cytokine administration and detection of circulating interleukin-6 in the tumor-bearing state. Ann NY Acad Sci 1989;557:157–160.

89. McNamara MJ, Alexander HR, Norton JA. Cytokines in their role in the pathophysiology of cancer cachexia. J Parenter Enteral Nutr 1992;16(Suppl 6):50S–55S.

90. Mule JJ, McIntosh JK, Jablons DM, Rosenberg SA. Antitumor activity of recombinant interleukin-6 in mice. J Exp Med 1990;171:629–636.

91. Suematsu S, Matsuda T, Aozasa K, et al. IgG1 plasmacytosis in interleukin-6 transgenic mice. Proc Natl Acad Sci USA 1989;86:7547–7551.

92. Patton JS, Shepard HM, Wilking H, et al. Interferon and tumor necrosis factors have similar catabolic effects on 3T3 L1 cells. Proc Natl Acad Sci USA 1986;83:8313–8317.

93. Matthys P, Heremans H, Opdenakker G, Billiau A. Anti-interferon- antibody treatment, growth of Lewis lung tumours in mice and tumour-associated cachexia. Eur J Cancer 1991;27:182–187.

94. Pisa P, Stenke L, Bernell P, et al. Tumor necrosis factor-a and interferon-g in serum of multiple myeloma patients. Anticancer Res 1990;10:817–820.

95. Puigserver P, Rhee J, Lin J, et al. Cytokine stimulation of energy expenditure through p38 MAP kinase activation of PPARgamma coactivator-1. Mol Cell 2001;8:971–982.

96. Masuno H, Yoshimura M, Ogawa N, Okuda H. Isolation of lipolytic factor (toxohormone-L) from ascites fluid of patients with hepatoma and its effects on feeding behavior. Eur J Cancer Clin Oncol 1984;20:1177–1185.

97. Kajimura N, Iseki H, Tanaka R, et al. Toxohormones are responsible for cancer cachexia syndrome in nude mice bearing human cancer cell lines. Cancer Chemother Pharmacol 1996;38(Suppl):S48–S52.

98. Mori M, Yamaguchi K, Honda S, et al. Cancer cachexia syndrome developed in nude mice bearing melanoma cells producing leukemia-inhibitory factor. Cancer Res l991;51:6656–6659.

99. Marshall MK, Doerrler W, Feingold KR, Grunfeld C. Leukemia inhibitory factor induces changes in lipid metabolism in cultured adipocytes. Endocrinology 1994;135:141–147.

100. Berg M, Fraker DL, Alexander HR. Characterization of differentiation factor/leukemia inhibitory factor effect on lipoprotein lipase activity and mRNA in 3T3-L1 adipocytes. Cytokine 1994;6:425–432.

101. Todorov PT, McDevitt TM, Meyer DJ, et al. Purification and characterization of a tumor lipid-mobilizing factor. Cancer Res 1998;58:2353–2358.

102. Hirai K, Hussey HJ, Barber MD, et al. Biological evaluation of a lipid-mobilizing factor isolated from the urine of cancer patients. Cancer Res 1998;58:2359–2365.

103. Lowell BB, Flier JS. Brown adipose tissue, beta 3-adrenergic receptors, and obesity. Annu Rev Med 1997;48:307–316.

104. Hyltander A, Daneryd P, Sandstrom R, et al. Beta-adrenoceptor activity and resting energy metabolism in weight losing cancer patients. Eur J Cancer 2000;36:330–334.

105. Bing C, Brown M, King P, et al. Increased gene expression of brown fat uncoupling protein (UCP)1 and skeletal muscle UCP2 and UCP3 in MAC16-induced cancer cachexia. Cancer Res 2000;60:2405–2410.

106. Bing C, Russell ST, Beckett EE, et al. Expression of uncoupling proteins-1, -2 and -3 mRNA is induced by an adenocarcinoma-derived lipid-mobilizing factor. Br J Cancer 2002;86:612–618.

107. Busquets S, Sanchis D, Alvarez B, et al. In the rat, tumor necrosis factor alpha administration results in an increase in both UCP2 and UCP3 mRNAs in skeletal muscle: a possible mechanism for cytokine-induced thermogenesis? FEBS Lett 1998;440:348–350.

108. Bing C, Bao Y, Jenkins J, et al. Zinc-alpha2-glycoprotein, a lipid mobilizing factor, is expressed in adipocytes and is up-regulated in mice with cancer cachexia. Proc Natl Acad Sci U S A 2004;101:2500–2505.

109. Russell ST, Tisdale MJ. The role of glucocorticoids in the induction of zinc-alpha2-glycoprotein expression in adipose tissue in cancer cachexia. Br J Cancer 2005;92:876–881.

110. Groundwater P, Beck SA, Barton C, et al. Alterations of serum and urinary lipolytic activity with weight loss in cachectic cancer patients. Br J Cancer 1990;62:816–821.

111. Beck SA, Groundwater P, Barton C, Tisdale MJ. Alteration in serum lipolytic activity in cancer patients with response to therapy. Br J Cancer 1990;62:822–825.

112. Belizario JE, Katz M, Chenker E, Raw I. Bioactivity of skeletal muscle proteolysis-inducing factors in the plasma proteins from cancer patients with weight loss. Br J Cancer 1991;63:705–710.

113. Cariuk P, Lorite MJ, Todorov PT, et al. Induction of cachexia in mice by a product isolated from the urine of cachectic cancer patients. Br J Cancer 1997;76:606–613.

114. Lorite MJ, Thompson MG, Drake JL, et al. Mechanism of muscle protein degradation induced by a cancer cachectic factor. Br J Cancer 1998;78:850–856.

115. Bossola M, Muscaritoli M, Costelli P, et al. Increased muscle proteasome activity correlates with disease severity in gastric cancer patients. Ann Surg 2003;237:384–389.

116. Wigmore SJ, Todorov PT, Barber MD, et al. Characteristics of patients with pancreatic cancer expressing a novel cancer cachectic factor. Br J Surg 2000;87:53–58.

117. Todorov PT, McDevitt TM, Cariuk P, et al. Induction of muscle protein degradation and weight loss by a tumor product. Cancer Res 1996;56:1256–1261.

118. Guttridge DC, Mayo MW, Madrid LV, et al. NF-kappaB-induced loss of MyoD messenger RNA: possible role in muscle decay and cachexia. Science 2000;289:2363–2366.

119. Acharyya S, Ladner KJ, Nelsen LL, et al. Cancer cachexia is regulated by selective targeting of skeletal muscle gene products. J Clin Invest 2004;114:370–378.

120. Wyke SM, Tisdale MJ. NF-kappaB mediates proteolysis-inducing factor induced protein degradation and expression of the ubiquitin-proteasome system in skeletal muscle. Br J Cancer 2005;92:711–721.

121. Watchorn TM, Dowidar N, Dejong CH, Waddell ID, Garden OJ, Ross JA. The cachectic mediator proteolysis inducing factor activates NF-kappaB and STAT3 in human Kupffer cells and monocytes. Int J Oncol 2005;27:1105–1111.

122. Jagoe RT, Redfern CP, Roberts RG, et al. Skeletal muscle mRNA levels for cathepsin B, but not components of the ubiquitin-proteasome pathway, are increased in patients with lung cancer referred for thoracotomy. Clin Sci (Lond) 2002;102:353–361.

123. Di Marco S, Mazroui R, Dallaire P, Chittur S, Tenenbaum SA, Radzioch D, Marette A, Gallouzi IE. NF-kappa B-mediated MyoD decay during muscle wasting requires nitric oxide synthase mRNA stabilization, HuR protein, and nitric oxide release. Mol Cell Biol 2005;25:6533–6545.

124. Acharyya S, Guttridge DC. Cancer cachexia signaling pathways continue to emerge yet much still points to the proteasome. Clin Cancer Res 2007;13:1356–1361.

125. Lee SJ. Regulation of muscle mass by myostatin. Annu Rev Cell Dev Biol 2004;20:61–86.

126. Acharyya S, Butchbach ME, Sahenk Z, et al. Dystrophin glycoprotein complex dysfunction: a regulatory link between muscular dystrophy and cancer cachexia. Cancer Cell 2005;8:421–432.

127. Mordes JP, Longcope C, Flatt JP, et al. The rat LTW (m) Leydig cell tumor: cancer cachexia due to estrogen. Endocrinology 1984;115:167–173.

128. Greenway B, Iqbal MJ, Johnson PJ, Williams R. Low serum testosterone concentrations in patients with carcinoma of the pancreas. Br Med J (Clin Res Ed) 1983;286:93–95.

129. Heber D, Tchekmedyian NS. Pathophysiology of cancer: hormonal and metabolic abnormalities. Oncology 1992;49(Suppl 2):28–31.

130. Schaur RJ, Fellier H, Gleispach, et al. Tumor host relations. I. Increased plasma cortisol in tumor-bearing humans compared with patients with benign surgical diseases. J Cancer Res Clin Oncol 1997;93:281–285.

131. Knapp ML, al-Sheibani S, Riches PG, et al. Hormonal factors associated with weight loss in patients with advanced breast cancer. Ann Clin Biochem 1991;28:480–486.

132. Tessitore L, Costelli P, Baccino FM. Humoral mediation for cachexia in tumour-bearing rats. Br J Cancer 1993;67:15–23.

133. Bennett A, Berstock DA, Carroll MA. Increased survival of cancer-bearing mice with inhibitors of prostaglandin synthesis, alone or with chemotherapy. Br J Cancer l982;45:762–768.

134. Noriki S, Imamura Y, Ikeda T, et al. Multi-organ damage (MOD) induced by cancer cachexia and its pathogenesis. Basic Appl Histochem 1989;33:337–346.

135. Wang W, Andersson M, Lõnnroth C, et al. Prostaglandin E and prostacyclin receptor expression in tumor and host tissues from MCG 101-bearing mice: a model with prostanoid-related cachexia. Int J Cancer 2005;115,582–590.

136. Radcliffe JD, Morrison SD. Histidine deficiency, food intake and growth in normal and Walker 256 carcinoma-bearing rats. Nutr Cancer 1981;3:40–45.

137. Torosian MH, Nguyen HQ. Tumors – effective nitrogen traps independent of protein intake. J Surg Res 1989;47:456–459.

138. Ulander K, Jeppsson B, Grahn G. Postoperative energy intake in patients after colorectal cancer surgery. Scand J Caring Sci 1998;12:131–138.

139. Ohnuma T, Holland JF. Nutritional consequences of cancer chemotherapy and immunotherapy. Cancer Res 1977;37:2395–2406.

140. Ohnuma T, Holland JF, Freeman A, Sinks LF. Biological and pharmacological studies with asparaginase in man. Cancer Res 1970;30:2297–2305.

141. Atkins MB, Robertson MJ, Gordon M, et al. Phase I evaluation of intravenous recombinant human interleukin 12 in patients with advanced malignancies. Clin Cancer Res 1997;3:409–417.

142. Scott HR, McMillan DC, Forrest LM, et al. The systemic inflammatory response, weight loss, performance status and survival in patients with inoperable non-small cell lung cancer. Br J Cancer 2002;87:264–267.

143. Bruera E, Roca E, Cedaro L, et al. Action of oral methylprednisolone in terminal cancer patients: a prospective randomized double-blind study. Cancer Treat Rep l985;69:751–754.

144. Popiela T, Lucchi R, Giongo F. Methylprednisolone as palliative therapy for female terminal cancer patients. The Methylprednisolone Female Preterminal Cancer Study Group. Eur J Cancer Clin Oncol l989;25:1823–1829.

145. Della Cuna GR, Pellegrini A, Piazzi M. Effect of methylprednisolone sodium succinate on quality of life in preterminal cancer patients: a placebo-controlled multicenter study. Eur J Cancer Clin Oncol 1989;25:1817–1821.

146. Loprinzi CL, Kugler JW, Sloan JA, et al. Randomized comparison of megestrol acetate versus dexamethasone versus fluoxymesterone for the treatment of cancer anorexia/cachexia. J Clin Oncol 1999;17:3299–3306.

147. Llovera M, Garcia-Martinez C, Costelli P, et al. Muscle hypercatabolism during cancer cachexia is not reversed by the glucocorticoid receptor antagonist RU38486. Cancer Lett 1996;99:7–14.

148. Rivadeneira DE, Naama HA, McCarter MD, et al. Glucocorticoid blockade does not abrogate tumor-induced cachexia. Nutr Cancer 1999;35:202–206.

149. Mantovani G, Maccio A, Bianchi A, et al. Megestrol acetate in neoplastic anorexia/cachexia: clinical evaluation and comparison with cytokine levels in patients with head and neck carcinoma treated with neoadjuvant chemotherapy. Int J Clin Lab Res 1995;25:135–141.

150. McCarthy HD, Crowder RE, Dryden S, Williams G. Megestrol acetate stimulates food and water intake in the rat: effects on regional hypothalamic neuropeptide Y concentrations. Eur J Pharmacol 1994;265:99–102.

151. Pascual Lopez A, Roque i Figuls M, Urrutia Cuchi G, et al. Systematic review of megestrol acetate in the treatment of anorexia-cachexia syndrome. J Pain Symptom Manage 2004;27:360–369.

152. Maltoni M, Nanni O, Scarpi E, et al. High-dose progestins for the treatment of cancer anorexia-cachexia syndrome: a systematic review of randomized clinical trials. Ann Oncol 2001;12:289–300.

153. Loprinzi CL, Schaid DJ, Dose AM, et al. Body-composition changes in patients who gain weight while receiving megestrol acetate. J Clin Oncol 1993;11:152–154.

154. McMillan DC, Simpson JM, Preston T, et al. Effect of megestrol acetate on weight loss, body composition and blood serum of gastrointestinal cancer patients. Clin Nutr 1994;13:85–89.

155. Nathanson L, Meelu MA, Losada R. Chemohormone therapy of metastatic melanoma with megestrol acetate plus dacarbazine, carmustine, and cisplatin. Cancer 1994;73:98–102.

156. Orme LM, Bond JD, Humphrey MS, et al. Megestrol acetate in pediatric oncology patients may lead to severe, symptomatic adrenal suppression. Cancer 2003;98:397–405.

157. Mantovani G, Maccio A, Esu S, et al. Medroxyprogesterone acetate reduces the in vitro production of cytokines and serotonin involved in anorexia/cachexia and emesis by peripheral blood mononuclear cells of cancer patients. Eur J Cancer 1997;33:602–607.

158. Downer S, Joel S, Allbright A, et al. A double-blind placebo-controlled trial of medroxyprogesterone acetate (MPA) in cancer cachexia. Br J Cancer 1993;67:1102–1105.

159. Simons JP, Aaronson NK, Vanateenkiste JF, et al. Effects of medroxyprogesterone acetate on appetite, weight and quality of life in advanced-stage non-hormone-sensitive cancer: a placebo-controlled multicenter study. J Clin Oncol 1996;14:1077–1084.

160. Lyden E, Cvetkovska E, Westin T, et al. Effects of nandrolone propionate on experimental tumor growth and cancer cachexia. Metabolism 1995;44:445–451.

161. Spiers AS, DeVita SF, Allar MJ, et al. Beneficial effects of an anabolic steroid during cytotoxic chemotherapy for metastatic cancer. J Med 1981;12:433–445.

162. Chlebowski RT, Herrold J, Ali I, et al. Influence of nandrolone decanoate in weight loss in advanced non-small cell lung cancer. Cancer 1986;58:183–186.

163. Plasse TF, Gorter RW, Krasnow SH, et al. Recent clinical experience with dronabinol. Pharmacol Biochem Behav 1991;40:695–700.

164. Nelson K, Walsh D, Deeter P, Sheehan F. A phase II study of delta-9-tetrahydrocannabinol for appetite stimulation in cancer-associated anorexia. J Palliat Care 1994;10:14–18.

165. Jatoi A, Windschitl HE, Loprinzi CL, et al. Dronabinol versus megestrol acetate versus combination therapy for cancer-associated anorexia: a North Central Cancer Treatment Group study. J Clin Oncol 2002;20:567–573.

166. Wolf RF, Ng B, Weksler B, et al. Effect of growth hormone on tumor and host in an animal model. Ann Surg Oncol 1994;1:314–320.

167. Fiebig HH, Dengler W, Hendriks HR. No evidence of tumor growth stimulation in human tumors in vitro following treatment with recombinant human growth hormone. Anticancer Drugs 2000;11:659–664.

168. Bartlett DL, Charland S, Torosian MH. Growth hormone, insulin, and somatostatin therapy of cancer cachexia. Cancer 1994;73:1499–1504.

169. Wolf RF, Pearlstone DB, Newman E, et al. Growth hormone and insulin reverse net whole body and skeletal muscle protein catabolism in cancer patients. Ann Surg 1992;216:280–288.

170. Berman RS, Harrison LE, Pearlstone DB, et al. Growth hormone, alone and in combination with insulin, increases whole body and skeletal muscle protein kinetics in cancer patients after surgery. Ann Surg 1999;229:1–10.

171. Tschop M, Statnick MA, Suter TM, Heiman ML. GH-releasing peptide-2 increases fat mass in mice lacking NPY: indication for a crucial mediating role of hypothalamic agouti-related protein. Endocrinology 2002;143:558–568.

172. Laferrere B, Abraham C, Russell CD, Bowers CY. Growth hormone releasing peptide-2 (GHRP-2), like ghrelin, increases food intake in healthy men. J Clin Endocrinol Metab 2005;90:611–614.

173. Tone CM, Cardoza DM, Carpenter RH, Draghia-Akli R. Long-term effects of plasmid-mediated growth hormone releasing hormone in dogs. Cancer Gene Ther 2004;11:389–396.

174. Froesch ER, Schmid C, Schwander J, Zapf J. Actions of insulin-like growth factors. Annu Rev Physiol 1985;47:443–467.

175. Florini JR. Hormonal control of muscle growth. Muscle Nerve 1987;10:577–598.

176. Ng EH, Rock CS, Lazarus DD, et al. Insulin-like growth factor I preserves host lean tissue mass in cancer cachexia. Am J Physiol 1992;262(3 Pt 2):R426–R431.

177. Lieberman SA, Butterfield GE, Harrison D, Hoffman AR. Anabolic effects of recombinant insulin-like growth factor-I in cachectic patients with the acquired immunodeficiency syndrome. J Clin Endocrinol Metab 1994;78:404–410.

178. Lee PD, Pivarnik JM, Bukar JG, et al. A randomized, placebo-controlled trial of combined insulin-like growth factor I and low dose growth hormone therapy for wasting associated with human immunodeficiency virus infection. J Clin Endocrinol Metab 1996;81:2968–2975.

179. Nelson KA, Walsh TD. Metoclopramide in anorexia caused by cancer-associated dyspepsia syndrome (CADS). J Palliat Care 1993;9:14–18.

180. Shivshanker K, Bennett RW Jr, Haynie TP. Tumor-associated gastroparesis: correction with metoclopramide. Am J Surg 1983;145:221–225.

181. Bruera ED, MacEachern J, Spachynski KA, et al. Comparison of the efficacy, safety, and pharmacokinetics of controlled release and immediate release metoclopramide for the management of chronic nausea in patients with advanced cancer. Cancer 1994;74:3204–3211.

182. Chen HC, Leung SW, Wang CJ, et al. Effect of megestrol acetate and propulside on nutritional improvement in patients with head and neck cancers undergoing radiotherapy. Radother Oncol 1997;43:75–79.

183. Ray PD, Hanson RL, Lardy HA. Inhibition by hydrazine of glyconeogenesis in the rat. J Biol Chem 1970;245:690–696.

184. Kosty MP, Fleischman SB, Herndon JE 2nd, et al. Cisplatin, vinblastine and hydrazine sulfate in advanced, non-small-cell lung cancer: a randomized placebo-controlled, double-blind phase III study of the Cancer and Leukemia Group B. J Clin Oncol 1994;12:1113–1120.

185. Loprinzi CL, Goldberg RM, Su JQ, et al. Placebo-controlled trial of hydrazine sulfate in patients with newly diagnosed non-small-cell lung cancer. J Clin Oncol 1994;12:1126–1129.

186. Loprinzi CL, Kuross SA, O'Fallon JR, et al. Randomized placebo-controlled evaluation of hydrazine sulfate in patients with advanced colorectal cancer. J Clin Oncol 1994;12:1121–1125.

187. Kikawa Y, Narumiya S, Fukushima M, et al. 9-Deoxy-delta 9, delta 12–13,14-dihydroprostaglandin D2, a metabolite of prostaglandin D2 formed in human plasma. Proc Natl Acad Sci U S A 1984;81:1317–1321.

188. Fischer SM, Furstenberger G, Marks F, Slaga TJ. Events associated with mouse skin tumor promotion with respect to arachidonic acid metabolism: a comparison between SENCAR and NMRI mice. Cancer Res 1987;47:3174–3179.

189. Bennett A, Houghton J, Leaper DJ, Stamford IF. Cancer growth, response to treatment and survival time in mice: beneficial effect of the prostaglandin synthesis inhibitor flurbiprofen. Prostaglandins 1979;17:179–191.

190. Homem-de-Bittencourt PI Jr, Pontieri V, Curi R, Lopes OU. Effects of aspirin-like drugs on Walker 256 tumor growth and cachexia in rats. Braz J Med Biol Res 1989;22:1039–1042.

191. McCarthy DO, Daun JM. The effects of cyclooxygenase inhibitors on tumor-induced anorexia in rats. Cancer 1993;71:486–492.

192. Davis TW, Zweifel BS, O'Neal JM, et al. Inhibition of cyclooxygenase-2 by celecoxib reverses tumor-induced wasting. J Pharmacol Exp Ther 2004;308:929–934.

193. Bredt AB, Girey GJ. Antipyretic effects of indomethacin in liver metastasis of solid tumors. Cancer 1982;50:1430–1433.

194. Romeu J, Chadha N, Fukilman O, et al. Indomethacin therapy in symptomatic hepatic neoplasms. Am J Gastroenterol 1982;77:655–659.

195. Preston T, Fearon KC, McMillan DC, et al. Effect of ibuprofen on the acute phase response and protein metabolism in patients with cancer and weight loss. Br J Surg 1995;82:229–234.

196. Wigmore SJ, Falconer JS, Plester CE, et al. Ibuprofen reduces energy expenditure and acute-phase protein production compared with placebo in pancreatic cancer patients. Br J Cancer 1995;72:185–188.

197. Lundholm K, Gelin J, Hyltander A, et al. Anti-inflammatory treatment may prolong survival in undernourished patients with metastatic solid tumors. Cancer Res 1994;54:5602–5606.

198. McMillan DC, Wigmore SJ, Fearon KC, et al. A prospective randomized study of megestrol acetate and ibuprofen in gastrointestinal cancer patients with weight loss. Br J Cancer 1999;79:495–500.

199. Daneryd P. Epoetin alfa for protection of metabolic and exercise capacity in cancer patients. Semin Oncol 2002;29(3 Suppl 8):69–74.

200. Daneryd P, Svanberg E, Korner U, et al. Protection of metabolic and exercise capacity in unselected weight-losing cancer patients following treatment with recombinant erythropoietin: a randomized prospective study. Cancer Res 1998;58:5374–5379.

201. Han J, Thompson P, Beutler B. Dexamethasone and pentoxifylline inhibit endotoxin-induced cachectin/tumor necrosis factor synthesis at separate points in the signaling pathway. J Exp Med 1990;172:391–394.

202. Combaret L, Ralliere C, Taillandier D, et al. Manipulation of the ubiquitin-proteasome pathway in cachexia: pentoxifylline suppresses the activation of 20S and 26S proteasomes in muscles from tumor-bearing rats. Mol Biol Rep 1999;26:95–101.

203. Bianco JA, Appelbaum FR, Nemunaitis J, et al. Phase I-II trial of pentoxifylline for prevention of transplant-related toxicities following bone marrow transplantation. Blood l991;78:1205–1211.

204. Goldberg RM, Loprinzi CL, Mailliard JA, et al. Pentoxifylline for treatment of cancer anorexia and cachexia? A randomized, double-blind, placebo-controlled trial. J Clin Oncol 1995;13:2856–2859.

205. Estey EH, Thall PF, Reed P, et al. Treatment of newly diagnosed AML, RAEB-t or RAEB with lisofylline or placebo in addition to chemotherapy. Leukemia 1999;13:850–854.

206. Margolin K, Atkins M, Sparano J, et al. Prospective randomized trial of lisofylline for the prevention of toxicities of high-dose interleukin 2 therapy in advanced renal cancer and malignant melanoma. Clin Cancer Res 1997;3:565–572.

207. Kwak KS, Zhou X, Solomon V, et al. Regulation of protein catabolism by muscle-specific and cytokine-inducible ubiquitin ligase E3alpha-II during cancer cachexia. Cancer Res 2004;64:8193–8198.

208. Busquets S, Carbo N, Almendro V, et al. Curcumin, a natural product present in turmeric, decreases tumor growth but does not behave as an anticachectic compound in a rat model. Cancer Lett 2001;167:33–38.

209. Wyke SM, Russell ST, Tisdale MJ. Induction of proteasome expression in skeletal muscle is attenuated by inhibitors of NF-kappaB activation. Br J Cancer 2004;91:1742–1750.

210. Kuroda K, Horiguchi Y, Nakashima J, et al. Prevention of cancer cachexia by a novel nuclear factor {kappa}B inhibitor in prostate cancer. Clin Cancer Res 2005;11:5590–5594.

211. Carbo N, Lopez-Soriano J, Tarrago T, et al. Comparative effects of beta 2-adrenergic agonists on muscle waste associated with tumour growth. Cancer Lett 1997;115:113–118.

212. Chance WT, Cao LQ, Zhang FS, et al. Clenbuterol treatment increases muscle mass and protein content of tumor-bearing rats maintained on total parenteral nutrition. J Parenter Enteral Nutr 1991;15:530–535.

213. Costelli P, Garcia-Martinez C, Llovera M, et al. Muscle protein waste in tumor-bearing rats is effectively antagonized by a b2-adrenergic agonist (clenbuterol). Role of the ATP-ubiquitin-dependent proteolytic pathway. J Clin Invest 1995;95:2367–2372.

214. Piffar PM, Fernandez R, Tchaikovski O, et al. Naproxen, clenbuterol and insulin administration ameliorates cancer cachexia and reduce tumor growth in Walker 256 tumor-bearing rats. Cancer Lett 2003;201:139–148.

215. Pinto JA Jr, Folador A, Bonato SJ, et al. Fish oil supplementation in F1 generation associated with naproxen, clenbuterol, and insulin administration reduce tumor growth and cachexia in Walker 256 tumor-bearing rats. J Nutr Biochem 2004;15:358–365.

216. Maltin CA, Delday MI, Watson JS, et al. Clenbuterol, a beta-adrenoceptor agonist, increases relative muscle strength in orthopaedic patients. Clin Sci 1993;84:651–654.

217. Kaplan G. Cytokine regulation of disease progression in leprosy and tuberculosis. Immunobiology 1994;191:564–568.

218. Tramontana JM, Utaipat U, Molloy A, et al. Thalidomide treatment reduces tumor necrosis factor alpha production and enhances weight gain in patients with pulmonary tuberculosis. Mol Med 1995;1:384–397.

219. Bruera E, Neumann CM, Pituskin E, et al. Thalidomide in patients with cachexia due to terminal cancer: preliminary report. Ann Oncol 1999;10:857–859.

220. Khan ZH, Simpson EJ, Cole AT, et al. Oesophageal cancer and cachexia: the effect of short-term treatment with thalidomide on weight loss and lean body mass. Aliment Pharmacol Ther 2003;17:677–682.

221. Gordon JN, Trebble TM, Ellis RD, et al. Thalidomide in the treatment of cancer cachexia: a randomised placebo controlled trial. Gut 2005;54:540–545.

222. Agteresch HJ, Dagnelie PC, van der Gaast A, et al. Randomized clinical trial of adenosine 5′-triphosphate in patients with advanced non-small-cell lung cancer. J Natl Cancer Inst 2000;92:321–328.

223. Agteresch HJ, Rietveld T, Kerkhofs LG, et al. Beneficial effects of adenosine triphosphate on nutritional status in advanced lung cancer patients: a randomized clinical trial. J Clin Oncol 2002;20:371–378.

224. Martin DS, Spriggs D, Koutcher JA. A concomitant ATP-depleting strategy markedly enhances anticancer agent activity. Apoptosis 2001;6:125–131.

225. Geschwind JF, Ko YH, Torbenson MS, et al. Novel therapy for liver cancer: direct intraarterial injection of a potent inhibitor of ATP production. Cancer Res 2002;62:3909–3913.

226. Eda H, Tanaka Y, Ishitsuka H. 5′-Deoxy-5-fluorouridine improves cachexia by a mechanism independent of its antiproliferative action in colon 26 adenocarcinoma-bearing mice. Cancer Chemother Pharmacol 1991;29:1–6.

227. Hussey HJ, Todorov PT, Field WN, et al. Effect of a fluorinated pyrimidine on cachexia and tumour growth in murine cachexia models: relationship with a proteolysis inducing factor. Br J Cancer 2000;83:56–62.

228. Sherry BA, Gelin J, Fong Y, et al. Anticachectin/tumor necrosis factor-a antibodies attenuate development of cachexia in tumor models. FASEB J 1989;3:1956–1962.

229. Costelli P, Carbo N, Tessitore L, et al. Tumor necrosis factor-alpha mediates changes in tissue protein turnover in a rat cancer cachexia model. J Clin Invest 1993;92:2783–2789.

230. Llovera M, Carbo N, Garcia-Martinez C, et al. Anti-TNF treatment reverts increased muscle ubiquitin gene expression in tumour-bearing rats. Biochem Biophys Res Commun 1996;221:653–655.

231. Reinhart K, Wiegand-Lohnert C, Grimminger F, et al. Assessment of the safety and efficacy of the monoclonal anti-tumor necrosis factor antibody-fragment, MAK 195F, in patients with sepsis and septic shock: a multicenter, randomized, placebo-controlled, dose-ranging study. Crit Care Med 1996;24:733–742.

232. Anker SD, Coats AJ. How to RECOVER from RENAISSANCE? The significance of the results of RECOVER, RENAISSANCE, RENEWAL and ATTACH. Int J Cardiol 2002;86:123–130.

233. Strassmann G, Fong M, Freter CE, et al. Suramin interferes with interleukin-6 receptor binding in vitro and inhibits colon-26-mediated experimental cancer cachexia in vivo. J Clin Invest 1993;92:2152–2159.

234. Bielefeldt-Ohmann H, Marzo AL, Himbeck RP, et al. Interleukin-6 involvement in mesothelioma pathobiology: inhibition by interferon alpha immunotherapy. Cancer Immunol Immunother 1995;40:241–250.

235. Emilie D, Wijdenes J, Gisselbrecht C, et al. Administration of an anti-interleukin-6 monoclonal antibody to patients with acquired immunodeficiency syndrome and lymphoma: effect on lymphoma growth and on B clinical symptoms. Blood 1994;84:2472–2479.

236. Shibata M, Nezu T, Kanou H, et al. Decreased production of interleukin-12 and type 2 immune responses are marked in cachectic patients with colorectal and gastric cancer. J Clin Gastroenterol 2002;34:416–420.

237. Mori K, Fujimoto-Ouchi K, Ishikawa T, et al. Murine interleukin-12 prevents the development of cancer cachexia in a murine model. Int J Cancer 1996;67:849–855.

238. Fujiki F, Mukaida N, Hirose K, et al. Prevention of adenocarcinoma colon 26-induced cachexia by interleukin 10 gene transfer. Cancer Res 1997;57:94–99.

239. Carbo N, Lopez-Soriano J, Costelli P, et al. Interleukin-15 antagonizes muscle protein waste in tumour-bearing rats. Br J Cancer 2000;83:526–531.

240. Figueras M, Busquets S, Carbo N, et al. Interleukin-15 is able to suppress the increased DNA fragmentation associated with muscle wasting in tumour-bearing rats. FEBS Lett 2004;569:201–206.

241. Tisdale MJ, Dhesi JK. Inhibition of weight loss by omega-3 fatty acids in an experimental cachexia model. Cancer Res 1990;50:5022–5026.

242. Dagnelie PC, Bell JD, Williams SC, et al. Effect of fish oil on cancer cachexia and host liver metabolism in rats with prostate tumors. Lipids 1994;29:195–203.
243. Wigmore SJ, Fearon KC, Maingay JP, Ross JA. Down-regulation of the acute-phase response in patients with pancreas cancer cachexia receiving oral eicosapentaenoic acid is mediated via suppression of interleukin-6. Clin Sci (Colch) 1997;92:215–221.
244. Whitehouse AS, Smith HJ, Drake JL, Tisdale MJ. Mechanism of attenuation of skeletal muscle protein catabolism in cancer cachexia by eicosapentaenoic acid. Cancer Res 2001;61:3604–3609.
245. Russell ST, Tisdale MJ. Effect of eicosapentaenoic acid (EPA) on expression of a lipid-mobilizing factor in adipose tissue in cancer cachexia. Prostaglandins Leukot Essent Fatty Acids 2005;72:409–414.
246. Belda-Iniesta C, de Castro Carpeno J, Fresno Vara JA, et al. Eicosapentaenoic acid as a targeted therapy for cancer cachexia. J Clin Oncol 2003;21:4657–4658.
247. Tisdale MJ, Beck SA. Inhibition of tumor-induced lipolysis in vitro and cachexia and tumour growth in vivo by eicosapentaenoic acid. Biochem Pharmacol 1991;41:103–107.
248. Hussey HJ, Tisdale MJ. Effect of a cachectic factor on carbohydrate metabolism and attenuation by eicosapentaenoic acid. Br J Cancer 1999;80:1231–1235.
249. Smith HJ, Lorite MJ, Tisdale MJ. Efect of a cancer cachectic factor on protein synthesis/degradation in murine C2C12 myoblasts. Modulation by eicosapentaenoic acid. Cancer Res 1999;59:5507–5513.
250. Wigmore SJ, Ross JA, Flaconer JS, et al. The effect of polyunsaturated fatty acids on the progress of cachexia in patients with pancreatic cancer. Nutrition 1996;12:527–530.
251. Barber MD, Ross JA, Voss AC, et al. The effect of an oral nutritional supplement enriched with fish oil on weight loss in patients with pancreatic cancer. Br J Cancer 1999;81:80–86.
252. Gogos CA, Ginopoulos P, Salsa B, et al. Dietary omega-3 polyunsaturated fatty acids plus vitamin E restore immunodeficiency and prolong survival for severely ill patients with generalized malignancy: a randomized control trial. Cancer 1998;82:395–402.
253. Bruera E, Strasser F, Palmer JL, et al. Effect of fish oil on appetite and other symptoms in patients with advanced cancer and anorexia/cachexia: a double-blind, placebo-controlled study. J Clin Oncol 2003;21:129–134.
254. Fearon KC, von Meyenfeldt MF, Moses AGW, et al. Effect of a protein and energy-dense n-3 fatty acid-enriched oral supplement on loss of weight and lean tissue in cancer cachexia: a randomised double blind rial. Gut 2003;52:1479–1486.
255. Jatoi A, Rowland K, Loprinzi CL, et al. An eicosapentaenoic acid supplement versus megestrol acetate versus both for patients with cancer-associated wasting: a North Central Cancer Treatment Group and National Cancer Institute of Canada collaborative effort. J Clin Oncol 2004;22:2469–2476.
256. Fearon KC, Barber MD, Moses AG, et al. Double-blind, placebo-controlled, randomized study of eicosapentaenoic acid diester in patients with cancer cachexia. J Clin Oncol 2006;24:3401–3407.
257. Panton LB, Rathmacher JA, Baier S, Nissen S. Nutritional supplementation of the leucine metabolite-hydroxy-methylbutyrate (HMB) during resistance training. Nutrition 2000;16:734–739.
258. Clark RH, Feleke G, Din M, et al. Nutritional treatment for acquired immunodeficiency virus-associated wasting using beta-hydroxy beta-methylbutyrate, glutamine, and arginine: a randomized, double-blind, placebo-controlled study. JPEN J Parenter Enteral Nutr 2000;24:133–139.
259. May PE, Barber A, D'Olimpio JT, et al. Reversal of cancer-related wasting using oral supplementation with a combination of beta-hydroxy-beta-methylbutyrate, arginine, and glutamine. Am J Surg 2002;183:471–479.
260. Detsky AS, Baker JP, O'Rourke K, Goel V. Perioperative parenteral nutrition: a meta-analysis. Ann Intern Med 1987;107:195–203.
261. Jensen S. Clinical effects of enteral and parenteral nutrition preceding cancer surgery. Med Oncol Tumor Pharmacother 1985;2:225–229.
262. Donaldson SS. Nutritional support as an adjunct to radiation therapy. J Parenter Enteral Nutr 1984;8:302–310.
263. McGeer AJ, Detsky AS, O'Rouke K. Parenteral nutrition in cancer patients undergoing chemotherapy: a meta-analysis. Nutrition 1990;6:233–240.
264. Barber MD, Fearon KC, Delmore G, Loprinzi CL. Should cancer patients with incurable disease receive parenteral or enteral nutritional support? Eur J Cancer 1998;34:279–285.

265. Copeland EM 3rd. Historical perspective on nutritional support of cancer patients. CA Cancer J Clin 1998;48:67–68.
266. Iestra JA, Fibbe WE, Zwinderman AH, et al. Parenteral nutrition following intensive cytotoxic therapy: an exploratory study on the need for parenteral nutrition after various treatment approaches for hematological malignancies. Bone Marrow Transplant 1999;23:933–939.
267. Lundholm K, Daneryd P, Bosaeus I, et al. Palliative nutritional intervention in addition to cyclooxygenase and erythropoietin treatment for patients with malignant disease: effects on survival, metabolism, and function. Cancer 2004;100:1967–1977.
268. Hunter DC, Weintraub M, Blackburn GL, Bistrian BR. Branched-chain amino acids as the protein component of parenteral nutrition in cancer cachexia. Br J Surg 1989;76:149–153.
269. Okada A, Mori S, Totsuka M, et al. Branched-chain amino acids metabolic support in surgical patients: a randomized, controlled trial in patients with subtotal or total gastrectomy in 16 Japanese institutions. J Parenter Enteral Nutr 1988;12:332–337.
270. Sandstedt S, Jorfeldt L, Larsson J. Randomized, controlled study evaluating effects of branched-chain amino acids and alpha-ketoisocaproate on protein metabolism after surgery. Br J Surg 1992;79:217–220.
271. Fernstrom JD. Dietary effects on brain serotonin synthesis: relationship to appetite regulation. Am J Clin Nutr 1985;42(5 Suppl):1072–1082.
272. Cangiano C, Laviano A, Meguid MM, et al. Effects of administration of oral branched-chain amino acids on anorexia and caloric intake in cancer patients. J Natl Cancer Inst 1996;88:550–552.
273. Rivera S, Azcon-Bieto J, Lopez-Soriano FJ, et al. Amino acid metabolism in tumour-bearing mice. Biochem J 1988;249:443–449.
274. Souba WW. Glutamine and cancer. Ann Surg 1993;218:715–728.
275. Ziegler TR, Young LS, Benfell K, et al. Clinical and metabolic efficacy of glutamine-supplemented parenteral nutrition after bone marrow transplantation. A randomized, double-blind, controlled study. Ann Intern Med 1992;116:821–828.
276. Moley JF, Morrison SD, Norton JA. Preoperative insulin reverses cachexia and decreases mortality in tumor-bearing rats. J Surg Res 1987;43:21–28.
277. Tessitore L, Costelli P, Baccino FM. Pharmacological interference with tissue hypercatabolism in tumour-bearing rats. Biochem J 1994;299(Pt 1):71–78.
278. Kabadi UM, Reust CS, Kabadi MU. Weight gain, improvement in metabolic profile, and CD4 count with insulin administration in an AIDS patient. AIDS Patient Care STDS 2000;14:575–579.
279. Hanada T, Toshinai K, Kajimura N, et al. Anti-cachectic effect of ghrelin in nude mice bearing human melanoma cells. Biochem Biophys Res Commun 2003;301:275–279.
280. Lissoni P, Barni S, Tancini G. Role of the pineal gland in the control of macrophage functions and its possible implementation in cancer: a study of interactions between tumor necrosis factor-alpha and the pineal hormone melatonin. J Biol Regul Homeost Agents 1994;8:126–129.
281. Lissoni P, Tancini G, Barni S, et al. Treatment of cancer chemotherapy-induced toxicity with the pineal hormone melatonin. Supportive Care Cancer 1997;5:126–129.
282. Lissoni P, Tancini G, Paolorossi F, et al. Chemoneuroendocrine therapy of metastatic breast cancer with persistent thrombocytopenia with weekly low dose epirubicin plus melatonin: a phase II study. J Pineal Res 1999;26:169–173.
283. Lissoni P, Paolorossi F, Tancini G, et al. Is there a role for melatonin in the treatment of neoplastic cachexia? Eur J Cancer 1996;32A:1340–1343.
284. Lissoni P, Barni S, Fossati V, et al. A randomized study of neuroimmunotherapy with low-dose subcutaneous interleuken-2 plus melatonin compared to supportive care alone in patients with untreated metastatic solid tumour. Supportive Care Cancer 1995;3:194–197.
285. Lissoni P, Paolorossi F, Ardizzoia A, et al. A randomized study of chemotherapy with cisplatin plus etoposide versus chemoendocrine therapy with cisplatin, etoposide and the pineal hormone melatonin as a first-line treatment of advanced non-small cell lung cancer patients in a poor clinical state. J Pineal Res 1997;23:15–19.
286. Persson C, Glimelius B, Ronnelid J, Nygren P. Impact of fish oil and melatonin on cachexia in patients with advanced gastrointestinal cancer: a randomized pilot study. Nutrition 2005;21:170–178.

287. Kardinal CG, Loprinzi CL, Schaid DJ, et al. A controlled trial of cyproheptadine in cancer patients with anorexia and/or cachexia. Cancer 1990;65:2657–2662.

288. Moody TW, Pert CB, Gazdar AF, et al. High levels of intracellular bombesin characterize human small cell lung cancer. Science 1981;214:1246–1248.

289. Jensen PB, Blume N, Mikkelsen JD, et al. Transplantable rat glucagonomas cause acute onset of severe anorexia and adiposia despite highly elevated NPY mRNA levels in the hypothalamic accuate nucleus. J Clin Invest 1998;101:503–510.

290. Bajorunas DR. Clinical manifestations of cancer-related hypercalcemia. Semin Oncol 1990;17(2 Suppl 5):16–25.

291. Baile CA, Zinn WM, Mayer J. Effects of lactate and other metabolites on food intake of monkeys. Am J Physiol 1970;219:1606–1613.

292. Knoll J. Endogenous anorectic agent-satietins. Annu Rev Pharmacol Toxicol 1988;28:247–268.

293. Hamilton J, Cabanac M, Lafrance L, Nagy J. Ingestive response shows absence of taste aversion after bovine satietin in rats. Physiol Behav 1995;57:125–128.

5 Fatigue

Michael J. Fisch

ABSTRACT

Fatigue is a highly prevalent, complex and poorly delineated symptom, which occurs before, during and after treatment for cancer. Difficulties in establishing a case definition of cancer-related fatigue have resulted in an absence of reliable and valid epidemiological data, and confound investigation into the etiology and pathogenesis of this problem. Among the possible predisposing and perpetuating factors underlying fatigue are female gender, personality factors such as neuroticism and/or a tendency toward catastrophizing, obesity, low level of activity, exposure to toxins, and prior infections. There is no evidence thus far to suggest that family history, genetic factors, or sociodemographic factors predominate. One of the most consistently evoked factors in describing the etiology of cancer fatigue is the role of cytokines. In cancer-related fatigue research, evidence and opinions support the role of cytokines, but there are also studies in which cytokine correlates were not found to be important. Anemia is a common underlying problem in cancer fatigue and can be due to cancer chemotherapy or the effects of the malignancy itself.

Various therapies may have efficacy for treating cancer-related fatigue. These include exercise, mind-body interventions such as Tai chi chuan and yoga, nutritional interventions, behavioral and psychoeducational interventions, the use of antidepressants, use of erythropoietic agents, and psychostimulants such as methylphenidate hydrochloride and modafinil. Most of the current understanding of fatigue in cancer has been influenced by and largely derived from the experience of patients with breast cancer. However,

From: *Cancer and Drug Discovery Development: Supportive Care in Cancer Therapy*
DOI: 10.1007/978-1-59745-291-5_5, Edited by: D. S. Ettinger © Humana Press, Totowa, NJ

in the absence of an established evidence-based standard of care for the assessment and management of cancer-fatigue, further research is clearly needed, including more randomized, controlled clinical trials, research in different cancer diagnoses and treatment settings (aside from breast and prostate cancer outpatient settings); more rigorous outcomes assessment and study methodology; and discernment of dose effects and optimal frequency for dosing.

Key Words: Cancer fatigue; Cytokines; Fatigue assessment; Fatigue etiology; Metabolic fatigue; Anemia.

INTRODUCTION

Fatigue is a highly prevalent symptom in patients who receive care for cancer, with reported prevalence exceeding 60% in many studies that include patients receiving active cancer treatment or living with advanced cancer *(1– 5)*, and in 15–40% of patients who are post cancer treatment *(6–11)*. It is a symptom that most people can relate to, having experienced it at some time due to illness (such as viral infection) or due to some other reason (injury, grief). Fatigue is a persistent, subjective sense of exhaustion, which is not proportional to recent activity. This sort of fatigue has been the subject of extensive research in the context of cancer, particularly during the past 5 years, along with the emergence and growth of symptom science. There have been, on average, 80 or more manuscripts published each year in the biomedical literature related to this topic in the past 5 years. Although attention to this topic still lags behind that given to cancer pain, the number of manuscripts focused on fatigue in cancer patients is similar to what is being produced from investigation of other common symptoms such as depression and nausea. In addition, during the past 20 years, there has been intense interest in chronic fatigue syndrome (CFS). Parallel to the situation in oncology, researchers, clinicians, and public health officials have struggled to agree upon a case definition, on the acceptability of making a discrete diagnosis of chronic fatigue, and understanding the pathophysiology underlying fatigue *(12)*.

THE COMPLEXITY OF FATIGUE

While it is tempting to plow ahead and describe various cross-sectional and prospective studies related to fatigue in cancer and what has been learned thus far, it is important to acknowledge that this symptom is exceedingly complex and poorly delineated. I suspect that each author of this textbook has significant experience and expertise in the assessment and management of fatigue, as well as other specific cancer-related symptoms. Nevertheless, there is no doubt that there would be tremendous variation in how fatigue is assessed and managed by these experts. As a general oncologist, I cannot describe a systematic approach to this symptom that would be rational and reproducible other than to suggest undertaking comprehensive, interdisciplinary care directed toward patients and their families, with attention given to managing the underlying cancer and other medical conditions as well as preventing and relieving suffering. In essence, this approach embraces the principles of palliative care rather than the principles of fatigue management, per se. What is missing in regard to fatigue is sufficient evidence-based information about predisposing conditions, related pathophysiologic insults, discriminating clinical features, and clinical consequences of this "diagnosis" so that expert clinicians can create a succinct mental abstraction of the problem (or "problem representation") as well as an "illness script" that facilitates the use of nonanalytical as well as analytical clinical reasoning as it applies to this problem *(13)*. The missing elements in the clinical reasoning process as it applies to fatigue are summarized in Fig. 3.

Understanding Fatigue Complexity Through Patient Vignettes

The basis for this very broad approach rather than the fatigue-specific approach may be best understood from the perspective of specific patient vignettes. Table 1 illustrates four patient vignettes where each patient expresses fatigue and manifests subjective and objective functional impairment. The patients vary in age, underlying disease, comorbidity, and other factors, including the method of fatigue assessment. This table reflects the variability that exists in clinical practice. Such heterogeneity is found in the fatigue literature, making the literature extremely difficult to interpret and apply to individual patients.

Practice guidelines related to fatigue resemble general principles of good palliative care. Consider the following sample of general standards for cancer-related fatigue paraphrased from the practice guidelines for the National Comprehensive Cancer Network (NCCN) *(14)*:

- Fatigue is subjective and should be assessed by self-report
- Patients should be screened, assessed, and managed at the initial visit and regular intervals
- Fatigue in patients of all ages should be evaluated, monitored, documented, and treated promptly
- Experts in fatigue management should be available for consultation
- There should be education and training programs as well as multidisciplinary institutional committees focused on aspects of fatigue management
- Fatigue management should be part of continuous quality improvement projects as well as health outcome studies
- Medical care contracts should reimburse for fatigue management, and disability insurance should include coverage for the effects of fatigue

Although these guidelines acknowledge that fatigue exists as an expressed symptom, they do little to reduce the variability in approaches (and outcomes) related to fatigue by different clinicians and institutions once it has been acknowledged. Fatigue is qualitatively different from other, more focused, symptoms as it is the least emotionally loaded, most nonspecific symptom that a person could offer to begin a discussion about his or her health status. In casual conversation, it is common for people to mention that they are "tired" or experiencing "fatigue." However, it is very difficult to ascertain, with any reasonable precision, the specific cause(s) of fatigue for any given person. When a patient comes to the clinic and reports significant fatigue (let's say greater than "4" on a scale ranging from 0 to 10, where "10" is the greatest imaginable level of fatigue), the meaning of that level of fatigue to that specific patient is not going to be immediately apparent. The physician might have to ask, "What does that mean to you?" Depending on the person's relationship with you, the presence or absence of family members, their cultural background, how communicative and self-aware they are, and other factors, you might find out that the patient is too weak, too sleepy, too frightened, too bored, too sore, too

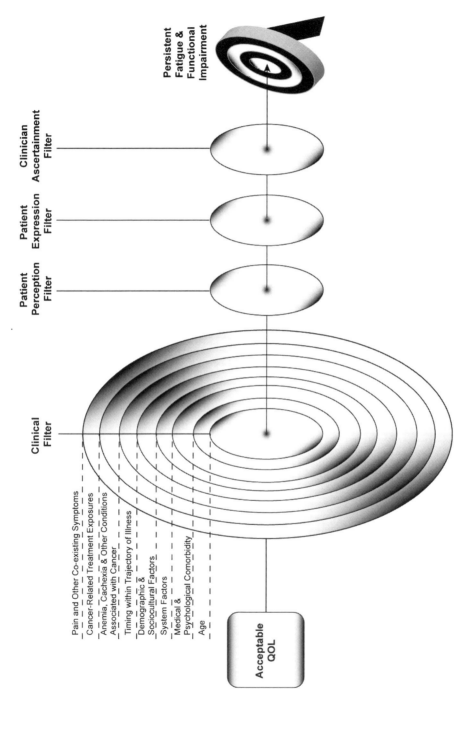

Fig. 1. The four filters that may confound fatigue assessment.

Table 1
Patient vignettes illustrating fatigue and functional impairment

Patient #1

27-year-old woman with a family history of ovarian cancer with newly diagnosed left breast cancer awaiting initiation of neoadjuvant chemotherapy. The patient reports fatigue level at 52 mm on a 100-mm visual analog scale

Patient #2

77-year-old Filipino man with a history of chronic obstructive pulmonary disease and mild cognitive impairment now with mild chronic dyspnea and hypercalcemia following his 3rd cycle of combination chemotherapy. The patient's daughter reports that he is persistently exhausted and that he is less active at home

Patient #3

51-year-old woman with a history of depression and fibromyalgia now 8 days status post her 2nd cycle of combination chemotherapy for stage III ovarian cancer. The fatigue item on the M.D. Anderson Symptom Inventory reveals a level of fatigue of 7 on a numerical rating scale where 10 represents the worst level of fatigue

Patient #4

An 18-year-old man is 4 months status post completion of cisplatin-based combination chemotherapy for intermediate risk nonseminomatous germ cell tumor. He remains in college, but he is taking fewer courses. He has experienced a worsening of 8 points on the General Fatigue Scale compared to his pretreatment baseline score

"poisoned", or too "cancer-laden" to be precise. The patient may have a combination of problems that are difficult to untangle and, thus, it is challenging to assign specific relative weights to them regarding their importance. Overall, your ability to optimally help the patient will depend largely on your ability to:

1. Specifically relate to the person
2. Assess the person in detail and across multiple dimensions
3. Evolve a strategy that strives to improve the situation over a series of visits or planned interventions to take place over a reasonable period of time

Fatigue Assessment: A Conceptual Model

A conceptual model that illustrates the complexity of fatigue assessment is shown in Fig. 2. The target of attention for understanding cancer-related fatigue (CRF) is cancer patients of all types who express fatigue in the presence of functional impairment. Acceptable quality of life (QOL) refers to individuals with intact QOL (with or without minor fatigue). Numerous parameters in the clinical "filter" may impact fatigue. The Patient Perception Filter refers to the individual patient's ability to discern the presence or absence of fatigue and impairment related to fatigue. The Patient Expression Filter refers to an ability and willingness to express the fatigue. This may vary depending on the target audience (friend, family, nurse, physician, social worker). The Clinician Ascertainment Filter refers to the various ways that fatigue expression may be elicited and categorized by clinicians. This may include (1) verbally responding to spontaneous complaints of fatigue, low energy, or tiredness, (2) asking about fatigue in follow-up to

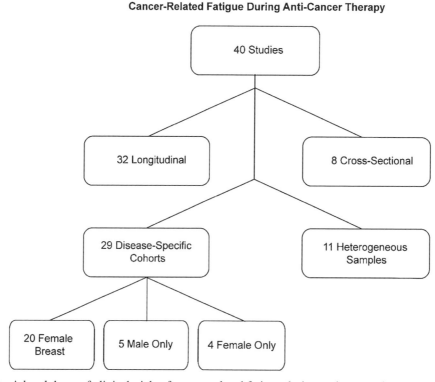

Fig. 2. A breakdown of clinical trials of cancer-related fatigue during anti-cancer therapy

a screening measure such as a distress thermometer *(15, 16)* or question about general health status or QOL, (3) including a fatigue item on a symptom checklist, symptom inventory, or multidimensional QOL instrument, (4) routine administration of a single-item measurement of fatigue, and (5) fatigue assessment using a multidimensional fatigue-specific instrument. Examples of fatigue measurement instruments are summarized in Table 2. A multitude of different instruments were developed in the 1990s. These instruments vary in the number of items and fatigue dimensions (physical fatigue, mental fatigue) that are included and emphasized. There is little research that compares these instruments, and the choice of instrument for research purposes varies with the purpose of the assessment, the appropriate response burden for the study population, the psychometric properties of the instrument, and the preference of the investigator. In general, the single-item scores correlate strongly with the multi-item, fatigue-specific instruments *(17, 18)*. It is rare to see anything other than a single item used in clinical settings, with multi-item instruments reserved for fatigue-related research. For some (but not all) of the available instruments, specific cutoff scores that are appropriate for diagnostic use are published, as well as investigations that establish the magnitude of change representing a minimally important clinical difference *(18–20)*. Item response theory and item banking is being explored as a way of selecting the most useful and parsimonious approach to fatigue measurement for specific patients *(21)*. The utility of item banking for this purpose remains unclear.

Table 2
Examples of fatigue measurements

Case definitions

ICD-10 definition of the cardinal symptom of fatigue in cancer

Significant fatigue, diminished energy, or increased need to rest,
    disproportionate to any recent change in activity level, and present
    every day or nearly every day during the same 2-week period
    in the past month

Single items on multidimensional symptom or quality of life instruments

M. D. Anderson symptom inventory fatigue item

Your fatigue (tiredness) at its WORST? [0–10 numerical rating scale,
    ranging from 0 ("not present") to 10 ("as bad as you can imagine")]

Edmonton symptom assessment scale (ESAS)

Visual analog assessment (100 mm) ranging from "No fatigue" to "Worst
    fatigue Imaginable"

EROTC QLQ-C30

Did you need to rest?

Were you tired?

Functional assessment of cancer therapy-general (FACT-G)

I have a lack of energy

Multi-item fatigue-specific instruments

Brief fatigue inventory	9 items
FACIT-F	13 items
Piper fatigue scale	22 items
Schwartz cancer fatigue scale	6 items
Lee fatigue scale	18 items
Fatigue questionnaire	11 items
Multidimensional fatigue inventory	20 items
Fatigue symptom inventory	13 items

Objective measurement of activity

Actigraphy

Limitations in the Existing Literature

With an appreciation of this complex conceptual model of CRF, it is much easier to understand how so much research could have been done without bringing this symptom into better focus. Each "filter" of the model shown in Fig. 1 (clinical factors, patient perception, patient expression, and clinician assessment) produces a significant source of variability. Thus, an estimate of the prevalence of fatigue in mixed cohorts of patients will vary depending on the nature of the patient mix rather than reflecting the essence of cancer fatigue. One approach to understanding the literature was applied by Prue and colleagues. They performed a critical appraisal of the literature evaluating cohort studies (interventional or noninterventional) that involved adult cancer patients with CRF while undergoing anticancer therapy who were assessed with a multidimensional CRF instrument *(3)*. This approach yielded 40 studies. Key features of these studies are summarized in Fig. 2. Only 32 of these studies were longitudinal, and 24 of 29 longitudinal studies involving disease-specific cohorts were limited to female patients. The prevalence of fatigue in these studies was high, sometimes more than 90%, but no specific proportion of these cohorts appropriately represents these data. Studies that involved only men were performed in prostate cancer clinics or veterans hospitals. The nature of the cancer therapy (radiation, conventional dose chemotherapy, high dose chemotherapy) was variable, as were the timing of the fatigue assessments, and the rate of missing follow-up data. A dozen different multidimensional fatigue instruments were utilized in these studies. The variability in the instruments is particularly problematic because (1) each instrument has a different cutoff point for clinically important fatigue and a different change score that might be considered clinically important, (2) the appropriate cutoff scores and clinically significant changes scores are not well described for each instrument, and (3) none of the instruments is widely used in clinical practice, thus limiting the generalizability of these data. Another source of information about the prevalence of fatigue is a large, cross-sectional study where adults over 65 years of age with newly diagnosed breast, colon, lung, or prostate cancer were followed over a 1-year period and asked about pain and fatigue in this fashion: "During the past 2 weeks, as a result of your cancer and its treatment, have you experienced any fatigue?" *(22)* In this study, 26–33% of patients experienced fatigue over a 1-year period. However, the single-item approach involved not only a judgment about fatigue, but also a patient judgment about attribution of the fatigue and it did not indicate any threshold for the functional consequences of the symptom. A systematic review of this literature reported by Lawrence and colleagues as part of the U. S. National Institutes of Health

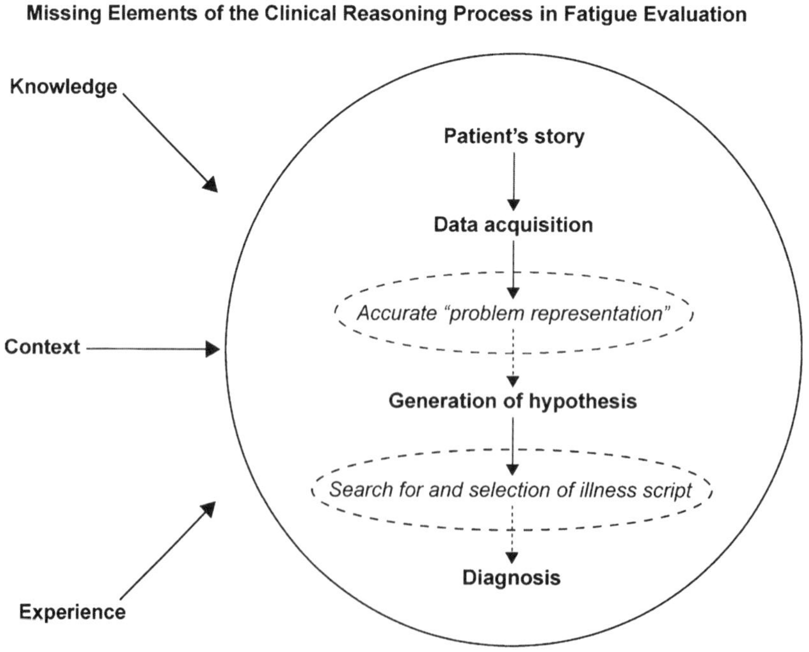

Missing Elements of the Clinical Reasoning Process in Fatigue Evaluation

Fig. 3. The missing elements of the clinical reasoning process in fatigue evaluation (adapted from ref. #13)

State-of-the-Science Conference on Symptom Management in Cancer in 2002 reported that the prevalence of CRF ranges from 4 to 91% depending on the population studied and the methods of assessment used *(23)*. That statistic summarizes how profoundly limited we are in our attempts to describe this symptom.

ETIOLOGY

Difficulties in establishing a case definition of CRF have resulted in an absence of reliable and valid epidemiologic data, and also confound investigation into the etiology and pathogenesis of this problem. In cancer, patients with breast cancer, particularly those who are undergoing or have completed adjuvant chemotherapy or radiation for early stage disease, are by far the most widely studied population. Thus, most of what is incorporated into the understanding of fatigue in cancer has been influenced by and largely derived from the experience of patients with breast cancer *(5, 6, 24–30)*. Similar to the situation with chronic fatigue syndrome (CFS), many different explanations for CRF have been proposed, with no dominant model emerging (Table 3). CRF is considered to have a multifactorial pathogenesis *(2, 5, 26, 30)*.

The Cytokine Hypothesis for Fatigue

One of the most consistently evoked factors in describing the etiology of cancer fatigue is the role of cytokines. Sickness behavior in animal models refers to the physiologic and behavioral responses observed in animals after the administration of infectious or inflammatory agents or certain proinflammatory cytokines. Symptoms

Table 3
Case definition for chronic fatigue syndrome (CFS)

Characterized by persistent or relapsing unexplained chronic fatigue
- Fatigue lasts for at least 6 months
- Fatigue is of new or definite onset
- Fatigue is not the result of an organic disease or of continuing exertion
- Fatigue is not alleviated by rest
- Fatigue results in a substantial reduction in previous occupational, educational, social, and personal activities
- Four or more of the following symptoms, concurrently present for ≥6 months: impaired memory or concentration, sore throat, tender cervical or axillary lymph nodes, muscle pain, pain in several joints, new headaches, unrefreshing sleep, or malaise after exertion

Exclusion criteria
- Medical condition explaining fatigue
- Major depressive disorder (psychotic features) or bipolar disorder
- Schizophrenia, dementia, or delusional disorder
- Anorexia nervosa, bulimia nervosa
- Alcohol or substance abuse
- Severe obesity

corresponding to sickness behavior in animal models reflect commonly co-occurring symptoms in cancer patients, such as fatigue, pain, cachexia, cognitive impairment, anxiety, and depression. Interdisciplinary collaboration among basic scientists doing preclinical work with animal models of cytokine-related "sickness behavior" and with oncologists, pain specialists, and psychiatrists led to the consensus that cancer symptoms in humans are similar to sickness behavior in animal models and that these similarities are related to cytokine exposure *(31)*. This may be called the "cytokine hypothesis" for fatigue and co-occurring symptoms. Cytokines are molecules produced by lymphocytes and macrophages in response to immune stimulation. Proinflammatory cytokines include interleukins 1, 2, 6, and 12 as well as tumor necrosis factor (alpha and beta) and interferon (alpha and gamma). The cytokine theory hypothesizes that when proinflammatory cytokines are released (peripheral immune activation in the setting of acute or chronic inflammation or tissue damage), cytokine receptors are activated in the central nervous system (CNS) and/or second messengers are activated and indirectly transfer chemical messages to the CNS *(32)*. The effects on the CNS include (1) changes in the transmission of monoamines such as dopamine, norepinephrine, and serotonin; (2) neuroendocrine effects on the hypothalamic–pituitary–adrenal (HPA) axis, which are reflected by changes in corticotrophin-releasing hormone and vasopressin; and (3) corticosteroid receptor and central inflammatory responses, including release of nitric oxide and prostaglandin E2.

A model incorporating the cytokine hypothesis in the understanding of fatigue is shown in Fig. 4. Precipitating events that result in tissue injury or immune activation can trigger a cascade of proinflammatory cytokines. Common precipitating events are (1) Underlying malignancy and its byproducts, (2) Infection, (3) Cancer therapy that induces cell death, (4) Comorbid medical and psychiatric disorders, and (5) Psychological stressors. When proinflammatory cytokines are produced in the periphery due to a precipitating event, cytokine receptors are activated in the CNS and/or second messengers are activated and indirectly transfer chemical messages to the CNS. Changes then occur in the transmission of monoamines, effects on the HPA axis, and corticosteroid receptor and central inflammatory responses, including release of nitric oxide and prostaglandin E2. Fatigue, and other symptoms, are essentially functional disturbances of the CNS, and result in mood and sleep alteration, changes in activity level, and changes in social interaction (obvious manifestations of sickness behavior). The somatic biologic impact of proinflammatory cytokines (outside of the CNS) along with effects on the CNS (neuroendocrine, inflammatory) result in a cascade of changes in the immune system and the autonomic nervous system, as well as other organ systems (bone marrow, musculoskeletal, gastrointestinal, and cardiopulmonary).

The cytokine interferon-alpha (IFN-α) has been administered to cancer patients for the treatment of malignant melanoma, renal cell carcinoma, and lymphoproliferative diseases. It is also used to treat hepatitis C infection. Neuropsychiatric problems are a well-described complication of IFN-α therapy. These range from fatigue, depression, and mental slowing to delirium and psychosis. One way to explore the cytokine hypothesis is to observe the effects of administering a cytokine-based therapy to a cohort of patients. In 2001, a group from Emory University showed that administering

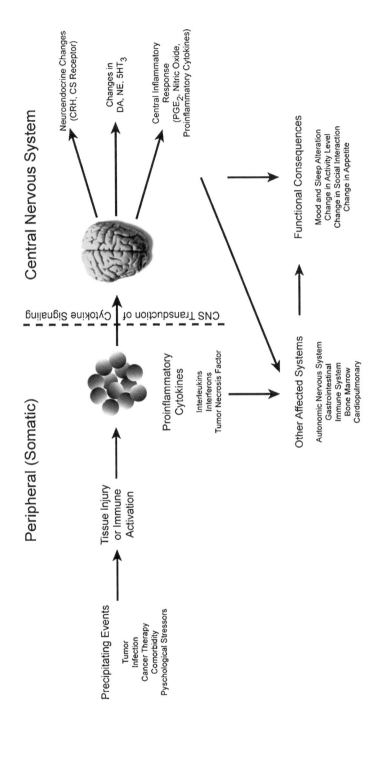

Fig. 4. A model of the cytokine hypothesis of fatigue

the serotonin reuptake inhibitor paroxetine could dramatically reduce the risk of major depression during IFN-α therapy and allowed patients to continue the treatment without disruption *(33)*. Building on that experience, a dimensional analysis was performed that distinguished the neurovegative symptoms (fatigue, anorexia, and psychomotor slowing) that occur early in the course of treatment from the depressive symptoms (anhedonia, depressed mood) that occur significantly later in the course of therapy and respond much better to antidepressant therapy *(34)*. In CRF research, there are both evidence and opinions in support of the role of cytokines *(6, 35–39)*, but there are also studies in which cytokine correlates were not found to be important *(40, 41)*.

PREDISPOSING AND PERPETUATING FACTORS

Ongoing exposure to the five precipitating factors outlined above, plus the presence of a high level of overall symptom burden *(42–44)*, predispose patients to CRF and also perpetuate the problem. Whereas CFS occurs most frequently in women *(12)*, no clear gender differences have emerged in CRF research *(45)*. Personality factors (such as neuroticism and/or a tendency toward catastrophism) are felt to have a predisposing influence *(46, 47)*. Other plausible predisposing factors that lack a substantial evidence basis include obesity *(48)*, low level of activity *(42)*, exposure to toxins (such as alcohol, environmental toxins, or prior cancer therapies), and prior infections with immune alteration. There is no evidence thus far to suggest that family history, genetic factors, or sociodemographic factors predominate.

THERAPY FOR CANCER FATIGUE

Most clinical research in CRF is based on the following logic:

1. Fatigue is an important problem in cancer
2. Intervention XX is considered promising based on anecdotal experience or uncontrolled studies or research in other patient populations
3. It is plausible that there is a biologic basis for an effect of Intervention X on fatigue
4. We can design a clinical trial and enroll patients on it

An example of ongoing randomized trials directed at cancer fatigue and approved through the U.S. Community Clinical Oncology Program (CCOP) is summarized in Table 4.

Any intervention directed at fatigue has a fair chance of being helpful to the patient. Regardless of the intervention, the result of any multidimensional assessment is usually the emergence of clinical insights regarding counseling approaches, changes in patient behavior(s), improved management of fatigue and nonfatigue symptoms, and improved management of comorbidities. The net result tends to be that patients achieve better health and less fatigue. Indeed, the National Comprehensive Cancer Network (NCCN) guidelines and most expert reviews suggest the multidimensional assessment as the starting point with clinicians using their judgment to identify and address problems that are amenable to specific treatment.

Specific causes of fatigue include anemia, infection, and metabolic disorders. These causes have specific treatments.

Table 4
Randomized trials targeting fatigue in the community clinical oncology program

Category	Intervention	Key factor in patient selection
Exercise	Exercise in patients undergoing curative-intent, combined-modality therapy	Nonsmall cell lung cancer
Nutritional/natural products	L-carnitine supplementation for fatigue	General cancer
	Valeriana officinalis (valerian) for improving sleep	Adjuvant therapy
	American ginseng to improve fatigue	General cancer
	Oral coenzyme Q-10 to relieve self-reported fatigue	Breast
Psychoeducational	Mindfulness relaxation	Chemotherapy
	Yoga for persistent sleep disturbance	Survivors
Antidepressants/ Anxiolytics	Buspirone for dyspnea associated with malignant disease	Shortness of breath
Psychostimulants	Modafinil for fatigue	Chemotherapy
Anti-inflammatory	Epoetin alfa with or without dexamethasone for the treatment of fatigue and anemia	Prostate
	Docetaxel with or without infliximab in elderly or poor performance status patients with wasting, anorexia and asthenia	Nonsmall cell lung cancer

Adapted from (97)

Anemia

The most commonly discovered underlying problem in cancer patients is the presence of anemia due to cancer chemotherapy or the effects of the malignancy itself. Anemia is the primary indication for transfusion of red blood cells, but the development and use of recombinant human erythropoietins such as epoetin alfa and darbopoetin alfa has been shown to reduce transfusion rates and increase hemoglobin response. Nonrandomized trials in community oncology patients have indicated that epoetins improve QOL (49, 50), but these agents have not been evaluated adequately for the purpose of treating fatigue specifically (that is, where fatigue is the primary endpoint of randomized, controlled trials). The use of these agents skyrocketed in the late 1990s, and by 2002 sales of epoietin alfa in the United States alone exceeded $3 billion (51). Erythropoietic agents remain widely used. However recent data demonstrate an increased risk of thromboembolism with aggressive use of these agents (52). There are provocative data concerning the expression and function of erythropoietin receptors in cancer cells, with unfavorable survival outcomes being noted in patients with breast and head and neck cancer possibly due to these agents affecting tumor growth *(52 –54)*. This area requires further investigation, and caution should be used when prescribing these agents. In the management of anemic patients, physicians should follow closely the dosing recommendations in product package inserts and/or the ASCO/American Society of Hematology guidelines *(55)*.

Infection

Both infection and malignancy are associated with tissue injury and the production of proinflammatory cytokines. It is therefore no surprise that infection is correlated with fatigue in cancer patients. It is common to treat acute or subacute infection that is readily discernible in patients presenting with CRF.

Metabolic Disorders

Patients with malignancy are susceptible to steroid-induced diabetes, as steroids may be part of the cancer-treatment regimen used to treat spinal cord compression, brain metastases or malignant bowel obstruction, or part of the antiemetic or pain treatment regimen. Hyperglycemia is a problem that can cause significant metabolic disarray as well as immune dysfunction, and it requires aggressive management *(56)*. Hypothyroidism and hypogonadism are also highly prevalent complications of cancer therapy. Hypothyroidism may be caused by malignancy involving the thyroid gland, or due to radiation therapy, biologic therapy such as interferon alfa, or by newer oral agents such as sunitinib *(57)*. Hypogonadism may be due to chemotherapy, surgery, radiation therapy, or hormonal therapy, as well as the effects of the underlying malignancy and associated proinflammatory cytokines *(58, 59)*. It is also associated with oral or intrathecal opioid analgesics *(60, 61)*. Each of these metabolic problems may present with significant fatigue and respond to appropriate treatment.

Specific Therapy for Fatigue

When there is no longer a discernible symptom masquerade, clinical trials of fatigue are good options for patients, for the care involved in the trial will be carefully implemented and monitored and health improvements often occur. The disappointing truth, however, is that most of these trials have been and will be negative trials; the remainder will be weakly positive or falsely positive. This is because the broad, basic principles related to fatigue management have a greater impact than amelioration by the specific interventions used in patient populations with substantial biologic and clinical heterogeneity *(62)*.

Exercise

It might seem counterintuitive to suggest an exercise program for cancer patients experiencing fatigue. Cancer patients have generally been advised to budget their level of activity carefully, and to rest when needed. Similar advice was previously given to patients who suffered from cardiac events, although cardiac rehabilitation is now firmly entrenched as an important aspect of cardiac care. Likewise, in cancer medicine, there is now a growing appreciation for the detrimental effects of a lack of physical activity and the functional consequences of deconditioning. Deconditioning causes patients to use greater effort than normal to perform daily activities, which may contribute to fatigue.

The best available evidence supporting aerobic or resistance exercise as an intervention for fatigue comes from studies of breast cancer patients and survivors. Meta-analyses of exercise interventions in breast cancer patients that reviewed 9–14 trials meeting specific methodologic criteria for inclusion confirm that exercise is an effective intervention to improve QOL, cardiorespiratory fitness, physical functioning, and fatigue (63). There are clinical data with similar findings in other cancer patients (particularly survivors), although those data are far less robust (64–69). Larger trials that have a greater focus on study quality and adverse effects and that examine the long-term benefits and risks of exercise are needed.

Mind–Body Interventions

Tai chi chuan and yoga have been used as mind–body practices in Asian cultures for centuries to improve wellness and reduce stress (70). These interventions are sometimes considered by researchers as a form of exercise intervention, and such interventions are being explored at major academic centers (71–74). Meditation and mindfulness relaxation techniques are other mind–body interventions that do not involve a physical activity component. These techniques are also the subject of increased interest by patients and researchers, with the preponderance of studies conducted in breast and prostate cancer patients, and with the intervention most commonly done in a clinic-based group setting. Consistent benefits including improved psychological functioning, reduction of stress symptoms, enhanced coping, and reduced fatigue in cancer outpatients have been seen (75). However, the evidence in favor of mind–body interventions remains somewhat limited. What is needed are more randomized, controlled designs; research in different cancer diagnoses and treatment settings (aside from breast and prostate cancer outpatient settings); more rigorous outcomes assessment and study methodology; and discernment of dose effects and optimal frequency.

Nutritional Interventions

It is clear to patients and clinicians that good nutrition is important for everyone, including cancer patients. Eating nutritiously can help people feel better, keep up strength and energy levels, decrease the risk of infection, and improve wound healing. Cancer patients may face impaired nutrition for a variety of reasons. Cachexia should be suspected in patients with cancer if an involuntary weight loss of greater than 5% of premorbid weight occurs within a six-month period of time. Cachexia arises from a complex interaction between the cancer and the host, a process that may include cytokine production, release of lipid-mobilizing and proteolysis-inducing factors, and other metabolic abnormalities (76). Cachexia is associated with fatigue and other major problems such as anorexia, fat and muscle tissue wasting, psychological distress, reduced quality of life, and disruption in function in general. Standard pharmacologic therapies for cachexia such as progestational agents, androgens, or corticosteroids are not recommended specifically to improve fatigue (77). Fatigue has innumerable associations with symptoms or syndromes that are treatable (anemia, psychological distress, sleep disturbance, cachexia, and others), and therapy directed at another entity sometimes improves fatigue expression in individual patients. However, treatment of a fatigue-associated symptom has not been shown to be generally efficacious for ameliorating CRF. Specifically, there is no evidence from well-controlled, randomized clinical trials that nutritional interventions such as parenteral or enteral supplementation, or nutritional counseling are effective for fatigue management. Recently, there has been interest in the micronutrient carnitine, which may play a role by reducing energy production through fatty acid oxidation. Administration of exogenous L-carnitine has been proven feasible (78), and it is now being compared to placebo for treatment of cancer-related fatigue in a multicenter trial.

Behavioral and Psychoeducational Interventions

Just as exercise is a broad-based intervention that can produce improvements in self-reported fatigue, psychoeducational interventions can also be beneficial. When a health professional is assigned to assist a patient on an individual basis across various domains of health (physical symptoms, psychological distress, social and family health) with the intent of improving the patient's level of energy, it is not surprising that improvements are more likely in such patients than in control groups that do not receive such an intervention. The improvements tend to be fairly minor (with unclear clinical significance) and short-term, and these types of interventions have been tested mostly in cohorts of women. Barsevick and colleagues compared a psychoeducational intervention related to energy conservation and activity management to a standard nutritional counseling strategy that involved the same length of time (telephone counseling with sessions 1 and 2 of 30 min and session 3 for 15 min) (79). The patients had solid tumors and were beginning chemotherapy or radiation, with 85% of the study population being female. The fatigue-specific intervention included homework assignments between sessions and daily journals to monitor various symptoms. Compared to controls, the intervention group had 10% more patients with stable or improved fatigue, and 15% fewer patients with worsening fatigue. Similarly, Yates and colleagues studied a comparable 3-session intervention in a cohort of women receiving adjuvant chemotherapy for breast cancer (80). In this case, the first session was face-to-face (rather than by telephone), and the control group received very general information about cancer rather than a fatigue-specific approach that included a personalized fatigue management plan. Once again, there were short-term decreases in self-reported fatigue intensity. Other investigators have demonstrated similar results in randomized controlled trials of nurse-driven interventions that are conceptually similar (81, 82).

Antidepressants

Fatigue is a cardinal symptom of depression, and both fatigue and depression are prevalent problems in cancer patients. Not surprisingly, the association between fatigue and depression in valid self-report measures of these symptoms is easy to demonstrate. For example, Tchekmedyian and colleagues showed correlations of changes in normal anxiety and depression subscale scores of the Brief Symptom Inventory with changes in Functional Assessment of Cancer Therapy (FACT). Fatigue scores had coefficients of −0.45 ($P < 0.001$) and −0.44 ($P < 0.001$), respectively (83). As mentioned earlier in the discussion about nutritional interventions, fatigue has innumerable associations with symptoms or syndromes that are treatable (such as depression), but therapy directed at another entity has not been shown to be generally efficacious for cancer-related fatigue. Another example of this general statement was shown by Morrow and colleagues in a large randomized controlled trial conducted through the Community Clinical Oncology Program (CCOP) of the National Cancer Institute, which compared the serotonin-reuptake inhibitor paroxetine at 20 mg/day to placebo in cancer patients undergoing chemotherapy for the first time (29). The intervention was for 8 weeks, and assessments of fatigue and depression were performed during cycles 3 and 4 of chemotherapy. A total of 244 patients treated with paroxetine and 235 patients treated with placebo provided assessable data, and no difference was detected in fatigue between patient groups.

Psychostimulants

Various psychostimulants have been explored for the treatment of fatigue in chronic illness, including methylphenidate, modafinil, and pemoline. Methylphenidate is the most widely studied psychostimulant in the context of cancer fatigue. Methylphenidate hydrochloride is a piperidine derivative that acts in the striatum to increase extracellular dopamine neurotransmission by blocking dopamine uptake in the presynaptic cell membrane (84). This drug is currently indicated for the treatment of conditions such as attention deficit disorder and narcolepsy. The most commonly used form of this medication in cancer patients is the short-acting formulation that is a racemic mixture comprised of D- and L-isomers, the former of which is the most active compound. It is sometimes prescribed with the intent of relieving depressive symptoms (particularly in dying patients with short expected survivals) (85), to offset sedation induced by opioid analgesics (86, 87), and to ameliorate cognitive difficulties (88–91).

Several phase II trials showed promise for methylphenidate in doses of 5–20 mg/day for the treatment of cancer fatigue (92, 93). Bruera and colleagues followed up with a randomized controlled trial evaluating the short-term effects of methylphenidate compared to placebo (94). Of 112 patients randomly assigned, 52 patients in the methylphenidate and 53 in the placebo group were assessable for analysis. Fatigue intensity improved significantly on day 8 in both the methylphenidate and placebo groups, with no significant differences found.

Modafinil is another oral agent used as a psychostimulant in cancer patients. The mechanism of action of this drug is not well understood; it may affect wakefulness by interacting with dopamine and norepinephrine transporters in the striatum (95). It is considered a promising agent (96, 97), and it is now being evaluated in randomized trials.

FUTURE DIRECTIONS

As there is currently no evidence-based standard of care for the assessment and management of cancer fatigue, further research is clearly needed. Fortunately, both explanatory and practical clinical trials addressing this topic are abundant. As of the

Spring of 2006, 76 National Institutes of Health-sponsored studies examining CRF were actively recruiting subjects, and 15% of these studies were being conducted through the National Cancer Institute (NCI) Community Clinical Oncology Program (CCOP).

What can be done in future clinical trials to improve the chances of designing meaningful positive trials that significantly impact patient care? Ideally, there will be clinical trials of fatigue where the patient assessment strategy is emphasized and applied uniformly across treatments arms, the patients enrolled are reasonably homogeneous in relation to some biologic attribute(s) as well as clinical characteristics, the intervention has specific intended clinical and biologic effects, and those clinical and biologic effects are appropriately measured and incorporated into the outcomes evaluation. There may also be a need for clinical studies that explore different doses of promising interventions before larger studies are implemented (i.e., phase I trials in symptom management). In essence, the methods and paradigms of cancer treatment research need to be applied to symptom research. Promising leads are abundant, as an increasing number of plausible drug targets as well as nonpharmacologic interventions are being discovered that impact cytokine release or action, inflammation, energy metabolism, and neuroendocrine pathways.

REFERENCES

1. Fernandes R, Stone P, Andrews P, Morgan R, Sharma S. Comparison between fatigue, sleep disturbance, and circadian rhythm in cancer inpatients and healthy volunteers: evaluation of diagnostic criteria for cancer-related fatigue. J Pain Symptom Manage 2006;32(3):245–54.
2. Morrow GR, Shelke AR, Roscoe JA, Hickok JT, Mustian K. Management of cancer-related fatigue. Cancer Invest 2005;23(3):229–39.
3. Prue G, Rankin J, Allen J, Gracey J, Cramp F. Cancer-related fatigue: a critical appraisal. Eur J Cancer 2006;42(7):846–63.
4. Stone P, Hardy J, Broadley K, Tookman AJ, Kurowska A, A'Hern R. Fatigue in advanced cancer: a prospective controlled cross-sectional study. Br J Cancer 1999;79(9–10):1479–86.
5. Wagner LI, Cella D. Fatigue and cancer: causes, prevalence and treatment approaches. Br J Cancer 2004;91(5):822–8.
6. Bower JE, Ganz PA, Desmond KA, et al. Fatigue in long-term breast carcinoma survivors: a longitudinal investigation. Cancer 2006;106(4):751–8.
7. Curt GA, Breitbart W, Cella D, et al. Impact of cancer-related fatigue on the lives of patients: new findings from the Fatigue Coalition. Oncologist 2000;5(5):353–60.
8. Fossa SD, Dahl AA, Loge JH. Fatigue, anxiety, and depression in long-term survivors of testicular cancer. J Clin Oncol 2003;21(7):1249–54.
9. Hjermstad MJ, Fossa SD, Oldervoll L, Holte H, Jacobsen AB, Loge JH. Fatigue in long-term Hodgkin's Disease survivors: a follow-up study. J Clin Oncol 2005;23(27):6587–95.
10. Nieboer P, Buijs C, Rodenhuis S, et al. Fatigue and relating factors in high-risk breast cancer patients treated with adjuvant standard or high-dose chemotherapy: a longitudinal study. J Clin Oncol 2005;23(33):8296–304.
11. Reyes-Gibby CC, Aday LA, Anderson KO, Mendoza TR, Cleeland CS. Pain, depression, and fatigue in community-dwelling adults with and without a history of cancer. J Pain Symptom Manage 2006;32(2):118–28.
12. Prins JB, van der Meer JW, Bleijenberg G. Chronic fatigue syndrome. Lancet 2006;367(9507):346–55.
13. Bowen JL. Educational strategies to promote clinical diagnostic reasoning. N Engl J Med 2006;355(21):2217–25.
14. Cancer-Related Fatigue. National Comprehensive Cancer Network (NCCN), 2006. (Accessed November 27, 2006.
15. Andrykowski MA, Schmidt JE, Salsman JM, Beacham AO, Jacobsen PB. Use of a case definition approach to identify cancer-related fatigue in women undergoing adjuvant therapy for breast cancer. J Clin Oncol 2005;23(27):6613–22.

16. Fleishman SB. Treatment of symptom clusters: pain, depression, and fatigue. J Natl Cancer Inst Monogr 2004(32):119–23.

17. Hwang SS, Chang VT, Kasimis BS. A comparison of three fatigue measures in veterans with cancer. Cancer Invest 2003;21(3):363–73.

18. Van Belle S, Paridaens R, Evers G, et al. Comparison of proposed diagnostic criteria with FACT-F and VAS for cancer-related fatigue: proposal for use as a screening tool. Support Care Cancer 2005;13(4):246–54.

19. Hwang SS, Chang VT, Cogswell J, Kasimis BS. Clinical relevance of fatigue levels in cancer patients at a Veterans Administration Medical Center. Cancer 2002;94(9):2481–9.

20. Schwartz AL, Meek PM, Nail LM, et al. Measurement of fatigue. Determining minimally important clinical differences. J Clin Epidemiol 2002;55(3):239–44.

21. Lai JS, Cella D, Chang CH, Bode RK, Heinemann AW. Item banking to improve, shorten and computerize self-reported fatigue: an illustration of steps to create a core item bank from the FACIT-Fatigue Scale. Qual Life Res 2003;12(5):485–501.

22. Given CW, Given B, Azzouz F, Kozachik S, Stommel M. Predictors of pain and fatigue in the year following diagnosis among elderly cancer patients. J Pain Symptom Manage 2001;21(6):456–66.

23. Lawrence DP, Kupelnick B, Miller K, Devine D, Lau J. Evidence report on the occurrence, assessment, and treatment of fatigue in cancer patients. J Natl Cancer Inst Monogr 2004(32):40–50.

24. Bower JE. Prevalence and causes of fatigue after cancer treatment: the next generation of research. J Clin Oncol 2005;23(33):8280–2.

25. Hickok JT, Roscoe JA, Morrow GR, Mustian K, Okunieff P, Bole CW. Frequency, severity, clinical course, and correlates of fatigue in 372 patients during 5 weeks of radiotherapy for cancer. Cancer 2005;104(8):1772–8.

26. Jacobsen PB. Assessment of fatigue in cancer patients. J Natl Cancer Inst Monogr 2004(32):93–7.

27. Jacobsen PB, Garland LL, Booth-Jones M, et al. Relationship of hemoglobin levels to fatigue and cognitive functioning among cancer patients receiving chemotherapy. J Pain Symptom Manage 2004;28(1):7–18.

28. Rodgers GM, 3rd, Cella D, Chanan-Khan A, et al. Cancer- and treatment-related anemia. J Natl Compr Canc Netw 2005;3(6):772–89.

29. Morrow GR, Hickok JT, Roscoe JA, et al. Differential effects of paroxetine on fatigue and depression: a randomized, double-blind trial from the University of Rochester Cancer Center Community Clinical Oncology Program. J Clin Oncol 2003;21(24):4635–41.

30. Stone P, Richards M, Hardy J. Fatigue in patients with cancer. Eur J Cancer 1998;34(11):1670–6.

31. Cleeland CS, Bennett GJ, Dantzer R, et al. Are the symptoms of cancer and cancer treatment due to a shared biologic mechanism? A cytokine-immunologic model of cancer symptoms. Cancer 2003;97(11):2919–25.

32. Raison CL, Miller AH. Depression in cancer: new developments regarding diagnosis and treatment. Biol Psychiatry 2003;54(3):283–94.

33. Musselman DL, Lawson DH, Gumnick JF, et al. Paroxetine for the prevention of depression induced by high-dose interferon alfa. N Engl J Med 2001;344(13):961–6.

34. Capuron L, Gumnick JF, Musselman DL, et al. Neurobehavioral effects of interferon-alpha in cancer patients: phenomenology and paroxetine responsiveness of symptom dimensions. Neuropsychopharmacology 2002;26(5):643–52.

35. Bower JE, Ganz PA, Aziz N, Fahey JL. Fatigue and proinflammatory cytokine activity in breast cancer survivors. Psychosom Med 2002;64(4):604–11.

36. Brown DJ, McMillan DC, Milroy R. The correlation between fatigue, physical function, the systemic inflammatory response, and psychological distress in patients with advanced lung cancer. Cancer 2005;103(2):377–82.

37. Collado-Hidalgo A, Bower JE, Ganz PA, Cole SW, Irwin MR. Inflammatory biomarkers for persistent fatigue in breast cancer survivors. Clin Cancer Res 2006;12(9):2759–66.

38. Kurzrock R. The role of cytokines in cancer-related fatigue. Cancer 2001;92(6 Suppl):1684–8.

39. Meyers CA, Albitar M, Estey E. Cognitive impairment, fatigue, and cytokine levels in patients with acute myelogenous leukemia or myelodysplastic syndrome. Cancer 2005;104(4):788–93.

40. Dimeo F, Schmittel A, Fietz T, et al. Physical performance, depression, immune status and fatigue in patients with hematological malignancies after treatment. Ann Oncol 2004;15(8):1237–42.

41. Geinitz H, Zimmermann FB, Stoll P, et al. Fatigue, serum cytokine levels, and blood cell counts during radiotherapy of patients with breast cancer. Int J Radiat Oncol Biol Phys 2001;51(3):691–8.

42. Berger AM, Higginbotham P. Correlates of fatigue during and following adjuvant breast cancer chemotherapy: a pilot study. Oncol Nurs Forum 2000;27(9):1443–8.

43. Bower JE, Ganz PA, Desmond KA, Rowland JH, Meyerowitz BE, Belin TR. Fatigue in breast cancer survivors: occurrence, correlates, and impact on quality of life. J Clin Oncol 2000;18(4):743–53.

44. Stone P, Richards M, A'Hern R, Hardy J. A study to investigate the prevalence, severity and correlates of fatigue among patients with cancer in comparison with a control group of volunteers without cancer. Ann Oncol 2000;11(5):561–7.

45. Miaskowski C. Gender differences in pain, fatigue, and depression in patients with cancer. J Natl Cancer Inst Monogr 2004(32):139–43.

46. Jacobsen PB, Andrykowski MA, Thors CL. Relationship of catastrophizing to fatigue among women receiving treatment for breast cancer. J Consult Clin Psychol 2004;72(2):355–61.

47. Sugawara Y, Akechi T, Okuyama T, et al. Occurrence of fatigue and associated factors in disease-free breast cancer patients without depression. Support Care Cancer 2005;13(8):628–36.

48. Meeske KA, Siegel SE, Globe DR, Mack WJ, Bernstein L. Prevalence and correlates of fatigue in long-term survivors of childhood leukemia. J Clin Oncol 2005;23(24):5501–10.

49. Demetri GD, Kris M, Wade J, Degos L, Cella D. Quality-of-life benefit in chemotherapy patients treated with epoetin-alpha is independent of disease response or tumor type: results from a prospective community oncology study. J Clin Oncol 1998;16:3412–25.

50. Glaspy J, Bukowski R, Steinberg D, Taylor C, Tchekmedyian S, Vadhan-Raj S. Impact of therapy with epoetin alfa on clinical outcomes in patients with nonmyeloid malignancies during cancer chemotherapy in community oncology practice. Procrit Study Group. J Clin Oncol 1997;15(3):1218–34.

51. Brower V. Epoetin for cancer patients: a boon or a danger? J Natl Cancer Inst 2003;95(24):1820–1.

52. Leyland-Jones B. Breast cancer trial with erythropoietin terminated unexpectedly. Lancet Oncol 2003;4(8):459–60.

53. Henke M, Laszig R, Rube C, et al. Erythropoietin to treat head and neck cancer patients with anaemia undergoing radiotherapy: randomised, double-blind, placebo-controlled trial. Lancet 2003;362(9392):1255–60.

54. Henke M, Mattern D, Pepe M, et al. Do erythropoietin receptors on cancer cells explain unexpected clinical findings? J Clin Oncol 2006;24(29):4708–13.

55. Bohlius J, Weingart O, Trelle S, Engert A. Cancer-related anemia and recombinant human erythropoietin – an updated overview. Nat Clin Pract Oncol 2006;3(3):152–64.

56. Oyer DS, Shah A, Bettenhausen S. How to manage steroid diabetes in the patient with cancer. J Support Oncol 2006;4(9):479–83.

57. Desai J, Yassa L, Marqusee E, et al. Hypothyroidism after sunitinib treatment for patients with gastrointestinal stromal tumors. Ann Intern Med 2006;145(9):660–4.

58. Garcia JM, Li H, Mann D, et al. Hypogonadism in male patients with cancer. Cancer 2006;106(12):2583–91.

59. Strasser F, Palmer JL, Schover LR, et al. The impact of hypogonadism and autonomic dysfunction on fatigue, emotional function, and sexual desire in male patients with advanced cancer: a pilot study. Cancer 2006;107(12):2949–57.

60. Rajagopal A, Vassilopoulou-Sellin R, Palmer JL, Kaur G, Bruera E. Hypogonadism and sexual dysfunction in male cancer survivors receiving chronic opioid therapy. J Pain Symptom Manage 2003;26(5):1055–61.

61. Rajagopal A, Vassilopoulou-Sellin R, Palmer JL, Kaur G, Bruera E. Symptomatic hypogonadism in male survivors of cancer with chronic exposure to opioids. Cancer 2004;100(4):851–8.

62. Fisch MJ. Fatigue trials in ambulatory cancer patients: where do we begin and where could it possibly end? J Support Oncol 2006;4(10):519–20.

63. Markes M, Brockow T, Resch KL. Exercise for women receiving adjuvant therapy for breast cancer. Cochrane Database Syst Rev 2006(4):CD005001.

64. Ladha AB, Courneya KS, Bell GJ, Field CJ, Grundy P. Effects of acute exercise on neutrophils in pediatric acute lymphoblastic leukemia survivors: a pilot study. J Pediatr Hematol Oncol 2006;28(10):671–7.

65. Karvinen KH, Courneya KS, Campbell KL, et al. Exercise preferences of endometrial cancer survivors: a population-based study. Cancer Nurs 2006;29(4):259–65.

66. Courneya KS, Friedenreich CM, Quinney HA, et al. A longitudinal study of exercise barriers in colorectal cancer survivors participating in a randomized controlled trial. Ann Behav Med 2005;29(2):147–53.

67. Jones LW, Courneya KS, Vallance JK, et al. Association between exercise and quality of life in multiple myeloma cancer survivors. Support Care Cancer 2004;12(11):780–8.

68. Segal RJ, Reid RD, Courneya KS, et al. Resistance exercise in men receiving androgen deprivation therapy for prostate cancer. J Clin Oncol 2003;21(9):1653–9.

69. Courneya KS, Friedenreich CM, Quinney HA, Fields AL, Jones LW, Fairey AS. A randomized trial of exercise and quality of life in colorectal cancer survivors. Eur J Cancer Care (Engl) 2003;12(4):347–57.

70. Mansky P, Sannes T, Wallerstedt D, et al. Tai chi chuan: mind-body practice or exercise intervention? Studying the benefit for cancer survivors. Integr Cancer Ther 2006;5(3):192–201.

71. Culos-Reed SN, Carlson LE, Daroux LM, Hately-Aldous S. A pilot study of yoga for breast cancer survivors: physical and psychological benefits. Psychooncology 2006;15(10):891–7.

72. Carlson LE, Speca M, Patel KD, Goodey E. Mindfulness-based stress reduction in relation to quality of life, mood, symptoms of stress and levels of cortisol, dehydroepiandrosterone sulfate (DHEAS) and melatonin in breast and prostate cancer outpatients. Psychoneuroendocrinology 2004;29(4):448–74.

73. Cohen L, Warneke C, Fouladi RT, Rodriguez MA, Chaoul-Reich A. Psychological adjustment and sleep quality in a randomized trial of the effects of a Tibetan yoga intervention in patients with lymphoma. Cancer 2004;100(10):2253–60.

74. Mustian KM, Katula JA, Zhao H. A pilot study to assess the influence of Tai Chi Chuan on functional capacity among breast cancer survivors. J Support Oncol 2006;4(3):139–45.

75. Ott MJ, Norris RL, Bauer-Wu SM. Mindfulness meditation for oncology patients: a discussion and critical review. Integr Cancer Ther 2006;5(2):98–108.

76. Inui A. Cancer anorexia-cachexia syndrome: current issues in research and management. CA Cancer J Clin 2002;52(2):72–91.

77. Strang P. The effect of megestrol acetate on anorexia, weight loss and cachexia in cancer and AIDS patients (review). Anticancer Res 1997;17(1B):657–62.v

78. Cruciani RA, Dvorkin E, Homel P, et al. L-carnitine supplementation for the treatment of fatigue and depressed mood in cancer patients with carnitine deficiency: a preliminary analysis. Ann N Y Acad Sci 2004;1033:168–76.

79. Barsevick AM, Dudley W, Beck S, Sweeney C, Whitmer K, Nail L. A randomized clinical trial of energy conservation for patients with cancer-related fatigue. Cancer 2004;100(6):1302–10.

80. Yates P, Aranda S, Hargraves M, et al. Randomized controlled trial of an educational intervention for managing fatigue in women receiving adjuvant chemotherapy for early-stage breast cancer. J Clin Oncol 2005;23(25):6027–36.

81. Given B, Given CW, McCorkle R, et al. Pain and fatigue management: results of a nursing randomized clinical trial. Oncol Nurs Forum 2002;29(6):949–56.

82. Godino C, Jodar L, Duran A, Martinez I, Schiaffino A. Nursing education as an intervention to decrease fatigue perception in oncology patients. Eur J Oncol Nurs 2006;10(2):150–5.

83. Sood A, Barton DL, Loprinzi CL. Use of methylphenidate in patients with cancer. Am J Hosp Palliat Care 2006;23(1):35–40.

84. Sarhill N, Walsh D, Nelson KA, Homsi J, LeGrand S, Davis MP. Methylphenidate for fatigue in advanced cancer: a prospective open-label pilot study. Am J Hosp Palliat Care 2001;18(3):187–92.

85. Bruera E, Miller MJ, Macmillan K, Kuehn N. Neuropsychological effects of methylphenidate in patients receiving a continuous infusion of narcotics for cancer pain. Pain 1992;48(2):163–6.

86. Wilwerding MB, Loprinzi CL, Mailliard JA, et al. A randomized, crossover evaluation of methylphenidate in cancer patients receiving strong narcotics. Support Care Cancer 1995;3(2):135–8.

87. Fillion L, Gelinas C, Simard S, Savard J, Gagnon P. Validation evidence for the French Canadian adaptation of the Multidimensional Fatigue Inventory as a measure of cancer-related fatigue. Cancer Nurs 2003;26(2):143–54.

88. Meyers CA, Weitzner MA, Valentine AD, Levin VA. Methylphenidate therapy improves cognition, mood, and function of brain tumor patients. J Clin Oncol 1998;16(7):2522–7.

89. Mulhern RK, Khan RB, Kaplan S, et al. Short-term efficacy of methylphenidate: a randomized, double-blind, placebo-controlled trial among survivors of childhood cancer. J Clin Oncol 2004;22(23):4795–803.

90. Thompson SJ, Leigh L, Christensen R, et al. Immediate neurocognitive effects of methylphenidate on learning-impaired survivors of childhood cancer. J Clin Oncol 2001;19(6):1802–8.

91. Bruera E, Driver L, Barnes EA, et al. Patient-controlled methylphenidate for the management of fatigue in patients with advanced cancer: a preliminary report. J Clin Oncol 2003;21(23):4439–43.

92. Hanna A, Sledge G, Mayer ML, et al. A phase II study of methylphenidate for the treatment of fatigue. Support Care Cancer 2006;14(3):210–5.

93. Bruera E, Valero V, Driver L, et al. Patient-controlled methylphenidate for cancer fatigue: a double-blind, randomized, placebo-controlled trial. J Clin Oncol 2006;24(13):2073–8.

94. Madras BK, Xie Z, Lin Z, et al. Modafinil occupies dopamine and norepinephrine transporters in vivo and modulates the transporters and trace amine activity in vitro. J Pharmacol Exp Ther 2006;319(2):561–9.

95. Morrow GR, Andrews PL, Hickok JT, Roscoe JA, Matteson S. Fatigue associated with cancer and its treatment. Support Care Cancer 2002;10(5):389–98.

96. Raison CL, Demetrashvili M, Capuron L, Miller AH. Neuropsychiatric adverse effects of interferon-alpha: recognition and management. CNS Drugs 2005;19(2):105–23.

97. Jean-Pierre P, Mustian K, Kohli S, Roscoe JA, Hickok JT, Morrow GR. Community-based clinical oncology research trials for cancer-related fatigue. J Support Oncol 2006;4(10):511–6.

6

Pathogenesis and Management of Venous Thromboembolism in Cancer Patients

Michael B. Streiff

CONTENTS

ABSTRACT

One hundred and forty one years have passed since Armand Trousseau's initial observation that venous thromboembolism (VTE) is a common manifestation of an underlying malignancy (1). Despite widespread recognition of this association and the availability of a multiple options for prevention and treatment of venous thrombosis, VTE remains a common cause of morbidity and mortality in cancer patients. The purpose of this chapter will be to review: (1) The epidemiology of VTE in cancer patients, (2) The pathogenesis of cancer-related thrombosis, (3) The prevention and treatment of VTE in the cancer patient, and (4) Special topics in VTE management including management of recurrent VTE and heparin-induced thrombocytopenia.

From: *Cancer and Drug Discovery Development: Supportive Care in Cancer Therapy*
DOI: 10.1007/978-1-59745-291-5_6, Edited by: D. S. Ettinger © Humana Press, Totowa, NJ

Key Words: Venous thromboembolism, Deep venous thrombosis, Pulmonary embolism, Prophylaxis, Treatment.

EPIDEMIOLOGY OF VENOUS THROMBOEMBOLISM
IN CANCER PATIENTS

Cancer is associated with a fourfold to sevenfold increase in the risk of VTE *(2, 3)*. An analysis of a prospective database of VTE among residents of Olmsted County, Minnesota, found that the annual incidence of a first episode of VTE among residents with active cancer was 0.5%, about fourfold higher than among residents without cancer. Residents receiving chemotherapy were at even higher risk of VTE, approximately sixfold higher than the general population *(2)*. A large population-based case control study conducted in anticoagulation clinics in the Netherlands had similar findings, noting a sevenfold increased risk of venous thrombosis among patients with cancer *(3)*. Over the course of cancer, it has been estimated that approximately 15% of cancer patients (range 3.8–30.7%) suffer an episode of VTE *(4)*.

It is important to note that the burden of VTE in cancer patients is not uniformly distributed. It varies depending upon primary tumor location, cell type, and the extent of disease. In a retrospective analysis of Medicare discharge data, Levitan et al. noted that VTE was more common in patients with ovarian, brain, and pancreatic tumors and less common among patients with head and neck, bladder, and breast tumors. Although a thrombophilic propensity is widely recognized in association with solid tumors, hematopoietic malignancies such as lymphoma and leukemia were also noted to be at significantly increased risk of VTE *(5)*. (Fig. 6.1) These trends have been confirmed in several subsequent studies *(6–9)*.

When considering the risk of VTE associated with a primary tumor site, it is also important to incorporate the prevalence of individual malignancies. While brain, ovarian, and pancreatic malignancies are associated with the highest risk of VTE, the high prevalence of lung, colon, and prostate cancers means that clinicians are more likely to

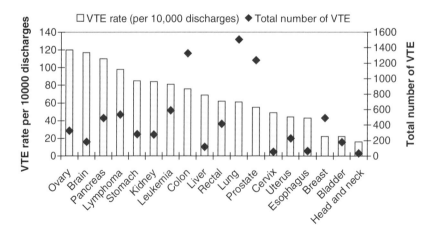

Fig. 6.1. Annual incidence and number of VTE in different malignancies (Adapted from Levitas N et al. and Luenberger ML and Wittkawsky AK Oncology 2005 19;853–61.

see patients with thromboembolism in association with these malignancies (Fig. 1). Among patients with the same primary tumor site, histology also has been shown to influence the risk of VTE. Patients with lung adenocarcinoma are at twofold to three-fold higher risk of VTE than patients with squamous cell carcinoma of the lung *(10, 11)*. Not surprisingly, disease extent also profoundly influences the thrombotic risk associated with malignancies. Patients with metastatic disease are at twice the risk of VTE as patients with localized or regional disease *(6, 9)*.

While clearly it is important to recognize that cancer places patients at high risk for VTE, it is also important to recognize that VTE is also a marker of an occult malignancy. Baron et al. found that incidence of cancer diagnosed at the time of a thromboembolic event and for a year afterward was fourfold higher than patients without thromboembolism. The risk of subsequent cancer among patients with thromboembolism remained 30% higher than patients without thromboembolism throughout the period from 2 to 25 years after diagnosis *(12)*. Sorensen et al. also found the risk of cancer was approximately threefold higher for patients with VTE during the first 6 months of follow-up. The risk of cancer is twice as high for patients with idiopathic versus triggered episodes of VTE *(13)*. Unfortunately, aggressive cancer screening among patients with idiopathic VTE has not been demonstrated to improve cancer mortality *(14)*, a reflection of the reality that cancers discovered during or soon after an episode of VTE are often advanced and associated with a poor prognosis *(15)*. Consequently, the possibility of an underlying malignancy should always be considered among patients presenting an idiopathic VTE but in the absence of obvious signs of an underlying malignancy, cancer screening should be limited to age-appropriate screening procedures.

PATHOGENESIS OF VTE IN CANCER PATIENTS

A multiplicity of factors contributes to the hypercoagulable state associated with cancer. The relevant factors can be categorized as being either endogenous tumor-specific or host-specific factors or exogenous environmental influences. As noted previously, tumor type, histology, and disease extent influence the risk of thrombosis. These factors clearly influence the impact of the tumor on the host's coagulation system. Numerous tumors including pancreatic adenocarcinoma and malignant glioma have been demonstrated to express tissue factor, the critical cofactor that activates factor VII triggering the activation of both factor X and factor IX and subsequent thrombin formation that results in fibrin clot formation *(16)*. Immunohistochemical studies support a link between increasing tissue factor expression and the risk of VTE in glioma patients *(17, 18)*. Similar studies have confirmed the presence of fibrin deposition on pancreatic cancer cells, demonstrating that tumor-expressed tissue factor is functional and associated with activation of the coagulation cascade *(19)*.

Cancer procoagulant is a 68-kDa cysteine protease that can activate factor X and has been identified in a wide variety of malignant cells *(20)*. Synthesis of a factor V receptor that facilitates assembly of the prothrombinase complex and a protein with fibrin crosslinking activity similar to factor XIII has been identified in tumor extracts *(21)*. Fibrinolytic proteins are also synthesized by cancer cells. Promyelocytic leukemia cells can express urokinase plasminogen activator receptor on their surface which binds and stimulates activation of urokinase and tissue plasminogen activator contributing to the fibrinolytic state manifested in some patients with acute promyelocytic leukemia *(22)*. Inhibitors of plasminogen activators, plasminogen activator inhibitor 1 and 2, are expressed by solid tumor cells and may contribute to a hypofibrinolytic and procoagulant state in affected patients *(23)*.

Tumor cells also impact the host's coagulation mechanism indirectly by production of proinflammatory cytokines such as interleukin-1 (IL-1), tumor necrosis factor alpha (TNF-α), and vascular endothelial growth factor (VEGF), all of which can induce tissue factor (by host monocytes and endothelial cells) and PAI-1 expression (by endothelial cells) and downregulate thrombomodulin expression (by endothelial cells). Thrombomodulin is an endogenous anticoagulant protein that binds and neutralizes thrombin's procoagulant activity and simultaneously facilitates thrombin's anticoagulant function in the activation of protein C. Consequently, downregulation of thrombomodulin could contribute to the prothrombotic state associated with cancer. In addition to its activation of endothelial and monocytic tissue factor production, VEGF also promotes tumor-associated activation of the coagulation cascade by inducing angiogenesis and increasing local vascular permeability facilitating the exposure of tissue factor to plasma coagulation factors. Inflammatory cytokines such as IL-1 and TNF-α also induce acute phase reactant proteins such as factor VIII and fibrinogen that tilt the balance of the hemostatic mechanism toward thrombosis. These biochemical mechanisms of thrombogenesis are supplemented by the local effect of tumor or nodal masses that compress vascular structures creating stagnant blood flow that favors local clot formation *(24, 25)*.

Host-specific factors influence the likelihood of VTE. In a retrospective cohort study of 125 patients with malignant gliomas, ABO blood group status and age were found to be significantly associated with VTE *(26)*. Previous studies have identified ABO blood group and age as risk factors for venous thromboembolism in the general population *(2, 27, 28)*. Since ABO blood group has a potent influence on von Willebrand factor and factor VIII levels and higher levels of factor VIII have been associated with an increased risk of initial and recurrent VTE in the general population *(29–32)*, it is plausible that the effect of ABO blood group on VTE rates may be mediated through its effect on factor VIII levels. Similarly, increasing age is associated with increasing coagulation factor levels that tip the hemostatic balance toward thrombosis.

The presence of thrombophilic mutations also modifies the risk of cancer patients developing VTE. Although conflicting results were noted in previously published smaller prospective cohort studies *(33, 34)*, the MEGA case control study of 3,220 participants identified a fourfold higher risk of VTE among carriers of the factor V Leiden and prothrombin gene mutation than cancer patients without these mutations *(3)*. Therefore, it is likely that the presence of underlying thrombophilia contributes to the overall risk of thromboembolism in cancer patients. Interestingly, the presence of factor V Leiden and the prothrombin mutation were not noted to be risk factors for VTE in participants in recent tamoxifen breast cancer prevention studies *(35)*. Increases in factor VIII, von Willebrand factor, fibrinogen, plasminogen activator inhibitor 1 and markers of coagulation activation such as prothrombin fragment 1.2, and D dimers are more common among patients with advanced cancer than those with localized disease *(36)*. Nevertheless, markers of activated coagulation have not proven useful in identifying cancer patients at higher risk of VTE who might benefit from primary anticoagulant prophylaxis *(4)*.

Environmental VTE risk factors likely play an important role in the development of venous thrombosis in cancer patients. Major surgery in a cancer patient is associated with a twofold greater risk of VTE than among patients without cancer (37). Although data are limited, radiation therapy alone has not been associated with an increased risk of venous thrombosis among early-stage ovarian cancer patients (38), while adjuvant radiation therapy combined with surgery or chemotherapy has been associated with an increased incidence of VTE (39, 40). In contrast, analysis of a large observational database was unable to identify radiotherapy as a risk factor for VTE (6).

Chemotherapy and hormonal therapy have been long associated with an increased risk of VTE. Increases in fibrinopeptide A, D dimer and thrombin–antithrombin complexes have been noted in association with chemotherapy administration (41, 42). Analysis of the Awareness of Neutropenia in Cancer (ANC) Registry noted an incidence of VTE of 0.8% per month among 3,003 cancer patients receiving chemotherapy (43). The best evidence for a prothrombotic effect of chemotherapy comes from analyses of prospective randomized trials of different chemotherapy and hormonal therapy regimens for breast cancer. Levine et al. noted that 6.8 percent of patients with stage II breast cancer receiving one of two chemotherapy regimens suffered a thrombotic event; all occurred during therapy (44). Goodnough noted a 17.6% incidence of thrombosis during CMFVP chemotherapy in 159 patients with breast cancer. Factor VIII activity was significantly increased in a subset of 10 patients during chemotherapy administration (45). In an analysis of 2,673 patients enrolled in ECOG studies of adjuvant therapy for breast cancer, Saphner et al. noted that the incidence of venous thromboembolism was lowest among postmenopausal patients assigned to observation (0.4%), intermediate among tamoxifen recipients (2.3%), and highest among those who received chemotherapy plus tamoxifen (8%). Premenopausal patients who received chemotherapy alone had fewer thrombotic events (0.8%) than those who received both chemotherapy and tamoxifen (2.8%). Postmenopausal patients were at higher risk for VTE than premenopausal patients (46). Pritchard et al. also found that combination chemo-hormonal therapy was associated with a greater risk of VTE than tamoxifen therapy alone in a RCT of adjuvant therapy for postmenopausal breast cancer patients (47). While the risk of VTE is less in patients receiving aromatase inhibitors compared with tamoxifen, anastrozole has been associated with a 1–2% incidence of VTE (48).

Exposure to cisplatin-based regimens has been associated with VTE in patients with germ cell tumors, lung, cervical, and ovarian cancer (49–51). L-asparaginase is associated with a 1–2% incidence of VTE in pediatric patients and a 4–14% incidence in adults with acute lymphoblastic leukemia (52, 53). The thrombotic potential of L-asparaginase has been ascribed to acquired protein C, protein S, and antithrombin deficiency as well as increases in factor VIII, IX, and XI levels (54, 55). 5-fluorouracil is commonly used in the adjuvant treatment of colorectal cancer where its use has been associated with an incidence of VTE of 15–17% (56). Potential mechanism to explain its thrombogenicity include the association of 5-fluorouracil with endothelial damage and reduced protein C levels (57).

Newer chemotherapy agents have also been associated with a significant risk of VTE. The immunomodulatory and antiangiogenic agent, thalidomide, has been used widely for the treatment of multiple myeloma, renal cell carcinoma, myelodysplastic syndromes, and idiopathic myelofibrosis. VTE rates as high as 20–40% have been noted among myeloma patients receiving thalidomide and dexamethasone- or doxorubicin-containing chemotherapy regimens *(58–60)*. Acquired resistance to activated protein C has been noted by some investigators as a potential mechanism for the prothrombotic potential of thalidomide *(61)*. Increases in von Willebrand factor antigen and platelet aggregation have also been noted *(62, 63)*. Prophylactic LMWH, warfarin, and aspirin have been shown to reduce the incidence of VTE in patients receiving thalidomide *(62, 64, 65)*. Preliminary reports suggest that lenalinomide, an analog of thalidomide, may also be thrombogenic when combined with high-dose dexamethasone *(66)*. Thus far, the humanized monoclonal antibody against VEGF, bevacizumab, has been associated with an increase in thrombotic complications in patients with metastatic colorectal cancer receiving chemotherapy but not among patients with advanced gastric cancer *(67, 68)*. Another angiogenesis inhibitor, SU5416, when combined with gemcitabine and cisplatin resulted in a thrombosis rate of 42% in a phase 1 study of patients with advanced malignancies *(69)*. Additional data are required to determine the impact of angiogenesis inhibitors on the frequency of thrombosis among cancer patients. Corticosteroids may also increase the risk of thrombosis in cancer patients. In one study of patients with germ cell tumors, patients receiving dexamethasone at doses exceeding 80mg per cycle were threefold to fivefold more likely to suffer an episode of VTE *(49)*. These findings are plausible given the positive influence of corticosteroids on factor VII, VIII, XI, and fibrinogen levels *(70)*.

Supportive care also plays a role in the development of thrombotic complications among cancer patients. Central venous catheters (CVC) have been instrumental in the supportive care of cancer patients since their introduction in the 1970s. Soon after the widespread use of CVC, it became evident that deep venous thrombosis (DVT) was a common complication of their use. Thirty-six prospective (31 adults, 5 children) and fifteen retrospective (14 adults, 1 child) studies have been conducted assessing the incidence of catheter-related deep venous thrombosis in cancer patients. The incidence of symptomatic CVC DVT varies from 0.3 to 28.3% among adult patients and 0 to 12% among children. Studies incorporating routine venography have identified CVC DVT in 27–66% of patients. Risk factors for CVC DVT include catheter diameter and lumen number (larger catheters and greater numbers of lumens are associated with a greater risk of DVT), side of insertion (left side higher risk than right side), catheter tip position (position at the right atrial superior vena caval junction associated with lower risk than more peripheral or central positions), history of a previous CVC, catheter-related infections, higher platelet counts, and presence of inherited thrombophilic mutations *(71)*.

Peripherally inserted central catheters (PICC) lines are associated with symptomatic CVC DVT in 1–4% of patients while as many as 23% have venographic evidence of venous thrombosis. Larger diameter PICC lines are associated with a higher risk of VTE (0% DVT for 3 French [F], 1% for 4 F, 6.6% for 5 F, and 9.8% for 6 F) *(71)*. Consequently, selection of the smallest CVC or PICC line necessary for the indication as well as careful attention to placement location are important to minimize catheter-related thrombotic complications. The utility of primary anticoagulant prophylaxis in the prevention and treatment of CVC and PICC-related DVT will be discussed below.

Use of hematopoietic growth factors has become an important supportive care tool in the treatment of patients with cancer. Their use has greatly reduced transfusion requirements for patients receiving chemotherapy and reduced the number of episodes of neutropenic infections. However, hematopoietic growth factors such as GCSF, GMCSG, and in particular, ecythcopoiesis-stimulatory agents (ESA) have also been recognized to increase the incidence of thrombotic complications. Use of erythropoietin during chemotherapy for cervical and vulvo-vaginal cancer and thalidomide for myelodysplastic syndrome was associated with a significant increase in thrombotic complications *(72, 73)*. Conversely, other studies have not found an increased incidence of thrombotic complication among patients receiving erythropoietin during thalidomide therapy for multiple myeloma or chemotherapy in patients with lung cancer *(74, 75)*. Erythropoietin use has also been associated with an increased risk of VTE in patients undergoing orthopedic surgery in some but not all studies *(76)*. Since erythropoietin has been associated with an increase of inflammatory markers and inhibitors of the fibrinolysis, accentuation of thrombosis during therapy is conceivable *(77)*. A recent metanalysis indicates that ESA increase the risk of VTE by 1.6 fold *(77a)* one small study suggested that low-dose warfarin (1–2mg daily) was ineffective in prevention of thrombosis in cervical and vulvo-vaginal cancer patients receiving chemoradiation therapy and erythropoietin *(78)*.

PREVENTION OF THROMBOEMBOLISM IN CANCER PATIENTS

Cancer patients are at fourfold higher risk of developing venous thrombosis than patients without cancer. The risk increases to sixfold higher in cancer patients receiving chemotherapy *(2)*. Compared with patients without cancer, cancer patients undergoing major surgery are at twofold increased risk of venous thrombosis *(37)*. Cancer patients who suffer an episode of thromboembolism are twice as likely to die *(8)*. Consequently, use of adequate prophylaxis for patients with cancer is essential to prevent unnecessary adverse outcomes.

Despite widespread recognition of the high thrombotic risk associated with cancer, VTE prophylaxis remains underutilized. Recent surveys of general medical and surgical inpatients have noted DVT prophylaxis in only 30–40% of patients *(79–81)*. The Frontline survey of almost 3,800 respondents conducted in 2003 found that only 52% of surgical oncologists and 5% of medical oncologists routinely used DVT prophylaxis in their patients *(82)*. These findings may partially explain the increasing incidence of VTE noted among cancer patients between 1979 and 1999 *(83)*.

All cancer patients should be prescribed risk-adjusted VTE prophylaxis at hospital admission. Compared with patients undergoing surgery for benign disease, patients with malignancies have twice the risk of VTE and a threefold higher risk of fatal pulmonary embolism *(84)*. Risk factors for venous thromboembolism and contraindications to pharmacologic and mechanical prophylaxis are listed in Tables 1 and 2. Pharmacologic and mechanical prophylaxis options are shown in Table 3. Several randomized controlled trials (RCT) have demonstrated the efficacy of unfractionated heparin, low molecular weight heparin, and fondaparinux in the prevention of VTE following major surgery in patients with cancer *(85–88)*.

It is important to note that in many of these trials, the first dose of anticoagulant prophylaxis was given before surgery and that prophylaxis was continued up to 10 days postoperatively. The Enoxacan study population was entirely composed of cancer surgery patients while in the Pegasus trial and the Canadian Colorectal Surgery Trial only

Table 1
Risk factors for venous thromboembolism in cancer patients

Risk Factor
Age
Type of cancer (Pancreas, brain, ovary > head and neck, breast, prostate)
Extent of cancer (metastatic > regional > localized)
Major surgery
Previous history of VTE
Thrombophilic disorder (e.g., Factor V Leiden, etc.)
Chemotherapy
Hormonal therapy
Immobility or limb paralysis
Acute medical illness (infection, cardiopulmonary failure, etc.)
Vascular compression (e.g., nodal/tumor masses, etc.)
Central venous catheters (Hickman catheter, PICC line, etc.)
Hematopoietic growth factors
Obesity

PICC peripherally inserted central venous catheter

Table 2
Contraindications to venous thromboembolism prophylaxis

Contraindications to pharmacologic prophylaxis
Active bleeding
High risk of bleeding
Recent (within 1 month) clinically significant bleeding
Thrombocytopenia (platelet count <50,000/μL)
Systemic coagulopathy (INR>1.4 or aPTT ratio> 1.2, excluding lupus inhibitors)
Known coagulation disorder (e.g., hemophilia A or B, von Willebrand disease)
Known platelet function disorder (e.g., Bernard-Soulier syndrome, uremic platelet dysfunction, etc.)
Heparin-induced thrombocytopenia (contraindication to use of unfractionated or low molecular weight heparin)

Contraindications to mechanical prophylaxis
Acute deep venous thrombosis (within 3 months)
Arterial insufficiency at placement location
Open extremity wound

INR international normalized ratio, *aPTT* activated partial thromboplastin time

approximately 60% and 30%, respectively, of patients had a malignancy. A metanalysis of DVT prophylaxis trials has indicated that any one of these pharmacological methods of VTE prophylaxis is effective *(85)*. Therefore, selection of prophylaxis agents should be based upon efficacy, cost, availability, the presence of comorbid diseases, ease of administration, and FDA approval status.

Table 3
Venous thromboembolism prophylaxis options for cancer patients

Pharmacologic prophylaxis options	Mechanical prophylaxis options
Unfractionated heparin 5,000 units SC q8–12 h	Sequential compression devices or intermittent pneumatic compression devices
Low molecular weight heparin	Graduated compression stockings
Dalteparin 5,000 units SC q24 h	
Enoxaparin 40 mg SC q24 h	
Tinzaparin 4,500 units (or 75 units /kg) SC q24 h	
Pentasaccharides	
Fondaparinux 2.5 mg SC q24 h	

SC subcutaneous, *h* hours, *mg* milligrams, *kg* kilograms

Similar to patients undergoing hip and knee arthroplasty, cancer surgery patients are at increased risk for VTE for more than a month after surgery. In a prospective observational study of 2,373 cancer surgery patients, Agnelli et al. noted that 40% of VTE occurred more than 21 days after surgery. In-hospital prophylaxis was given to 82% of patients and 31% received prophylaxis after hospital discharge. Risk factors for VTE included a previous history of VTE (Odds Ratio (OR) 6.0 [95% Confidence Interval (CI), 2.1–16.8]), anesthesia time ≥ 2 h (OR 4.5 [95% CI, 1.1–19.0]), bed rest ≥ 4 days (OR 4.4 [95% CI, 2.5–7.8]), advanced-stage disease (OR 2.7 [95% CI, 1.4–5.2]), and patient age ≥ 60 years (OR 2.6 [95% CI, 1.2–5.7]) *(89)*. These data have prompted several studies of extended VTE prophylaxis after major surgery *(90, 91)*. Enoxacan II demonstrated a 60% reduction in objectively documented VTE (12% to 4.8%) by extending prophylaxis with enoxaparin 40 mg SC once daily from 6–10 days to 28 days *(90)*. Similar efficacy (55% relative risk reduction of VTE) has been demonstrated for extended duration dalteparin VTE prophylaxis in patients after major abdominal surgery *(91)*. Therefore, extended VTE prophylaxis should be strongly considered for cancer surgery patients, particularly in patients with risk factors for VTE.

In patients with contraindications to pharmacologic VTE prophylaxis, mechanical prophylaxis should be employed until the contraindication is no longer present. Sequential compression devices and intermittent pneumatic compression devices appear to be more effective modes of mechanical prophylaxis in general surgery patients than elastic stockings; therefore these modalities should be used preferentially *(92, 93)*. For optimal results, mechanical prophylaxis should be used continuously. Several studies have demonstrated that mechanical prophylaxis is applied continuously in less than 50% of patients in routine practice, explaining inferior results compared with those obtained in randomized clinical trials *(94, 95)*. This observation, the smaller study populations (and thus less precise estimates of efficacy), and the unmasked design of mechanical prophylaxis studies support preferential use of pharmacologic prophylaxis when possible. When mechanical prophylaxis modalities must be employed, it is important for institutions to have established guidelines regarding their use to ensure optimal results. Combined mechanical and pharmacologic prophylaxis has been demonstrated to be superior to pharmacologic or mechanical prophylaxis alone in several different patient populations *(96, 97)*. Therefore, combined modality prophylaxis is a reasonable option in high-risk surgical patients, particularly in surgical patient populations for whom clinical trial data exists supporting the efficacy of combined prophylaxis.

Medical oncology patients are at high risk of venous thromboembolism and the risk increases as the number of VTE risk factors increases *(98)*. Although no randomized controlled trials of VTE prophylaxis have been conducted in medical oncology patient populations, some information on the effectiveness of VTE prevention strategies can be inferred from studies conducted in medical inpatients that have included a small proportion of cancer patients (between 5 and 15%) *(99–104)*. All medical oncology patients who are not ambulatory should receive pharmacologic VTE prophylaxis regimens appropriate for high-risk medical patients (Table 3). If contraindications exist to pharmacologic VTE prophylaxis, mechanical prophylaxis should be employed until the contraindication is no longer present. When employing VTE prophylaxis in medical oncology patients, it is important to note several limitations of the current literature. Oncology patients make up a small proportion of the study populations in the currently published RCTs of VTE prophylaxis in medical inpatients. Therefore, the benefits of prophylaxis identified in these studies may not be accurate estimates of benefit in oncology patients. This limitation should be kept firmly in mind when designing institutional prophylaxis guidelines for medical oncology patients. Similar concerns apply to mechanical prophylaxis, which has been studied in only a small population of medical patients without malignancies *(92)*. Nevertheless, until medical oncology-specific data are available, VTE prophylaxis strategies used in medical inpatients should be applied to medical oncology patients as well.

Although a substantial number of medical oncology patients may be at a long-term risk for VTE as outpatients, particularly patients with pancreatic adenocarcinoma and malignant gliomas *(105, 26)*, limited information exists to support extended duration VTE prophylaxis. In a placebo-controlled RCT in patients with stage IV breast cancer undergoing chemotherapy, Levine et al. demonstrated that low-dose warfarin (1 mg daily adjusted to an INR 1.3–1.9) was associated with 85% reduction in the incidence of VTE ($p = 0.03$) without an increase in bleeding *(44)*. Despite these results, primary prophylaxis in cancer patients is not practiced because of concerns for bleeding complications, the applicability of these data to other patient populations, and questions regarding the appropriate duration of prophylaxis for patients.

PREVENTION OF CENTRAL VENOUS CATHETER THROMBOSIS

Central venous catheters are a common cause of DVT in cancer patients. Prospective studies employing routine radiologic surveillance have identified catheter-associated venous thrombosis in 28–66% of adult cancer patients. Symptomatic thrombosis has been noted in 0.3–26% of patients *(71)*. In addition to the morbidity associated with anticoagulation and additional invasive procedures to establish vascular access at other sites, catheter-associated DVT is associated with a significant risk of pulmonary embolism (15–25%) *(106)*. Consequently, anticoagulant prophylaxis with warfarin and low molecular weight heparin has been studied in a number of clinical trials *(107–110)*.

Bern et al. conducted an open randomized clinical trial of low-dose warfarin (1 mg daily starting 3 days before catheter insertion and adjusted to keep the pro-thrombin time below 15 s) in oncology patients receiving a central venous catheter. All patients underwent venography at the onset of thrombotic symptoms or at 90 days post insertion. Warfarin-treated patients had significantly fewer thrombotic events (4/42, 9.5%) than control patients (15/40, 37.5%; $p < 0.001$) *(107)*. Using dalteparin 2,500 units daily and routine venography, Monreal et al. demonstrated significantly fewer catheter-associated thrombi in the active treatment group (1/16, 6%) than in controls (8/13, 62%; $p = 0.03$) *(108)*. However, several more recent large open-label as well as randomized placebo-controlled double-blind studies of low molecular weight heparin and low-dose warfarin have failed to demonstrate significant efficacy of active prophy-laxis for CVC-associated DVT *(109–110)*. While subpopulations of cancer patients at especially high risk for CVC-associated DVT may exist, in which pharmacologic prophylaxis is warranted, routine use of catheter prophylaxis should not be employed until these data are available.

DIAGNOSIS OF VENOUS THROMBOEMBOLISM IN CANCER PATIENTS

Cancer patients are at high risk for thromboembolic events; therefore, physicians should always consider the possibility of thromboembolism when evaluating cancer patients. Assessing the pre-test probability of thrombotic disease prior to diagnostic imaging studies is important to determine subsequent management when study results are available. Clinical prediction models such as the Wells criteria for DVT and PE have proven useful in identifying patients at higher risk for thrombotic disease, although their utility in this task has not been demonstrated in all management settings *(111, 112)*. Diagnostic algorithms based upon these clinical prediction models have been proposed *(111)*. Initiation of anticoagulation should be considered in patients judged to be at high risk of VTE. Signs or symptoms that may suggest the presence of an underlying throm-bosis include unexplained swelling or pain in a lower or upper extremity, the neck or supraclavicular space, catheter dysfunction, or new onset fatigue. Duplex ultrasound remains the primary imaging modality for detection of venous clots although CT venog-raphy and magnetic resonance venography are very useful for identification of thrombi particularly in less accessible sites (pelvis, iliac and inferior and superior vena cava, abdominal and intracranial vasculature). Development of increasingly sensitive and rapid multidetector spiral CT scanners has made CT the imaging modality of choice for identification of pulmonary emboli. Ventilation perfusion scanning and/or lower/upper extremity duplex examination, or rarely, pulmonary angiography may provide supple-mental diagnostic information in selected cases. Although D dimer testing has been shown to play a useful role in VTE diagnosis in patients without malignancies, D dimer levels are often elevated in cancer patients and, therefore, it is considerably less useful in the cancer patient with suspected VTE *(113)*. Sohne et al. used the Wells Clinical prediction rule in conjunction with D dimer testing to exclude PE in a series of 3,306 outpatients including 474 cancer patients. Spiral CT scans were obtained in patients with likely PE by the Wells' clinical prediction rule or an abnormal D dimer result. Although only 2% of cancer patients considered not to have a PE developed a VTE during the three-month follow-up period, the confidence intervals for this estimate were wide (0.05–10.9%) *(114)*. Therefore, use of D dimer testing and clinical prediction rules to exclude VTE in cancer patients should await further investigation.

TREATMENT OF VENOUS THROMBOEMBOLISM IN CANCER PATIENTS: INITIAL THERAPY

In most cancer patients, initial therapy for venous thromboembolism should consist of anticoagulation with weight-based doses of unfractionated heparin (UFH) (adjusted to achieve a therapeutic activated partial thromboplastin time), low molecular weight heparin, or fondaparinux (Table 4). Choice of initial therapy should be based upon efficacy, cost, ease of administration, need for monitoring, need for hospitalization, presence of comorbid conditions (e.g., renal insufficiency), reversibility, and FDA approval status. In patients with a high likelihood of DVT/PE, initiation of therapy should be considered before objective radiologic confirmation. When using UFH, it is important to use a weight-based dosage nomogram to ensure rapid achievement of therapeutic levels. Since the therapeutic range for unfractionated heparin depends upon the particular aPTT reagent and coagulometer used to perform the test, use of arbitrary fixed therapeutic ranges (e.g., aPTT 60–80 s or aPTT ratio 1.5–2.5) should be avoided. Instead, each laboratory should establish the therapeutic range for their reagent-coagulometer combination using amidolytic assays of factor Xa activity in the presence of known concentrations of heparin. The therapeutic range of heparin as measured by the aPTT should correspond to anti-Xa heparin levels of 0.3–0.7 units/mL *(115)*.

Table 4
Venous thromboembolism treatment regimens for cancer patients

Acute VTE treatment options
    Unfractionated heparin – 80 unit/kg IV bolus followed by 18 units/kg/h infusion adjusted
        to aPTT results
    Low molecular weight heparin
        Dalteparin 200 units/kg SC q24 h
        Enoxaparin 1 mg/kg SC q12 h
        Tinzaparin 175 units/kg SC q24 h
    Pentasaccharide
        Fondaparinux 5–10 mg SC q24 h (5 mg for weight < 50 kg, 7.5 mg for weight 50–100
        kg and 10 mg for weight > 100 kg)
    Vena caval filter
Chronic VTE treatment options
    Low molecular weight heparin
        Dalteparin 200 units/kg SC q24 h for month 1 then 150 units/kg SC q24 h
        Enoxaparin 1–1.5 mg/kg SC q24 h
        Tinzaparin 175 units/kg SC q24 h
    Vitamin K antagonist adjusted to an INR of 2–3
    Vena caval filter

VTE venous thromboembolism, *kg* kilograms, *h* hour, *SC* subcutaneous, *INR* international normalized ratio

Advantages of UFH include its short half-life and complete reversibility with protamine and reticuloendothelial system-based clearance. Therefore, UFH is probably the agent of choice for hospitalized patients at high risk for bleeding, those with abnormal renal function (creatinine clearance < 30 mL/min), or those with planned invasive procedures. The acquisition cost of UFH is also lower than LMWH or fondaparinux, although some economic analyses have noted that LMWH may be more cost effective if all the costs associated with UFH therapy are taken into account *(116)*. The disadvantages of UFH are the requirement for close laboratory monitoring (at least daily), ready intravenous access for administration and laboratory monitoring, and a higher incidence of heparin-induced thrombocytopenia (HIT) (approximately 1% in medical patients, up to 5% in surgical patients) *(117)*. For a more complete discussion of HIT, see section on HIT below. Although a recent RCT demonstrated the feasibility of using subcutaneous UFH to treat outpatients with VTE, this study enrolled a limited number of cancer patients (~16%); therefore, routine use of UFH in this fashion should await further investigation *(118)*.

Weight-adjusted doses of low molecular weight heparin (LMWH) or fondaparinux are convenient attractive options for treatment of venous thromboembolism in cancer patients. Unlike UFH, LMWH and fondaparinux do not require routine laboratory monitoring and therefore they are attractive agents for the outpatient management of VTE in cancer patients. LMWH and fondaparinux are also much less likely to induce HIT. The incidence of HIT with LMWH appears to be about 0.3% while HIT is very rare with fondaparinux *(119, 120a)*. Disadvantages of LMWH and fondaparinux include their renal clearance, longer half-life, and lower reversibility. LMWH typically have a half-life between 3–5 h, which increases significantly with renal dysfunction (creatinine clearance < 30 ml/min). FDA-approved dosage guidelines have been developed for enoxaparin in renal insufficiency (1 mg/kg SC q24 h) but caution should be exercised in patients with severe renal dysfunction (creatinine clearance < 20 ml/min) and patients anticipated to be on LMWH for a prolonged period of time. Measurement of LMWH levels should be considered in patients in these situations. Although a once-daily dosage enoxaparin regimen (1.5 mg/kg SC q24 h) has been tested for acute therapy of VTE in patients with normal renal function, it is important to note that this regimen was less effective in cancer patients and, therefore, standard twice-daily dosing (1 mg/kg SC q12 h) should be used initially *(121)*. Fondaparinux, which has a half-life of 17–21 h, should not be used in patients with creatinine clearances less than 30 ml/min. While protamine can be used to partially reverse LMWH (60–80%), it is ineffective in reversal of fondaparinux *(122)*. Recombinant human factor VIIa has been shown to reverse the anticoagulant effects of fondaparinux *(123)*.

Several studies have documented the feasibility of outpatient management of VTE in cancer patients *(124, 125, 126)*. When considering outpatient management, it is important to select patients appropriately to limited adverse events. Contraindications to outpatient management are listed in Table 5. Although patients with stable pulmonary embolism have been managed as outpatients in several clinical studies *(125–127)*, since this patient population has a mean 3-month mortality rate of 15% *(128)*, it is important to risk-stratify patients to avoid adverse outcomes in this potentially high-risk patient

Table 5
Contraindications to outpatient treatment of venous thromboembolism

Contraindications
Active bleeding or high risk of bleeding
Recent surgery (within 7 days)
Cardiopulmonary instability
Severe symptomatic venous obstruction
High-risk pulmonary embolism[a]*
Thrombocytopenia (platelets < 50,000/μL)
Medical/surgical condition requiring inpatient management
Medical noncompliance
Geographical or telephone inaccessibility
Poor hepatic function (INR ≥ 1.5)
Unstable renal function (e.g., rising serum creatinine)
Poor home health care support environment

List may not be all inclusive
INR international normalized ratio
[a]See Table 6 for Geneva risk score

Table 6
Geneva PE risk stratification score

Risk factors
Active cancer (2 points on Geneva risk scale)
Systolic blood pressure < 100 mmHg (2 points on Geneva risk scale)
Concomitant DVT at diagnosis (1 point on Geneva risk scale)
History of VTE (1 point on Geneva risk scale)
Heart failure (1 point on Geneva risk scale)
Hypoxia (arterial PaO2 < 60 mmHg)

Geneva risk score – low risk = 2 or fewer points, high risk = 3 or more points

group. Wicki et al. used the Geneva PE risk score (see Table 6) to risk-stratify patients with pulmonary embolism. When used prospectively, the Geneva risk score subdivided the entire population of PE patients into a low-risk group that had a subsequent adverse outcome rate of 2% compared with the high-risk group that had an adverse outcome rate of 26% *(129)*. Findings consistent with right ventricular overload on echocardiography or spiral CT have also been used to identify higher risk populations of PE patients who have a twofold to fourfold higher risk of adverse outcomes *(130, 131)*. Low-risk PE patients, particularly those with asymptomatic PE, potentially could be managed as outpatients after a short initial inpatient stay while higher risk patients' initial treatment should be managed predominantly as inpatients. The development of increasingly sensitive multislice CT scanners has led to the discovery of more patients with "asymptomatic" pulmonary embolism. A recent study, however, indicates that many of these "asymptomatic" patients on close examination are not asymptomatic, reinforcing the notion that all patients with PE regardless of the circumstances of detection warrant therapy *(132)*.

Thrombolytic therapy should be strongly considered for initial therapy of any cancer patient presenting with massive pulmonary embolism associated with cardiopulmonary instability. Thrombolytic therapy results in more rapid clot lysis than anticoagulation alone which can be life-saving in patients with high clot burdens. This benefit must be weighed against the twofold to threefold higher bleeding risk associated with thrombolytic therapy compared with anticoagulation alone *(115)*. Since patients with submassive pulmonary embolism have worse outcomes than patients with less severe hemodynamic compromise, some have advocated for application of thrombolytic therapy in this patient population. A recent RCT of patients with submassive PE demonstrated that patients receiving tissue plasminogen activator (tPA) were significantly less likely to require escalation of therapy (e.g., thrombolysis, mechanical ventilation, catecholamine infusion, etc.) than patients receiving anticoagulation alone. Unfortunately, no mortality benefit was realized as a result of thrombolytic therapy; therefore, the application of thrombolytic therapy to this population remains controversial and should be made on a case-by-case basis *(133)*. Although streptokinase and urokinase are effective thrombolytic agents for the treatment of PE, tPA has emerged as the agent of choice given its comparable effectiveness and convenient 2-h dosage regimen (tPA 10-mg intravenous bolus followed by 90-mg intravenous infusion over 2 h).

Thrombolytic therapy is also a useful alternative for patients with massive lower extremity DVT particular patients at risk for limb compromise. Compared with anticoagulation alone, thrombolytic therapy results in greater complete and partial clot lysis rates (complete lysis 45%, partial lysis 18%) than anticoagulation alone (complete lysis 4%, partial lysis 14%) *(134)*. In recent years, systemic thrombolysis has been replaced with catheter-directed thrombolysis, which allows more efficient delivery of thrombolytic agents to the surface of the clot. A national registry of catheter-directed thrombolysis has demonstrated the value of this approach (complete lysis 31%, partial lysis 52%). Nevertheless, CDT is still associated with a significant risk of major bleeding (11%) which exceeds that associated with standard anticoagulation *(135)*. While combination of CDT with catheter-based mechanical thrombectomy devices offers the potential to improve results by decreasing lytic treatment time and total dose, this hypothesis has yet to be demonstrated in randomized trials *(136)*. Consequently, catheter-directed thrombolysis should be reserved for cancer patients with massive DVT where restoration of venous blood flow is essential to outcome.

Vena caval filter placement should be considered in any cancer patient with acute venous thromboembolism who cannot be treated with anticoagulation. In selected circumstances, IVC filters may be worthwhile intervention in patients who have suffered recurrent thromboembolism despite anticoagulation. In these instances, it is important to rule out the possibility of Trousseau's syndrome, heparin-induced thrombocytopenia, and anatomic abnormalities such as the May-Thurner syndrome or vascular compression by tumor or nodal masses as the patient with these conditions will not be benefited by placement of an IVC filter that may exacerbate rather than ameliorate the underlying thrombotic disorder. Although strong supportive evidence of benefit is lacking, vena caval filters are also considered commonly in patients with poor cardiopulmonary reserve and in patients undergoing pulmonary artery thromboembolectomy. In patients with potentially transient contraindications to anticoagulation, retrievable vena caval filters should be strongly considered as they appear to function as well as permanent filters (137). Since filters are associated with an increased risk of IVC and lower extremity venous thrombosis, filter recipients should be treated with anticoagulation whenever possible (138).

Similar to other forms of VTE in the cancer patient, initial therapy for catheter-associated DVT relies upon anticoagulation, with initial anticoagulation options including unfractionated heparin, low molecular weight heparin, and fondaparinux. Although not infrequently recommended in routine practice, catheter removal is not necessary in most instances of catheter thrombosis and it may be associated with worse outcomes particularly when done in the absence of anticoagulation. In most cases, thrombotic symptoms resolve with anticoagulation alone. In the event of persistent symptoms, thrombolytic therapy may be considered. Thrombolytic therapy is also a useful option in the event of massive CVC-associated thrombosis when limb viability or future function is in question. Since thrombolytic therapy has been associated with a higher incidence of major bleeding, its risks and benefits should be carefully weighed before employing it. Small doses of thrombolytic agents are the therapy of choice for patients with dysfunctional catheters due to intraluminal clots or fibrin sheaths. TPA (2 mg IV), urokinase (5,000 units IV), and reteplase (0.4 units/ml IV) have all been used to treat occluded catheters. Although no randomized trials are available to guide therapy, the duration of anticoagulation for catheter thrombosis should be at least 3 months or for the lifespan of the catheter, whichever is longer (71, 139).

TREATMENT OF VENOUS THROMBOEMBOLISM IN CANCER PATIENTS: CHRONIC THERAPY

Options for chronic therapy for VTE in cancer patients include vitamin K antagonists (VKA) such as warfarin and low molecular weight heparin. Traditionally, VKA are used for chronic therapy of VTE. Vitamin K antagonists can be initiated as soon as therapeutic acute therapy with UFH, LMWH, or fondaparinux is achieved. Loading doses of warfarin should be avoided as they do not result in more rapid achievement of therapeutic anticoagulation and increase the chances of supratherapeutic INR values. Instead, clinicians should select a dose of warfarin that they think will be the patient's maintenance dose (usually 5–7.5 mg daily). Low initial doses of warfarin (e.g., 2.5 mg daily) should be employed in elderly patients, postoperative patients, or patients with liver disease or taking medications that interact with warfarin (Table 7). Prothrombin times should be obtained daily in hospitalized patients and at least three times a week in outpatients transitioning to warfarin therapy. Acute therapy with heparin or LMWH should continue for at least 5–7 days and until a prothrombin time International Normalized Ratio (INR) greater than or equal to 2 is achieved. Failure to adhere to these standards can precipitate early recurrent VTE (140, 141).

Vitamin K antagonists have several advantages including oral administration, complete reversibility with vitamin K and fresh frozen plasma and a long half-life that means a missed dose will not result in sudden declines in drug concentrations and

Table 7
Medications that can influence vitamin K antagonists

Increase in the INR	Decrease in the INR
Alcohol	Azathioprine (Imuran)
Amiodarone	Barbiturates
Anabolic steroids	Carbamazepine (Tegretol)
Broad-spectrum antibiotics	Chlordiazepoxide
Capecitabine	Cholestyramine
Cimetidine	Griseofulvin
Erlotinib	Methimazole
Erythromycin	Mitotane
Fluorouracil	Nafcillin
Fluconazole and other azole antifungals	Phenytoin
Flutamide	Rifampin
Gefitinib	Rifabutin
Gemcitabine	Spironolactone
Ifosfamide	Sucralfate
Imatinib	Vitamin K and vitamin K-rich foods
Isoniazid	
Metronidazole (Flagyl)	
Omeprazole	
Piroxicam (Feldene)	
Propafenone	
Propranolol	
Quinidine	
Sulfinpyrazone	
Trastuzumib	
Trimethoprim/sulfamethoxazole (Bactrim/Septra)	

anticoagulant activity that might precipitate recurrent episodes of thromboembolism. These favorable characteristics of warfarin are balanced and perhaps overshadowed by a number of disadvantages including its narrow therapeutic window, substantial interindividual differences in dose response, and a significant potential for dietary and drug–drug interactions. Consequently, close monitoring of warfarin therapy is essential to prevent recurrent thromboembolism or bleeding. In addition, the long half-life of warfarin can also complicate management in the setting of thrombocytopenia or around invasive procedures (140, 141).

Despite these shortcomings, with optimal management, warfarin therapy has been associated with excellent results with an incidence of recurrent thromboembolism and major bleeding less than 1 per 100 patient years (142). However, the results of VKA therapy have been less favorable in cancer patients. Palareti et al. noted a twofold to sevenfold higher incidence of recurrent VTE and a sixfold higher incidence of major bleeding in cancer patients compared to patients without malignancies (143). Prandoni et al. and Hutten et al. have noted similar results (144, 145). Cancer patients experienced more episodes of bleeding and thrombosis regardless of INR level or quality of antico-agulation control *(143–145)*. Therefore, optimization of anticoagulation management is unlikely to result in improved outcomes.

These limitations have increased interest in using LMWH for chronic therapy of VTE in cancer patients. Low molecular weight heparin has several advantages over vitamin K antagonists. LMWH do not bind in appreciable quantities to cell membranes or plasma proteins endowing them with predictable pharmacokinetics allowing weight-based dosing without the need for laboratory monitoring. LMWH are not affected by changes in diet or medications and have short half-lives. The latter characteristic is particularly attractive in cancer patients who often experience thrombocytopenia and the need for invasive procedures that require transient interruptions in therapy.

LMWH and warfarin have been compared for chronic therapy of VTE in cancer patients in several randomized trials *(146–149)*. The CATHANOX trial randomized 146 patients to three months of warfarin adjusted to an INR of 2–3 or enoxaparin 1.5 mg/kg daily. Fifteen warfarin patients (21.2%) and seven enoxaparin patients (10.5%) experienced an episode of VTE or major bleeding ($p = 0.09$). Seventeen warfarin patients (22.7%) and eight enoxaparin patients (11.3%) died during the three-month study ($p = 0.07$). Fatal hemorrhages occurred in six warfarin patients and no patients in the enoxaparin group *(146)*.

The ONCENOX study enrolled 102 cancer patients into a three-arm trial comparing warfarin (INR 2–3) with enoxaparin 1.5 mg/kg daily or enoxaparin 1 mg/kg daily for 180 days. Only 3.3% of enoxaparin patients suffered a recurrent VTE compared with 6.7% of warfarin patients. Similar to the CATHANOX study, these results were not statistically significant due to the limited study enrollment *(147)*.

Tinzaparin was investigated as an alternative to warfarin for the secondary prevention of VTE in the LITE study. This RCT compared three months of tinzaparin monotherapy with UFH followed by warfarin (INR 2–3) in 737 patients with proximal DVT. Two-hundred six participants (28%) had cancer. Recurrent VTE occurred in six tinzaparin recipients (5.9%) and eleven warfarin patients (10.5%) (95% CI of difference −12% to 2.9%, $p = $ NS) *(148)*.

The strongest evidence supporting LMWH for chronic therapy of VTE in cancer patients comes from the results of the CLOT trial. Lee et al. randomized 676 cancer patients with VTE to six months of dalteparin or VKA adjusted to achieve an INR of 2–3. Of 1,303 cancer patients presenting with VTE to study centers, 676 were enrolled in the study. Ninety percent of participants had solid tumors and sixty-seven percent had metastatic disease. Dalteparin patients received 200 IU/kg once daily for the first month followed by 150 IU/kg for months two through six. VKA patients received acute therapy with once daily dalteparin 200 IU/kg for at least 5–7 days until their INR reached 2 or more on two consecutive days after which they were treated with INR-adjusted VKA therapy. Recurrent VTE occurred in 27 dalteparin patients (9%) and 53 VKA patients (17%) for a VTE hazard ratio of 0.48 (95% CI 0.30–0.77, $p = 0.002$). Twenty of 53 recurrent VTE (38%) in the warfarin group occurred when the INR was less than two. Major bleeding (dalteparin 6% vs. VKA 4%, $p = 0.27$) and six-month mortality (dalteparin 39% vs. VKA 41%, $p = 0.57$) were similar *(149)*.

In response to these data, the American College of Chest Physicians consensus conference as well as the National Comprehensive Cancer Center Network guidelines have recommended use of a LMWH for chronic therapy of VTE in cancer patients for the first 3–6 months of therapy. Although it is possible that all LMWH will prove to have similar efficacy, the strongest evidence supports dalteparin for chronic therapy of VTE in cancer patients and so it should be used preferentially for this purpose. Aside from the results of RCT, providers should also take cost into consideration when deciding upon chronic therapy for VTE. Some insurers will not cover the costs of chronic LMWH therapy for VTE. A recent decision analysis found that while LMWH resulted in an average increased quality-adjusted life expectancy surplus of 19 days it achieved this result at an additional cost of $7,609 per patient treated *(150)*. Therefore, physicians and cancer patients must carefully weigh the greater efficacy and cost of LMWH when making decisions on secondary prevention of VTE. Patient preferences, current drug therapy, and co-morbidities and drug acquisition cost must all be considered. One strategy to maximize the benefits of LMWH would be to focus its use in patients at the highest risk for VKA-associated complications (e.g., patients with advanced disease, poor hepatic function, etc.). Another strategy would be to utilize LMWH preferentially in the first 3 months of therapy when the risk of recurrent VTE is highest.

Cancer and its treatment are associated with a significant and persistent risk of recurrent VTE. Therefore, although studies of chronic therapy of VTE in cancer patients have focused on the first three to six months of therapy, cancer patients should be treated for as long as their disease is active or for a period appropriate for the patient's specific thrombotic event, whichever duration is longer *(115)*. An important chronic complication of DVT is post-thrombotic syndrome. Post-thrombotic syndrome is characterized by the development of persistent brawny edema, pain, varicose veins and in severely affected patients, skin ulcerations. Post-thrombotic syndrome is caused by chronic venous hypertension due to venous obstruction and valvular dysfunction that result from an episode of deep venous thrombosis *(151)*. Prospective studies indicate that 25% of patients will develop signs and symptoms of PTS within 2 years of their thrombotic event *(152)*. Routine use of graduated compression stockings (30–40 mmHg) has been shown to reduce the incidence of PTS by 50% *(153, 154)*. Therefore, all cancer patients suffering an episode of DVT should be prescribed compression stockings to prevent this avoidable complication of VTE.

MANAGEMENT OF CANCER PATIENTS WITH RECURRENT VTE

Cancer patients have a high incidence of recurrent VTE. Management of patients with recurrent VTE should be guided by the patient's particular clinical situation. Diagnostic possibilities that must be considered in any cancer patient with recurrent thromboembolism include subtherapeutic anticoagulation, heparin-induced thrombocytopenia, Trousseau's syndrome, and anatomic abnormalities impeding venous flow. Subtherapeutic anticoagulation is common among cancer patients on VKA. In RCTs of chronic therapy of VTE, cancer patients were in the therapeutic range less than 50% of the time *(146, 149)*, significantly lower than noted in studies of chronic therapy conducted in patients without cancer *(142)*. Contributing factors include chemotherapy-induced thrombocytopenia and nausea that result in held or reduced doses and frequent invasive procedures that require discontinuation of therapy. Options for treatment following a course of acute therapy with UFH or LMWH include targeting a higher INR goal (e.g., 2.5–3.5) or using a LMWH for chronic therapy. Although higher INR targets are often used for patients with recurrent VTE, there are no data to support the efficacy of this practice and higher INR goals in at least one RCT were not associated with fewer thrombotic events (155). Alternatively, chronic LMWH therapy could be considered, particularly if VKA control has been suboptimal. One study noted a low recurrence rate in cancer patients with recurrent VTE treated with LMWH (156).

In cancer patients who return to the hospital with a recurrent VTE soon after discharge, it is important to rule out the possibility of heparin-induced thrombocytopenia (HIT). Heparin-induced thrombocytopenia results from the development of antibodies directed against a neoepitope formed by complexes of heparin and platelet factor 4, a constituent of platelet alpha granules. These antibodies activate platelets causing a consumptive form of thrombocytopenia that is associated with a profound hypercoagulable state. Monocytes and endothelial cells are also activated by these antibodies inducing the expression of tissue factor on their surface, which further contributes to activation of the coagulation cascade. Although most patients with HIT develop thrombocytopenia within 5–10 days of heparin therapy, delayed presentations of HIT occurring as late as several weeks after heparin exposure have been published. Therefore, any patient who presents with a new thrombotic event in association with thrombocytopenia (or a 50% reduction in platelet count from baseline) should be evaluated for HIT with objective laboratory testing (HIT PF4 antibody ELISA assay and/or the ^{14}C-labeled serotonin release assay). All patients with a suspected HIT should be treated with a direct thrombin inhibitor (either argatroban or lepirudin adjusted to an aPTT ratio of 1.5–2.5 or 1.5–2.0, respectively) until the results of laboratory testing are available. All heparin (and LMWH) exposure (bonded catheters etc.) should be eliminated. Platelet transfusions should be avoided unless major bleeding develops as platelets may precipitate progressive thrombosis. Since as many as 50% of HIT patients may have asymptomatic VTE, screening duplex ultrasound of the extremities should be performed. In patients with HIT, DTI treatment should continue until the platelet count has normalized and the patient has achieved an INR of 2–3 on VKA therapy. Warfarin should not be initiated until the platelet count has returned to the normal range as early and rapid transition of HIT patients to warfarin alone has been associated with development of venous gangrene. Warfarin should be continued for at least one month (for patients without thrombosis) or for as long as dictated by the underlying thrombotic episode (DVT, at least 3 months; PE, at least 6 months) (157).

Another important cause of recurrent thromboembolism in cancer patients is Trousseau's syndrome. Trousseau's syndrome, named after the renowned nineteenth century French physician who noted the association of cancer with VTE, is characterized by recurrent episodes of venous and/or arterial thromboembolism despite adequate anticoagulation with VKA, migratory superficial thrombophlebitis, nonbacterial thrombotic endocarditis, and often evidence of disseminated intravascular coagulation on laboratory testing (158). Control of the thrombotic process can only be achieved by therapeutic anticoagulation with unfractionated or low molecular weight heparin. LMWH is generally employed initially because it can be administered in weight-based doses without any requirement for laboratory monitoring. I would recommend using twice daily dosing for LMWH given the higher recurrence rate seen in one study in cancer patients receiving once daily enoxaparin dosing *(159)*. In the event of a recurrent episode of VTE despite LMWH therapy, it is important to objectively document recurrent thrombosis and establish whether noncompliance or inadequate dosing may have contributed to the event. Rarely, patients with Trousseau's syndrome will demonstrate resistance to LMWH. In this case, continuous infusion or subcutaneous UFH therapy has been effective in preventing further thrombotic events. Therapy for Trousseau's syndrome should be continued as long as active cancer is present. Since patients with Trousseau's syndrome generally have metastatic disease on presentation, life-long therapy is indicated as cessation of therapy will invariably be associated with recurrent thromboembolism.

Anatomic vascular compression is another important cause of recurrent thromboembolism that should be investigated in cancer patients with recurrent thrombotic events. While hypercoagulable alterations in the blood of cancer patients contribute significantly to their thrombotic phenotype, stasis and turbulent blood flow can also play an important role in the development of venous thrombosis. Tumor or lymph node masses can compress vessels and contribute to thrombosis. It is important to consider these anatomic risk factors for thrombosis as relief of vascular obstructions/stenosis is often more effective than more intensive anticoagulation.

IMPACT OF ANTICOAGULATION ON CANCER MORTALITY

Aside from reducing the morbidity and mortality due to VTE, anticoagulation may have a beneficial impact on the overall clinical course of cancer patients. Growing evidence suggests a link between the coagulation proteins and cancer biology *(25)*. The first clinical support for the potential role of anticoagulation in modifying cancer outcome comes from the landmark Veterans Administration Cooperative Study #75. This randomized clinical trial demonstrated a significant improvement in median survival among the subgroup of patients with small-cell lung cancer receiving chemotherapy and warfarin compared with patients receiving chemotherapy alone (50 weeks vs. 24 weeks, $p = 0.03$). No differences in mortality were noted in other subgroups of cancer patients *(160)*. However, subsequent randomized studies of the impact of warfarin therapy on outcomes in cancer patients have been mixed *(161–163)*.

Substantial experimental evidence has accumulated that heparins, in particular low molecular weight heparins, possess antineoplastic properties that include inhibition of angiogenesis, cancer and endothelial cell growth, oncogene expression, and metastasis *(164)*. Corroboration of the biological applicability of these findings is available in the results of clinical trials of heparins in the treatment of VTE. Metanalyses of randomized clinical trials of unfractionated and LMWH in the treatment of VTE have identified a survival advantage for patients treated with LMWH that is attributable to reduced mortality among cancer patients *(165)*. Several subsequent studies have tested the impact of low molecular weight heparin on the clinical course of cancer patients. The Fragmin Advanced Malignancy Outcome Study (FAMOUS study) randomized 385 patients with advanced solid tumors to once daily dalteparin (5,000 IU per day) or placebo for up to one year. While one-year survival was not different in the group as a whole (dalteparin 46% vs. placebo 41%, $p = 0.19$), median survival was significantly longer among dalteparin recipients (43.5 months vs. 24.3 months, $p = 0.03$) in a subgroup of patients, not defined a priori, with a better prognosis (survival beyond 17 months) *(166)*.

Two subsequent trials have identified similar results *(167–169)*. The MALT trial randomized 302 patients with advanced solid tumors to 6 weeks of nadroparin (2 weeks full dose, 4 weeks half dose) or placebo. The median survival was 8 months for the nadroparin group compared with 6.6 months for the placebo group (Hazard Ratio (HR) 0.75 [95% CI 0.59–0.96]). As with the FAMOUS study, the difference was even more pronounced in patients with a better prognosis (HR 0.64 [95% CI 0.45–0.90]) *(167)*. In a randomized study of combination chemotherapy with or without dalteparin in patients with small-cell lung cancer, Altinbas et al. noted improved response rates and overall survival in patients receiving LMWH *(169)*. In a secondary analysis of the CLOT trial, Lee et al. noted reduced mortality at 12 months among patients without metastatic disease receiving dalteparin compared with VKA ($p = 0.03$) *(168)*. Despite using different regimens in diverse patient populations, these studies all provide tantalizing evidence of a mortality benefit to the use of LMWH in cancer patients. While additional information is needed to identify the cancer patients most likely to benefit and the most effective regimens, these studies provide further evidence of potential added benefits of anticoagulation, in particular LMWH, in the management of cancer patients.

REFERENCES

1. Trousseau A. Phlegmasia alba dolens. In: Trouuseau A, editor. Clinique Medicale de l'Hotel-Dieu de Paris. Paris: Balliere, 1865: 654–712.
2. Heit JA, Silverstein MD, Mohr DN et al. Risk factors for deep vein thrombosis and pulmonary embolism: a population-based case-control study. *Arch Intern Med.* 2000;160(6):809–815.
3. Blom JW, Doggen CJ, Osanto S, Rosendaal FR. Malignancies, prothrombotic mutations, and the risk of venous thrombosis. *JAMA.* 2005;293(6):715–722.
4. Deitcher SR. Cancer and thrombosis: mechanisms and treatment. *J Thromb Thrombolysis.* 2003;16(1–2):21–31.
5. Levitan N, Dowlati A, Remick SC et al. Rates of initial and recurrent thromboembolic disease among patients with malignancy versus those without malignancy. Risk analysis using Medicare claims data. *Medicine (Baltimore).* 1999;78(5):285–291.
6. Blom JW, Vanderschoot JP, Oostindier MJ et al. Incidence of venous thrombosis in a large cohort of 66,329 cancer patients: results of a record linkage study. *J Thromb Haemost.* 2006;4(3):529–535.
7. Stein PD, Beemath A, Meyers FA et al. Incidence of venous thromboembolism in patients hospitalized with cancer. *Am J Med.* 2006;119(1):60–68.
8. Khorana AA, Francis CW, Culakova E et al. Thromboembolism in hospitalized neutropenic cancer patients. *J Clin Oncol.* 2006;24(3):484–490.
9. Chew HK, Wun T, Harvey D et al. Incidence of venous thromboembolism and its effect on survival among patients with common cancers. *Arch Intern Med.* 2006;166(4):458–464.
10. Ogren M, Bergqvist D, Wahlander K et al. Trousseau's syndrome - what is the evidence? A population-based autopsy study. *Thromb Haemost.* 2006;95(3):541–545.
11. Blom JW, Osanto S, Rosendaal FR. The risk of a venous thrombotic event in lung cancer patients: higher risk for adenocarcinoma than squamous cell carcinoma. *J Thromb Haemost.* 2004;2(10):1760–1765.
12. Baron JA, Gridley G, Weiderpass E et al. Venous thromboembolism and cancer. *Lancet.* 1998;351(9109):1077–1080.
13. Sorensen HT, Mellemkjaer L, Steffensen FH et al. The risk of a diagnosis of cancer after primary deep venous thrombosis or pulmonary embolism. *N Engl J Med.* 1998;338(17):1169–1173.
14. Piccioli A, Lensing AW, Prins MH et al. Extensive screening for occult malignant disease in idiopathic venous thromboembolism: a prospective randomized clinical trial. *J Thromb Haemost.* 2004;2(6):884–889.
15. Sorensen HT, Mellemkjaer L, Olsen JH, Baron JA. Prognosis of cancers associated with venous thromboembolism. *N Engl J Med.* 2000;343(25):1846–1850.

16. Semeraro N, Colucci M. Tissue factor in health and disease. *Thromb Haemost.* 1997;78(1):759–764.

17. Rong Y, Post DE, Pieper RO et al. PTEN and hypoxia regulate tissue factor expression and plasma coagulation by glioblastoma. *Cancer Res.* 2005;65(4):1406–1413.

18. Hamada K, Kuratsu J, Saitoh Y et al. Expression of tissue factor correlates with grade of malignancy in human glioma. *Cancer.* 1996;77(9):1877–1883.

19. Wojtukiewicz MZ, Rucinska M, Zacharski LR et al. Localization of blood coagulation factors in situ in pancreatic carcinoma. *Thromb Haemost.* 2001;86(6):1416–1420.

20. Gordon SG. Cancer cell procoagulants and their role in malignant disease. *Semin Thromb Hemost.* 1992;18(4):424–433.

21. Hettasch JM, Bandarenko N, Burchette JL et al. Tissue transglutaminase expression in human breast cancer. *Lab Invest.* 1996;75(5):637–645.

22. Barbui T, Finazzi G, Falanga A. The impact of all-trans-retinoic acid on the coagulopathy of acute promyelocytic leukemia. *Blood.* 1998;91(9):3093–3102.

23. Kwaan HC, Keer HN, Radosevich JA et al. Components of the plasminogen-plasmin system in human tumor cell lines. *Semin Thromb Hemost.* 1991;17(3):175–182.

24. Falanga A, Rickles FR. Pathophysiology of the thrombophilic state in the cancer patient. *Semin Thromb Hemost.* 1999;25(2):173–182.

25. Nash GF, Walsh DC, Kakkar AK. The role of the coagulation system in tumour angiogenesis. *Lancet Oncol.* 2001;2(10):608–613.

26. Streiff MB, Segal J, Grossman SA et al. ABO blood group is a potent risk factor for venous thromboembolism in patients with malignant gliomas. *Cancer.* 2004;100(8):1717–1723.

27. Jick H, Porter J. Thrombophlebitis of the lower extremities and ABO blood type. *Arch Intern Med.* 1978;138(10):1566–1567.

28. Talbot S, Wakley EJ, Ryrie D, Langman MJ. ABO blood groups and venous thromboembolic disease. *Lancet.* 1970;1(7659):1257–1259.

29. O'Donnell J, Laffan MA. The relationship between ABO histo-blood group, factor VIII and von Willebrand factor. *Transfus Med.* 2001;11(4):343–351.

30. O'Donnell J, Mumford AD, Manning RA, Laffan M. Elevation of FVIII: C in venous thromboembolism is persistent and independent of the acute phase response. *Thromb Haemost.* 2000;83(1):10–13.

31. Kraaijenhagen RA, in't Anker PS, Koopman MM et al. High plasma concentration of factor VIIIc is a major risk factor for venous thromboembolism. *Thromb Haemost.* 2000;83(1):5–9.

32. Kyrle PA, Minar E, Hirschl M et al. High plasma levels of factor VIII and the risk of recurrent venous thromboembolism. *N Engl J Med.* 2000;343(7):457–462.

33. Ramacciotti E, Wolosker N, Puech-Leao P et al. Prevalence of factor V Leiden, FII G20210A, FXIII Val34Leu and MTHFR C677T polymorphisms in cancer patients with and without venous thrombosis. *Thromb Res.* 2003;109(4):171–174.

34. Pihusch R, Danzl G, Scholz M et al. Impact of thrombophilic gene mutations on thrombosis risk in patients with gastrointestinal carcinoma. *Cancer.* 2002;94(12):3120–3126.

35. Abramson N, Costantino JP, Garber JE et al. Effect of factor V Leiden and prothrombin G20210 A mutations on thromboembolic risk in the national surgical adjuvant breast and bowel project breast cancer prevention trial. *J Natl Cancer Inst.* 2006;98(13):904–910.

36. Beer JH, Haeberli A, Vogt A et al. Coagulation markers predict survival in cancer patients. *Thromb Haemost.* 2002;88(5):745–749.

37. White RH, Zhou H, Romano PS. Incidence of symptomatic venous thromboembolism after different elective or urgent surgical procedures. *Thromb Haemost.* 2003;90(3):446–455.

38. Jhingran A, Eifel PJ. Perioperative and postoperative complications of intracavitary radiation for FIGO stage I-III carcinoma of the cervix. *Int J Radiat Oncol Biol Phys.* 2000;46(5):1177–1183.

39. Holm T, Singnomklao T, Rutqvist LE, Cedermark B. Adjuvant preoperative radiotherapy in patients with rectal carcinoma. Adverse effects during long-term follow-up of two randomized trials. *Cancer.* 1996;78(5):968–976.

40. Silvani A, Salmaggi A, Eoli M et al. Venous thromboembolism in malignant glioma patients treated by chemoradiotherapy. *Neurol Sci.* 2003;24(4):272.

41. Weitz IC, Israel VK, Waisman JR et al. Chemotherapy-induced activation of hemostasis: effect of a low molecular weight heparin (dalteparin sodium) on plasma markers of hemostatic activation. *Thromb Haemost.* 2002;88(2):213–220.

42. Edwards RL, Klaus M, Matthews E et al. Heparin abolishes the chemotherapy-induced increase in plasma fibrinopeptide A levels. *Am J Med.* 1990;89(1):25–28.

43. Khorana AA, Francis CW, Culakova E, Lyman GH. Risk factors for chemotherapy-associated venous thromboembolism in a prospective observational study. *Cancer.* 2005;104(12):2822–2829.

44. Levine MN, Gent M, Hirsh J et al. The thrombogenic effect of anticancer drug therapy in women with stage II breast cancer. *N Engl J Med.* 1988;318(7):404–407.

45. Goodnough LT, Saito H, Manni A et al. Increased incidence of thromboembolism in stage IV breast cancer patients treated with a five-drug chemotherapy regimen. A study of 159 patients. *Cancer.* 1984;54(7):1264–1268.

46. Saphner T, Tormey DC, Gray R. Venous and arterial thrombosis in patients who received adjuvant therapy for breast cancer. *J Clin Oncol.* 1991;9(2):286–294.

47. Pritchard KI, Paterson AH, Paul NA et al. Increased thromboembolic complications with concurrent tamoxifen and chemotherapy in a randomized trial of adjuvant therapy for women with breast cancer. National Cancer Institute of Canada Clinical Trials Group Breast Cancer Site Group. *J Clin Oncol.* 1996;14(10):2731–2737.

48. Bonneterre J, Buzdar A, Nabholtz JM et al. Anastrozole is superior to tamoxifen as first-line therapy in hormone receptor positive advanced breast carcinoma. *Cancer.* 2001;92(9):2247–2258.

49. Weijl NI, Rutten MF, Zwinderman AH et al. Thromboembolic events during chemotherapy for germ cell cancer: a cohort study and review of the literature. *J Clin Oncol.* 2000;18(10):2169–2178.

50. Numico G, Garrone O, Dongiovanni V et al. Prospective evaluation of major vascular events in patients with nonsmall cell lung carcinoma treated with cisplatin and gemcitabine. *Cancer.* 2005;103(5):994–999.

51. Jacobson GM, Kamath RS, Smith BJ, Goodheart MJ. Thromboembolic events in patients treated with definitive chemotherapy and radiation therapy for invasive cervical cancer. *Gynecol Oncol.* 2005;96(2):470–474.

52. Priest JR, Ramsay NK, Steinherz PG et al. A syndrome of thrombosis and hemorrhage complicating L-asparaginase therapy for childhood acute lymphoblastic leukemia. *J Pediatr.* 1982;100(6):984–989.

53. Alberts SR, Bretscher M, Wiltsie JC et al. Thrombosis related to the use of L-asparaginase in adults with acute lymphoblastic leukemia: a need to consider coagulation monitoring and clotting factor replacement. *Leuk Lymphoma.* 1999;32(5–6):489–496.

54. Priest JR, Ramsay NK, Bennett AJ et al. The effect of L-asparaginase on antithrombin, plasminogen, and plasma coagulation during therapy for acute lymphoblastic leukemia. *J Pediatr.* 1982;100(6):990–995.

55. Liebman HA, Wada JK, Patch MJ, McGehee W. Depression of functional and antigenic plasma antithrombin III (AT-III) due to therapy with L-asparaginase. *Cancer.* 1982;50(3):451–456.

56. Otten HM, Mathijssen J, ten Cate H et al. Symptomatic venous thromboembolism in cancer patients treated with chemotherapy: an underestimated phenomenon. *Arch Intern Med.* 2004;164(2):190–194.

57. Edwards RL, Klaus M, Matthews E et al. Heparin abolishes the chemotherapy-induced increase in plasma fibrinopeptide A levels. *Am J Med.* 1990;89(1):25–28.

58. Zangari M, Anaissie E, Barlogie B et al. Increased risk of deep-vein thrombosis in patients with multiple myeloma receiving thalidomide and chemotherapy. *Blood.* 2001;98(5):1614–1615.

59. Rajkumar SV, Hayman S, Gertz MA et al. Combination therapy with thalidomide plus dexamethasone for newly diagnosed myeloma. *J Clin Oncol.* 2002;20(21):4319–4323.

60. Zangari M, Siegel E, Barlogie B et al. Thrombogenic activity of doxorubicin in myeloma patients receiving thalidomide: implications for therapy. *Blood.* 2002;100(4):1168–1171.

61. Zangari M, Saghafifar F, Anaissie E et al. Activated protein C resistance in the absence of factor V Leiden mutation is a common finding in multiple myeloma and is associated with an increased risk of thrombotic complications. *Blood Coagul Fibrinolysis.* 2002;13(3):187–192.

62. Minnema MC, Fijnheer R, De Groot PG, Lokhorst HM. Extremely high levels of von Willebrand factor antigen and of procoagulant factor VIII found in multiple myeloma patients are associated with activity status but not with thalidomide treatment. *J Thromb Haemost.* 2003;1(3):445–449.

63. Baz R, Li L, Kottke-Marchant K et al. The role of aspirin in the prevention of thrombotic complications of thalidomide and anthracycline-based chemotherapy for multiple myeloma. *Mayo Clin Proc.* 2005;80(12):1568–1574.

64. Zangari M, Barlogie B, Anaissie E et al. Deep vein thrombosis in patients with multiple myeloma treated with thalidomide and chemotherapy: effects of prophylactic and therapeutic anticoagulation. *Br J Haematol.* 2004;126(5):715–721.

65. Ikhlaque N, Seshadri V, Kathula S, Baumann MA. Efficacy of prophylactic warfarin for prevention of thalidomide-related deep venous thrombosis. *Am J Hematol.* 2006;81(6):420–422.

66. Knight R, DeLap RJ, Zeldis JB. Lenalidomide and venous thrombosis in multiple myeloma. *N Engl J Med.* 2006;354(19):2079–2080.

67. Kabbinavar F, Hurwitz HI, Fehrenbacher L et al. Phase II, randomized trial comparing bevacizumab plus fluorouracil (FU)/leucovorin (LV) with FU/LV alone in patients with metastatic colorectal cancer. *J Clin Oncol.* 2003;21(1):60–65.

68. Shah MA, Ilson D, Kelsen DP. Thromboembolic events in gastric cancer: high incidence in patients receiving irinotecan- and bevacizumab-based therapy. *J Clin Oncol.* 2005;23(11):2574–2576.

69. Kuenen BC, Rosen L, Smit EF et al. Dose-finding and pharmacokinetic study of cisplatin, gemcitabine, and SU5416 in patients with solid tumors. *J Clin Oncol.* 2002;20(6):1657–1667.

70. Brotman DJ, Girod JP, Posch A et al. Effects of short-term glucocorticoids on hemostatic factors in healthy volunteers. *Thromb Res.* 2006;118(2):247–252.

71. Verso M, Agnelli G. Venous thromboembolism associated with long-term use of central venous catheters in cancer patients. *J Clin Oncol.* 2003;21(19):3665–3675.

72. Wun T, Law L, Harvey D et al. Increased incidence of symptomatic venous thrombosis in patients with cervical carcinoma treated with concurrent chemotherapy, radiation, and erythropoietin. *Cancer.* 2003;98(7):1514–1520.

73. Steurer M, Sudmeier I, Stauder R, Gastl G. Thromboembolic events in patients with myelodysplastic syndrome receiving thalidomide in combination with darbepoietin-alpha. *Br J Haematol.* 2003; 121(1):101–103.

74. Vansteenkiste J, Pirker R, Massuti B et al. Double-blind, placebo-controlled, randomized phase III trial of darbepoetin alfa in lung cancer patients receiving chemotherapy. *J Natl Cancer Inst.* 2002; 94(16):1211–1220.

75. Galli M, Elice F, Crippa C et al. Recombinant human erythropoietin and the risk of thrombosis in patients receiving thalidomide for multiple myeloma. *Haematologica.* 2004;89(9):1141–1142.

76. Feagan BG, Wong CJ, Kirkley A et al. Erythropoietin with iron supplementation to prevent allogeneic blood transfusion in total hip joint arthroplasty. A randomized, controlled trial. *Ann Intern Med.* 2000;133(11):845–854.

77. Smith KJ, Bleyer AJ, Little WC, Sane DC. The cardiovascular effects of erythropoietin. *Cardiovasc Res.* 2003;59(3):538–548.

77a. Bennett CL, Silver SM, Djulbegovic B et al. Venous thromboembolism and mortality associated with recombinant erythropoietin and darbepoetin administration for the treatment of cancer-associated anemia. JAMA. 2008;299(8):914–924.

78. Lin A, Ryu J, Harvey D et al. Low-dose warfarin does not decrease the rate of thrombosis in patients with cervix and vulvo-vaginal cancer treated with chemotherapy, radiation, and erythropoeitin. *Gynecol Oncol.* 2006;102(1):98–102.

79. Bratzler DW, Raskob GE, Murray CK et al. Underuse of venous thromboembolism prophylaxis for general surgery patients: physician practices in the community hospital setting. *Arch Intern Med.* 1998;158(17):1909–1912.

80. Rahim SA, Panju A, Pai M, Ginsberg J. Venous thromboembolism prophylaxis in medical inpatients: a retrospective chart review. *Thromb Res.* 2003;111(4–5):215–219.

81. Goldhaber SZ, Tapson VF. A prospective registry of 5,451 patients with ultrasound-confirmed deep vein thrombosis. *Am J Cardiol.* 2004;93(2):259–262.

82. Kakkar AK, Levine M, Pinedo HM et al. Venous thrombosis in cancer patients: insights from the FRONTLINE survey. *Oncologist.* 2003;8(4):381–388.

83. Stein PD, Beemath A, Meyers FA et al. Incidence of venous thromboembolism in patients hospitalized with cancer. *Am J Med.* 2006;119(1):60–68.

84. Kakkar AK, Williamson RC. Prevention of venous thromboembolism in cancer patients. *Semin Thromb Hemost.* 1999;25(2):239–243.

85. Mismetti P, Laporte S, Darmon JY et al. Meta-analysis of low molecular weight heparin in the prevention of venous thromboembolism in general surgery. *Br J Surg.* 2001;88(7):913–930.

86. Efficacy and safety of enoxaparin versus unfractionated heparin for prevention of deep vein thrombosis in elective cancer surgery: a double-blind randomized multicentre trial with venographic assessment. ENOXACAN Study Group. *Br J Surg.* 1997;84(8):1099–1103.

87. McLeod RS, Geerts WH, Sniderman KW et al. Subcutaneous heparin versus low-molecular-weight heparin as thromboprophylaxis in patients undergoing colorectal surgery: results of the Canadian colorectal DVT prophylaxis trial: a randomized, double-blind trial. *Ann Surg.* 2001;233(3):438–444.

88. Agnelli G, Bergqvist D, Cohen AT et al. Randomized clinical trial of postoperative fondaparinux versus perioperative dalteparin for prevention of venous thromboembolism in high-risk abdominal surgery. *Br J Surg.* 2005;92(10):1212–1220.

89. Agnelli G, Bolis G, Capussotti L et al. A clinical outcome-based prospective study on venous thromboembolism after cancer surgery: the @RISTOS project. *Ann Surg.* 2006;243(1):89–95.

90. Bergqvist D, Agnelli G, Cohen AT et al. Duration of prophylaxis against venous thromboembolism with enoxaparin after surgery for cancer. *N Engl J Med.* 2002;346(13):975–980.

91. Rasmussen MS, Jorgensen LN, Wille-Jorgensen P et al. Prolonged prophylaxis with dalteparin to prevent late thromboembolic complications in patients undergoing major abdominal surgery: a multicenter randomized open-label study. *J Thromb Haemost.* 2006;4(11):2384–2390.

92. Roderick P, Ferris G, Wilson K et al. Towards evidence-based guidelines for the prevention of venous thromboembolism: systematic reviews of mechanical methods, oral anticoagulation, dextran and regional anaesthesia as thromboprophylaxis. *Health Technol Assess.* 2005;9(49):iii–x, 1.

93. Geerts WH, Heit JA, Clagett GP et al. Prevention of venous thromboembolism. *Chest.* 2001;119(1 Suppl):132S–175S.

94. Comerota AJ, Katz ML, White JV. Why does prophylaxis with external pneumatic compression for deep vein thrombosis fail? *Am J Surg.* 1992;164(3):265–268.

95. Cornwell EE, III, Chang D, Velmahos G et al. Compliance with sequential compression device prophylaxis in at-risk trauma patients: a prospective analysis. *Am Surg.* 2002;68(5):470–473.

96. Agnelli G, Piovella F, Buoncristiani P et al. Enoxaparin plus compression stockings compared with compression stockings alone in the prevention of venous thromboembolism after elective neurosurgery. *N Engl J Med.* 1998;339(2):80–85.

97. Ramos R, Salem BI, De Pawlikowski MP et al. The efficacy of pneumatic compression stockings in the prevention of pulmonary embolism after cardiac surgery. *Chest.* 1996;109(1):82–85.

98. Kroger K, Weiland D, Ose C et al. Risk factors for venous thromboembolic events in cancer patients. *Ann Oncol.* 2006;17(2):297–303.

99. Mismetti P, Laporte-Simitsidis S, Tardy B et al. Prevention of venous thromboembolism in internal medicine with unfractionated or low-molecular-weight heparins: a meta-analysis of randomised clinical trials. *Thromb Haemost.* 2000;83(1):14–19.

100. Samama MM, Cohen AT, Darmon JY et al. A comparison of enoxaparin with placebo for the prevention of venous thromboembolism in acutely ill medical patients. Prophylaxis in Medical Patients with Enoxaparin Study Group. *N Engl J Med.* 1999;341(11):793–800.

101. Lechler E, Schramm W, Flosbach CW. The venous thrombotic risk in non-surgical patients: epidemiological data and efficacy/safety profile of a low-molecular-weight heparin (enoxaparin). The Prime Study Group. *Haemostasis.* 1996;26(Suppl 2):49–56.

102. Kleber FX, Witt C, Vogel G et al. Randomized comparison of enoxaparin with unfractionated heparin for the prevention of venous thromboembolism in medical patients with heart failure or severe respiratory disease. *Am Heart J.* 2003;145(4):614–621.

103. Leizorovicz A, Cohen AT, Turpie AG et al. Randomized, placebo-controlled trial of dalteparin for the prevention of venous thromboembolism in acutely ill medical patients. *Circulation.* 2004;110(7): 874–879.

104. Cohen AT, Davidson BL, Gallus AS et al. Efficacy and safety of fondaparinux for the prevention of venous thromboembolism in older acute medical patients: randomised placebo controlled trial. *BMJ.* 2006;332(7537):325–329.

105. Blom JW, Osanto S, Rosendaal FR. High risk of venous thrombosis in patients with pancreatic cancer: a cohort study of 202 patients. *Eur J Cancer.* 2006;42(3):410–414.

106. Monreal M, Raventos A, Lerma R et al. Pulmonary embolism in patients with upper extremity DVT associated to venous central lines--a prospective study. *Thromb Haemost.* 1994;72(4):548–550.

107. Bern MM, Lokich JJ, Wallach SR et al. Very low doses of warfarin can prevent thrombosis in central venous catheters. A randomized prospective trial. *Ann Intern Med.* 1990;112(6):423–428.

108. Monreal M, Alastrue A, Rull M et al. Upper extremity deep venous thrombosis in cancer patients with venous access devices--prophylaxis with a low molecular weight heparin (Fragmin). *Thromb Haemost.* 1996;75(2):251–253.

109. Karthaus M, Kretzschmar A, Kroning H et al. Dalteparin for prevention of catheter-related complications in cancer patients with central venous catheters: final results of a double-blind, placebo-controlled phase III trial. *Ann Oncol.* 2006;17(2):289–296.

110. Verso M, Agnelli G, Bertoglio S et al. Enoxaparin for the prevention of venous thromboembolism associated with central vein catheter: a double-blind, placebo-controlled, randomized study in cancer patients. *J Clin Oncol.* 2005;23(18):4057–4062.

111. Wells PS. The role of qualitative D-dimer assays, clinical probability, and noninvasive imaging tests for the diagnosis of deep vein thrombosis and pulmonary embolism. *Semin Vasc Med.* 2005;5(4):340–350.

112. Oudega R, Hoes AW, Moons KG. The Wells rule does not adequately rule out deep venous thrombosis in primary care patients. *Ann Intern Med.* 2005;143(2):100–107.

113. Lee AY, Julian JA, Levine MN et al. Clinical utility of a rapid whole-blood D-dimer assay in patients with cancer who present with suspected acute deep venous thrombosis. *Ann Intern Med.* 1999;131(6):417–423.

114. Sohne M, Kruip MJ, Nijkeuter M et al. Accuracy of clinical decision rule, D-dimer and spiral computed tomography in patients with malignancy, previous venous thromboembolism, COPD or heart failure and in older patients with suspected pulmonary embolism. *J Thromb Haemost.* 2006;4(5): 1042–1046.

115. Buller HR, Agnelli G, Hull RD et al. Antithrombotic therapy for venous thromboembolic disease: the Seventh ACCP Conference on Antithrombotic and Thrombolytic Therapy. *Chest.* 2004;126(3 Suppl): 401S–428S.

116. Segal JB, Bolger DT, Jenckes MW et al. Outpatient therapy with low molecular weight heparin for the treatment of venous thromboembolism: a review of efficacy, safety, and costs. *Am J Med.* 2003;115(4): 298–308.

117. Warkentin TE, Greinacher A. Heparin-induced thrombocytopenia: recognition, treatment, and prevention: the Seventh ACCP Conference on Antithrombotic and Thrombolytic Therapy. *Chest.* 2004;126(3 Suppl):311S–337S.

118. Kearon C, Ginsberg JS, Julian JA et al. Comparison of fixed-dose weight-adjusted unfractionated heparin and low-molecular-weight heparin for acute treatment of venous thromboembolism. *JAMA.* 2006;296(8):935–942.

119. Martel N, Lee J, Wells PS. Risk for heparin-induced thrombocytopenia with unfractionated and low-molecular-weight heparin thromboprophylaxis: a meta-analysis. *Blood.* 2005;106(8):2710–2715.

120. Kuo KH, Kovacs MJ. Fondaparinux: a potential new therapy for HIT. *Hematology.* 2005;10(4): 271–275.

120a. Warkentin TE, Maurer BT, Aster RH. Heparin-Induced Thrombocytopenia Associated with Fondaparinux. New Eng J Med. 2007;356(25):2653–2655.

121. Merli G, Spiro TE, Olsson CG et al. Subcutaneous enoxaparin once or twice daily compared with intravenous unfractionated heparin for treatment of venous thromboembolic disease. *Ann Intern Med.* 2001;134(3):191–202.

122. Crowther MA, Berry LR, Monagle PT, Chan AK. Mechanisms responsible for the failure of protamine to inactivate low-molecular-weight heparin. *Br J Haematol.* 2002;116(1):178–186.

123. Bijsterveld NR, Moons AH, Boekholdt SM et al. Ability of recombinant factor VIIa to reverse the anticoagulant effect of the pentasaccharide fondaparinux in healthy volunteers. *Circulation.* 2002;106(20):2550–2554.

124. Ageno W, Grimwood R, Limbiati S et al. Home-treatment of deep vein thrombosis in patients with cancer. *Haematologica.* 2005;90(2):220–224.

125. Siragusa S, Arcara C, Malato A et al. Home therapy for deep vein thrombosis and pulmonary embolism in cancer patients. *Ann Oncol.* 2005;16(Suppl 4):iv136–iv139.

126. Dager WE, King JH, Branch JM et al. Tinzaparin in outpatients with pulmonary embolism or deep vein thrombosis. *Ann Pharmacother.* 2005;39(7–8):1182–1187.

127. Kovacs MJ, Anderson D, Morrow B et al. Outpatient treatment of pulmonary embolism with dalteparin. *Thromb Haemost.* 2000;83(2):209–211.

128. Goldhaber SZ, Visani L, De Rosa M. Acute pulmonary embolism: clinical outcomes in the International Cooperative Pulmonary Embolism Registry (ICOPER). *Lancet.* 1999;353(9162):1386–1389.

129. Wicki J, Perrier A, Perneger TV et al. Predicting adverse outcome in patients with acute pulmonary embolism: a risk score. *Thromb Haemost.* 2000;84(4):548–552.

130. Kucher N, Rossi E, De Rosa M, Goldhaber SZ. Prognostic role of echocardiography among patients with acute pulmonary embolism and a systolic arterial pressure of 90 mmHg or higher. *Arch Intern Med.* 2005;165(15):1777–1781.

131. Schoepf UJ, Kucher N, Kipfmueller F et al. Right ventricular enlargement on chest computed tomography: a predictor of early death in acute pulmonary embolism. *Circulation.* 2004;110(20):3276–3280.

132. O'Connell CL, Boswell WD, Duddalwar V et al. Unsuspected pulmonary emboli in cancer patients: clinical correlates and relevance. *J Clin Oncol.* 2006;24(30):4928–4932.

133. Konstantinides S, Geibel A, Heusel G et al. Heparin plus alteplase compared with heparin alone in patients with submassive pulmonary embolism. *N Engl J Med.* 2002;347(15):1143–1150.

134. Comerota AJ, Aldridge SC. Thrombolytic therapy for deep venous thrombosis: a clinical review. *Can J Surg.* 1993;36(4):359–364.

135. Mewissen MW, Seabrook GR, Meissner MH et al. Catheter-directed thrombolysis for lower extremity deep venous thrombosis: report of a national multicenter registry. *Radiology.* 1999;211(1):39–49.

136. Kim HS, Patra A, Paxton BE et al. Adjunctive percutaneous mechanical thrombectomy for lower-extremity deep vein thrombosis: clinical and economic outcomes. *J Vasc Interv Radiol.* 2006;17(7):1099–1104.

137. Hann CL, Streiff MB. The role of vena caval filters in the management of venous thromboembolism. *Blood Rev.* 2005;19(4):179–202.

138. Eight-year follow-up of patients with permanent vena cava filters in the prevention of pulmonary embolism: the PREPIC (Prevention du Risque d'Embolie Pulmonaire par Interruption Cave) randomized study. *Circulation.* 2005;112(3):416–422.

139. Linenberger ML. Catheter-related thrombosis: risks, diagnosis, and management. *J Natl Compr Canc Netw.* 2006;4(9):889–901.

140. Streiff MB. Long-term therapy of venous thromboembolism in cancer patients. *J Natl Compr Canc Netw.* 2006;4(9):903–910.

141. Ansell J, Hirsh J, Poller L et al. The pharmacology and management of the vitamin K antagonists: the Seventh ACCP Conference on Antithrombotic and Thrombolytic Therapy. *Chest.* 2004;126(3 Suppl):204S–233S.

142. Streiff MB, Segal JB, Tamariz LJ et al. Duration of vitamin K antagonist therapy for venous thromboembolism: a systematic review of the literature. *Am J Hematol.* 2006;81(9):684–691.

143. Palareti G, Legnani C, Lee A et al. A comparison of the safety and efficacy of oral anticoagulation for the treatment of venous thromboembolic disease in patients with or without malignancy. *Thromb Haemost.* 2000;84(5):805–810.

144. Prandoni P, Lensing AW, Piccioli A et al. Recurrent venous thromboembolism and bleeding complications during anticoagulant treatment in patients with cancer and venous thrombosis. *Blood.* 2002;100(10):3484–3488.

145. Hutten BA, Prins MH, Gent M et al. Incidence of recurrent thromboembolic and bleeding complications among patients with venous thromboembolism in relation to both malignancy and achieved international normalized ratio: a retrospective analysis. *J Clin Oncol.* 2000;18(17):3078–3083.

146. Meyer G, Marjanovic Z, Valcke J et al. Comparison of low-molecular-weight heparin and warfarin for the secondary prevention of venous thromboembolism in patients with cancer: a randomized controlled study. *Arch Intern Med.* 2002;162(15):1729–1735.

147. Deitcher SR, Kessler CM, Merli G et al. Secondary prevention of venous thromboembolic events in patients with active cancer: enoxaparin alone versus initial enoxaparin followed by warfarin for a 180-day period. *Clin Appl Thromb Hemost.* 2006;12(4):389–396.

148. Hull RD, Pineo GF, Brant RF, et al. Long-term low molecular weight heparin versus usual care in proximal-vein thrombosis patients with cancer. Am J Med 2006;119(12):1062–1072.

149. Lee AY, Levine MN, Baker RI et al. Low-molecular-weight heparin versus a coumarin for the prevention of recurrent venous thromboembolism in patients with cancer. *N Engl J Med.* 2003;349(2):146–153.

150. Aujesky D, Smith KJ, Cornuz J, Roberts MS. Cost-effectiveness of low-molecular-weight heparin for secondary prophylaxis of cancer-related venous thromboembolism. *Thromb Haemost.* 2005;93(3):592–599.

151. Bernardi E, Bagatella P, Frulla M et al. Postthrombotic syndrome: incidence, prevention, and management. *Semin Vasc Med.* 2001;1(1):71–80.

152. Prandoni P, Villalta S, Bagatella P et al. The clinical course of deep-vein thrombosis. Prospective long-term follow-up of 528 symptomatic patients. *Haematologica.* 1997;82(4):423–428.

153. Prandoni P, Lensing AW, Prins MH et al. Below-knee elastic compression stockings to prevent the post-thrombotic syndrome: a randomized, controlled trial. *Ann Intern Med.* 2004;141(4):249–256.

154. Brandjes DP, Buller HR, Heijboer H et al. Randomised trial of effect of compression stockings in patients with symptomatic proximal-vein thrombosis. *Lancet.* 1997;349(9054):759–762.

155. Crowther MA, Ginsberg JS, Julian J et al. A comparison of two intensities of warfarin for the prevention of recurrent thrombosis in patients with the antiphospholipid antibody syndrome. *N Engl J Med.* 2003;349(12):1133–1138.

156. Luk C, Wells PS, Anderson D, Kovacs MJ. Extended outpatient therapy with low molecular weight heparin for the treatment of recurrent venous thromboembolism despite warfarin therapy. *Am J Med.* 2001;111(4):270–273.

157. Warkentin TE, Greinacher A. Heparin-induced thrombocytopenia: recognition, treatment, and prevention: the Seventh ACCP Conference on Antithrombotic and Thrombolytic Therapy. *Chest.* 2004;126(3 Suppl):311S–337S.

158. Sack GH, Jr., Levin J, Bell WR. Trousseau's syndrome and other manifestations of chronic disseminated coagulopathy in patients with neoplasms: clinical, pathophysiologic, and therapeutic features. *Medicine (Baltimore).* 1977;56(1):1–37.

159. Merli G, Spiro TE, Olsson CG et al. Subcutaneous enoxaparin once or twice daily compared with intravenous unfractionated heparin for treatment of venous thromboembolic disease. *Ann Intern Med.* 2001;134(3):191–202.

160. Zacharski LR, Henderson WG, Rickles FR et al. Effect of warfarin anticoagulation on survival in carcinoma of the lung, colon, head and neck, and prostate. Final report of VA Cooperative Study #75. *Cancer.* 1984;53(10):2046–2052.

161. Aisner J, Goutsou M, Maurer LH et al. Intensive combination chemotherapy, concurrent chest irradiation, and warfarin for the treatment of limited-disease small-cell lung cancer: a Cancer and Leukemia Group B pilot study. *J Clin Oncol.* 1992;10(8):1230–1236.

162. Maurer LH, Herndon JE, Hollis DR et al. Randomized trial of chemotherapy and radiation therapy with or without warfarin for limited-stage small-cell lung cancer: a Cancer and Leukemia Group B study. *J Clin Oncol.* 1997;15(11):3378–3387.

163. Chahinian AP, Propert KJ, Ware JH et al. A randomized trial of anticoagulation with warfarin and of alternating chemotherapy in extensive small-cell lung cancer by the Cancer and Leukemia Group B. *J Clin Oncol.* 1989;7(8):993–1002.

164. Smorenburg SM, Van Noorden CJ. The complex effects of heparins on cancer progression and metastasis in experimental studies. *Pharmacol Rev.* 2001;53(1):93–105.

165. Dolovich LR, Ginsberg JS, Douketis JD et al. A meta-analysis comparing low-molecular-weight heparins with unfractionated heparin in the treatment of venous thromboembolism: examining some unanswered questions regarding location of treatment, product type, and dosing frequency. *Arch Intern Med.* 2000;160(2):181–188.

166. Kakkar AK, Levine MN, Kadziola Z et al. Low molecular weight heparin, therapy with dalteparin, and survival in advanced cancer: the fragmin advanced malignancy outcome study (FAMOUS). *J Clin Oncol.* 2004;22(10):1944–1948.

167. Klerk CP, Smorenburg SM, Otten HM et al. The effect of low molecular weight heparin on survival in patients with advanced malignancy. *J Clin Oncol.* 2005;23(10):2130–2135.

168. Lee AY, Rickles FR, Julian JA et al. Randomized comparison of low molecular weight heparin and coumarin derivatives on the survival of patients with cancer and venous thromboembolism. *J Clin Oncol.* 2005;23(10):2123–2129.

169. Altinbas M, Coskun HS, Er O et al. A randomized clinical trial of combination chemotherapy with and without low-molecular-weight heparin in small cell lung cancer. *J Thromb Haemost.* 2004;2(8):1266–1271.

7

Depression in Cancer Patients

Jimmie C. Holland and Yesne Alici-Evcimen

ABSTRACT

Oncologists commonly encounter patients with depressive symptoms. It is important for the clinician to recognize and treat these symptoms in cancer patients, since they can occur for both physical and psychological reasons. This chapter describes assessment of depression, differentiating between types and causes of depressive disorders, and treatment interventions. Risk factors for suicide, assessment and management of suicide are also reviewed.

Key Words: Depression; Cancer; Suicide; Psycho-oncology.

INTRODUCTION

Depressive symptoms are common in the oncology setting. Evaluating their nature and intensity is important. Cancer patients are vulnerable to these symptoms at all stages of the illness, from appearance of the first symptoms of cancer to the time of diagnosis, during treatment, palliative care, and even after remission or cure. Sadness and worry for the future are normal responses, partly because of the meaning attached to cancer, such as the fear of disability or death. For the oncologist, the relevant clinical

From: *Cancer and Drug Discovery Development: Supportive Care in Cancer Therapy*
DOI: 10.1007/978-1-59745-291-5_7, Edited by: D. S. Ettinger © Humana Press, Totowa, NJ

question is how to identify the point when normal sadness or distress associated with the cancer has become a depressive disorder which demands treatment or referral for evaluation to a mental health professional. It is important to remember that depression responds to treatment and should not be left untreated "based on reality."

PREVALENCE OF DEPRESSION IN CANCER PATIENTS

Many studies have documented the prevalence of depression in cancer patients. The prevalence estimates of current major depression in cancer patients have varied widely in different studies, from a low of 1% to a high of 50% (1–3). Comparably, the current (30-day) prevalence of major depression in the general United States population is estimated to be 4.9% (4). The use of different diagnostic measures and cutoff criteria impacts prevalence estimates. In a study of terminally ill cancer patients, a symptom threshold consistent with DSM-IV criteria was associated with a depression diagnosis in 13.0% of patients (5). A relatively minor reduction in the symptom severity threshold elevated the depression diagnosis to 26.1% of patients. Other factors that contribute to differences in prevalence are the site of cancer(s), the physical symptoms, and the stage of cancer (6).

EVALUATION AND DIAGNOSIS OF DEPRESSION IN CANCER PATIENTS

Diagnosis of depression is challenging in cancer patients due to the neurovegetative symptoms, which are the same as many symptoms caused by cancer: loss of appetite, fatigue, sleep disturbances, psychomotor retardation, apathy, and poor concentration (7). These may represent symptoms of depression, or the result of cancer and/or its treatment. The assessment of depressive symptoms related to psychological issues should focus on the presence of dysphoria, anhedonia, hopelessness, worthlessness, excessive or inappropriate guilt, and suicidal ideation (Table 1). Presence of these symptoms help distinguish depression from cancer-related symptoms (6). Poor memory and impaired concentration are more likely to be the initial chief complaints in elderly depressed patients. Although rare, delusions or hallucinations may accompany depression. In medically ill patients, this combination of symptoms is usually reflective of a diagnosis of delirium, which should be ruled out first. If present, the diagnosis of delirium precludes the diagnosis of mood disorder with depressive features. Depressed patients with psychotic features should be referred to a psychiatrist for further assessment and management.

Cohen-Cole and colleagues (8) reviewed four conceptual approaches to evaluate depression in the medically ill, namely inclusive, exclusive, etiological, and substitutive approaches. No single approach is inherently superior to the others (8). When selecting a conceptual approach, it is important to consider whether a diagnosis of depression is being made for clinical or research purposes (8). The inclusive approach, in which all symptoms of depression are counted regardless of their suspected etiology, is highly sensitive, making its use more appropriate for diagnoses in clinical settings. The exclusive approach eliminates the somatic symptoms from the diagnostic criteria. The high specificity associated with the exclusive approach makes it valuable for research purposes, but it is not desirable in clinical practice due to the risk of denying treatment to patients who may

Table 1
Evaluation of depression

Psychological
　　Dysphoric mood (e.g., sad, depressed, anxious, tearful, diurnal mood changes)
　　Feelings of hopelessness, helplessness
　　Loss of interest and pleasure, anhedonia
　　Guilt, burden on others, worthlessness
　　Mood congruent delusions (poverty, nihilistic delusions)
　　Mood incongruent delusions
　　Suicidal thoughts or plans

Somatic (difficult to interpret in physically impaired patients)
　　Insomnia or hypersomnia
　　Anorexia and weight loss
　　Fatigue
　　Psychomotor retardation or agitation
　　Poor concentration
　　Decreased libido

Adapted from *(16)*

benefit. The etiological approach requires that the clinician include a symptom as part of a clinical depression only if it is clearly not a result of medical illness. While it is theoretically sound, it is difficult to apply this reliably in oncology due to the overlap of symptoms. The substitutive approach *(9)* replaces somatic symptoms of depression (i.e., fatigue, sleep disturbance, change in weight or appetite, difficulty concentrating) with psychological symptoms such as depressed appearance, social withdrawal, brooding, self-pity, pessimism, and anhedonia. While this approach is conceptually reasonable, there is little evidence for its superiority *(5)*.

Several subcategories of DSM-IV (Diagnostic and Statistical Manual of Mental Disorders *(10)*) depression diagnoses are found in the context of cancer. A diagnosis of "mood disorder with depressive features due to cancer" is the appropriate diagnosis when the depressive disorder is due to an underlying cancer, such as pancreatic cancer. When a medication (such as interferon) is the underlying cause of a depressive disorder, the diagnosis of "substance-induced mood disorder" is used. However, establishing the etiology of symptoms of depression in cancer patients is difficult, and usually multiple factors contribute to depressive symptoms in most of these patients. A diagnosis of "adjustment disorder with depressed mood" is used in patients who have emotional or behavioral symptoms that significantly impair role (e.g., job, academic, social), functioning, or that are accompanied by a level of distress in excess of what one would normally expect. In the context of cancer, one can reasonably expect patients to experience a level of sadness and problems with sleep, appetite, and concentration. Thus, the clinician must use clinical judgment as when these symptoms exceed a "normal sadness" to become "adjustment disorder with depressed mood." Major depression, the most severe level, is defined as an episode of clinically significant persistent and pervasive depressed mood and/or anhedonia, accompanied by cognitive and behavioral symptoms. The DSM-IV criteria for major depression are consistent with the etiological approach in which symptoms that are deemed to be due to a medical condition or medication do not count toward the diagnosis. Patients may have a preexisting chronic depression called dysthymia, which may become more manifest or worse in cancer patients. Patients who have had a major depressive episode in the past are at risk of a recurrence in the context of cancer.

RISK FACTORS FOR DEPRESSION IN CANCER PATIENTS

There are several risk factors for depression in cancer patients (Table 2). The site of cancer and several chemotherapy regimens tend to raise the risk. Vinblastine, vincristine, interferon, procarbazine, asparaginase, tamoxifen, cyproterone, and corticosteroids are associated with greater risk (11). A higher prevalence of depression has been found among patients with pancreatic, oropharyngeal, breast, and lung cancer, with lower rates observed among those with lymphoma, colon, and gynecological cancers (3, 12). Depression is a common symptom of pancreatic cancer, with some early data that the mood disturbance is mediated by alteration of brain serotonergic function through proinflammatory cytokines (13–16).

Depression may also relate to organ failure, or nutritional, endocrine, and neurological complications of cancer (Table 3). Other risk factors for depression, not specific to cancer patients are advanced disease stage and physical disability, presence of other chronic illnesses (1), a previous history of depression (17), family history of depression, uncontrolled pain (18), younger age (19), low social support, social isolation, recent experience of a significant loss (20), low self-esteem (20). Although it is well established that depression is more prevalent among women than men in the general population (21), the gender difference is not evident among cancer patients (22). Older individuals are at greater risk for depression even in the absence of medical illness due to multiple losses through the years, such as death of loved ones, retirement, physical deconditioning, etc.

Table 2
Risk factors for depression in cancer patients

Family history of depression, suicide

Personal history of previous depression, bipolar disorder, suicide attempts, alcohol abuse or
    dependence, other substance abuse or dependence

Recent losses/bereavement

Prior experience with cancer

Pessimistic outlook on life

Multiple obligations, responsibilities

Absence of a belief or a value system

Rigid and inflexible coping style

Social isolation

Low socioeconomic status

Adapted from (16)

Table 3
Medical conditions that cause depression

Metabolic abnormalities
    Hypercalcemia
    Sodium, potassium imbalance
    Other electrolyte disturbances
    Vitamin B12, folate, or other vitamin deficiencies
Cancer-related
    Primary CNS tumors
    CNS metastasis
    Paraneoplastic syndromes
    Pancreatic cancer, small-cell lung cancer, breast cancer
    Neurological diseases
    Cerebrovascular disease
    Dementia
    Cerebral trauma
    CNS infections
Systemic disorders
    Autoimmune disorders
    Inflammatory disorders
    Infections
Endocrine abnormalities
Hyper- or Hypothyroidism
Adrenal insufficiency
Medications
    Corticosteroids
    Interferon and interleukin 2
    Cardiac and antiarrhythmic drugs
    Antibiotics, antivirals
    Psychotropic drugs (antipsychotics, benzodiazepines, other sedative/hypnotics)
    Opiates
    Cimetidine
    Levodopa, methyldopa
    Pentazocine
    Tamoxifen
    Analgesics, and anti-inflammatory drugs
    Some chemotherapeutic agents: vincristine, vinblastine, procarbazine, asparaginase,
        tamoxifen, cyproterone, mithramycin, L-asparaginase
Other diseases
    Cardiorespiratory disease
    Renal disease
    Anemia
    Uncontrolled pain

Adapted from *(6, 16)*

SUICIDE ASSESSMENT AND MANAGEMENT IN CANCER PATIENTS

The incidence of suicide is higher in cancer patients compared with the general population. Studies suggest that although a small number of cancer patients commit suicide, the relative risk of suicide in this population is twice that of the general population *(23–26)*. Suicide is more likely to occur in advanced disease with escalating depression, hopelessness, and the presence of poorly controlled symptoms, particularly pain *(16)*. Suicidal thoughts in patients with advanced disease, poor prognosis, or poorly controlled symptoms are likely viewed as rational by physicians *(27)*. It is important to note that those patients may have a treatable major depressive episode precipitating their suicidal ideation. Clinicians should evaluate for hopelessness and a diagnosis of depression in terminally ill patients with persistent desire for death or suicidal intention *(28–30)*.

Prior history of psychiatric illness, previous history of depression or suicide attempts, recent bereavement, history of alcohol or other substance abuse or dependence, male gender, family history of depression or suicide and lack of family or social support, and recent losses are common risk factors for suicide. Older patients in the sixth and seventh decade of life, individuals with head and neck, lung, breast, urogenital, gastrointestinal cancers, and myeloma seem to have an increased risk of suicide *(23–26, 31–33)*. An international population-based study from Denmark, Finland, Norway, Sweden, and the United States showed a small, but statistically significant, increased long-term risk of suicide, 25 or more years after a breast cancer diagnosis *(34)*.

Establishing rapport with the patient is the most important initial step in evaluation of suicidal risk. Evaluation of suicidal thoughts should take into account the disease stage and prognosis. It is helpful to consider the issue of suicidality from four perspectives: (1) the suicidal thoughts that occur transiently in all patients with cancer, (2) suicidal thoughts in patients who are in remission with a good prognosis, (3) suicidal thoughts in patients with poor prognosis/poor symptom control, and (4) patients in terminal stages *(35)*. Suicidal ideation, or plans to commit suicide in cancer patients with good prognosis or those in remission, requires careful assessment *(30)*. A Finnish survey of suicides in one year revealed that 4.3% had cancer *(36)*. Half of the patients were in remission at the time of suicide. Patients were noted to have a history of psychiatric illness prior to cancer diagnosis, in particular substance abuse.

It is important to recognize and aggressively treat high-risk patients for depression and address suicidal risk with psychiatric hospitalization, if necessary. Untreated delirium may lead to unpredictable suicide attempts due to impaired judgment and impulse control *(37)*. The presence of a 24-h companion or a family member and treatment of delirium would help protect these patients from self-harm. Maintaining a supportive relationship, symptom control (e.g., pain, nausea, depression), and involving the family or friends are the initial steps in management of a suicidal patient. A recent study examining the suicidal ideation and past suicidal attempt in adult survivors of childhood cancer found a strong correlation between physical health and suicidality, which underscores the importance of symptom control in cancer patients *(38)*. Early psychiatric involvement with high-risk individuals can often avert suicide in cancer patients *(39)*. Psychiatrists or other mental health care professionals are helpful in assessing depression. A careful evaluation includes an exploration of the reasons for suicidal thoughts and the seriousness of the risk. The clinician should listen empathically, without appearing critical or judgmental. Allowing the patient to discuss suicidal thoughts often decreases the risk of suicide despite common belief to the contrary. Patients often reconsider and reject the idea of suicide when the physician acknowledges the legitimacy of their option and the need to retain a sense of control over aspects of their death *(32)*.

If a patient expresses suicidal intent in the hospital, a 24-h companion should be provided to ensure constant observation. Consultation with the psychiatry team helps the oncologists in assessment and management of the suicidal patient. Psychiatric hospitalization is usually not a good option for a seriously ill patient. The medical hospital or home is usually the setting in which the management takes place *(32)*. When the patient is at home, it is helpful to work with the family, to maintain vigilance, while encouraging the patient to agree to call if suicidal thoughts become overwhelming.

MANAGEMENT OF DEPRESSION IN CANCER PATIENTS

Managing depression requires a comprehensive approach that addresses the evaluation, treatment, and follow-up of cancer patients. The initial management begins with the establishment of a therapeutic alliance with the oncologist and the recruiting of support from family or friends. The relationship with the oncologist is the key component of support. Maintaining ongoing contact with the depressed cancer patient, especially terminally ill patients, ensures that continual evaluation and caring are available to the patient without fear of being abandoned *(40)*.

The APA (American Psychiatric Association) has created practice guidelines for the treatment of depressive disorders in physically healthy individuals *(41)*. This same comprehensive approach has been applied to the treatment of depression in cancer patients by the National Comprehensive Cancer Network. (NCCN *(42)*). There are several pharmacologic and psychotherapeutic strategies available. Prior to selecting an appropriate treatment, attention should be paid to the site of cancer, current cancer treatment, comorbid medical conditions, and medications, any of which may contribute to depressive symptoms. The evaluation of medical, neurologic, and endocrinologic factors may reveal reversible causes of depression, particularly thyroid function abnormalities, or medications that can be eliminated or substituted. If the depressive disorder is believed to be caused by a medical condition or by a drug, the clinician should treat the underlying condition or change the drug. Antidepressants are usually started concurrently to relieve patient's suffering more quickly.

Pharmacologic Treatments

The use of antidepressant medications in cancer patients poses unique challenges. A rapid onset of action is preferable in cancer patients; however, antidepressants may take several weeks to have a therapeutic effect due to their delayed onset of action *(43)*. An appropriate antidepressant should be selected based on the potential side effects of each antidepressant, a consideration of each patient's prognosis, primary symptoms of depression, and comorbid symptoms or conditions. Drug–drug interactions through inhibiton of cytochrome P450 isoenzymes are important to note *(44)*. Antidepressants should be started at low doses and titrated up slowly in medically frail cancer patients, especially in the elderly *(45)*. Table 4 lists the commonly used antidepressants.

Table 4
Medications used to treat depression in cancer patients

Medication	Brand name	Starting dose/therapeutic range	Common side effects/comments
Selective serotonin reuptake inhibitors:			
Fluoxetine[a]	Prozac	10–20 mg/20–60 mg	Varying degrees of gastrointestinal distress, nausea, headache, insomnia, increased anxiety, sexual dysfunction. Sertraline, citalopram, and escitalopram produce the least p450 system interactions
Sertraline[a]	Zoloft	25–50 mg/50–200 mg	
Paroxetine	Paxil, Paxil CR	10–20 mg/20–50 mg	
Fluvoxamine	Luvox	50 mg/100–300 mg	
Citalopram[a]	Celexa	10–20 mg/20–60 mg	
Escitalopram[a]	Lexapro	10 mg/10–20 mg	
Tricyclic antidepressants:			
Amitriptyline	Elavil	10–25 mg/50–150 mg	Sedation, anticholinergic effects, orthostasis
Imipramine	Tofranil	10–25 mg/50–300 mg	
Desipramine	Norpramin	25 mg/75–200 mg	Minimal sedation or orthostasis; moderate anticholinergic effects
Nortriptyline[a]	Pamelor	10–25 mg/50–150 mg	Sedation, minimal anticholinergic effects or orthostasis
Doxepin[a]	Sinequan	25 mg/75–300 mg	Sedating, anticholinergic effects, orthostasis
Monoamine oxidase inhibitors:			
Phenelzine	Nardil	15 mg/30–60 mg	Orthostasis, drug–drug interactions, requires avoidance of certain foods (can cause hypertensive crisis)
Tranylcypromine	Parnate	10 mg/20–40 mg	
Newer antidepressants:			
Bupropion	Wellbutrin, Wellbutrin SR and XL	75 mg/150–450 mg	Activating, seizures if predisposed, no sexual dysfunction
Trazodone	Desyrel	50 mg/150–200 mg	Sedation, useful as a sleep aid, priapism
Nefazodone	Serzone	100/150–300 mg	Risk of liver failure, sedation, dizziness, constipation, sexual dysfunction unlikely
Venlafaxine	Effexor and Effexor XR	37.5 mg bid/75–225 mg	Activating, nausea, anxiety, sedation, sweating, hypertension
Duloxetine	Cymbalta	20–30 mg/30–60 mg	Activating, anxiety, nausea
Mirtazapine	Remeron	7.5–15 mg/15–45 mg	Sedation, weight gain; dissolvable tablet form available

(continued)

Table 4
(continued)

Medication	Brand name	Starting dose/thera-peutic range	Common side effects/ comments
Stimulants and wakefulness promoting agents:			
Dextroamphetamine	Dexedrine	2.5 mg/5–30 mg	Possible cardiac complica-
Methylphenidate	Ritalin	2.5 mg/5–15 mg bid	tions, agitation, anxiety, agitation, nausea
Modafinil	Provigil	50 mg/100–400 mg	Activating, nausea, cardiac side effects, usually well-tolerated

Adapted from (6, 16)

[a] Available in liquid form

SELECTIVE SEROTONIN REUPTAKE INHIBITORS (SSRIs)

SSRIs have become the first line of treatment for depression and anxiety disorders, replacing tricyclic antidepressants. They are efficacious, generally well tolerated, and are not as toxic in overdose as tricyclic antidepressants. Some SSRIs, such as fluoxetine and fluvoxamine, are inhibitors of cytochrome P450 isoenzymes. It is therefore important to monitor for the possibility of drug–drug interactions. Sertraline, citalopram, and escitalopram are less protein-bound and may have a lower risk of drug interactions with the P450 system *(46, 47)*. Many of the SSRIs now come in liquid forms, making it easier for patients who cannot swallow pills. SSRIs with a short half-life, such as paroxetine, have occasionally been associated with flu-like withdrawal symptoms if stopped abruptly. Fluoxetine has the longest half-life of all SSRIs. Common side effects of SSRIs are headache, palpitations, nausea, and sexual dysfunction, most of which disappear with continued use of the medication *(48)*.

TRICYCLIC ANTIDEPRESSANTS

These medications have been around for many years and are therefore less expensive than many of the SSRIs. The tricyclics are also used as adjunct pain medications, especially for neuropathic pain. Because of their anticholinergic, antiadrenergic, and antihistaminergic side effects, they are less frequently used in cancer patients. The anticholinergic side effects of urinary retention, constipation, blurred vision, and dry mouth, as well as orthostatic hypotension and arrhythmias, make them less desirable. Tricyclic antidepressants are highly cardiotoxic in overdose.

MONOAMINE OXIDASE INHIBITORS (MAOIs)

MAOIs are rarely used as treatment for cancer patients with depression. Patients must adhere to a strict diet while on these medications, as concurrent intake of foods rich in tyramine or the use of sympathomimetic drugs can cause a potentially fatal hypertensive crisis. In addition, there are numerous other potentially severe drug–drug interactions, such as the interaction between MAOIs and meperidine.

NEWER ANTIDEPRESSANTS

This category of antidepressants includes medications with a range of therapeutic mechanisms. Examples are buproprion, nefazodone, trazodone, venlafaxine, duloxetine, mirtazapine.

Buproprion acts primarily on the dopamine system and may have a mild stimulant effect, which can be beneficial for individuals with fatigue or psychomotor retardation. It is generally not associated with weight gain or sexual dysfunction and has an additional application for use in the pharmacotherapy of smoking cessation. It is generally tolerated well. Buproprion is associated with an increased risk of seizures at higher doses and should not be used in individuals with central nervous system disorders or seizure disorders. Newer extended release forms of buproprion allow for dosing once or twice daily.

Both nefazodone and trazodone block postsynaptic serotonin 5-HT$_2$ receptors.

Nefazodone has been associated with less sexual dysfunction than the SSRIs, although it has recently received a black box warning concerning cases of hepatic failure. Trazodone is often used as a nonaddictive sleep aid, rather than a primary antidepressant because of its main side effect of sedation. Other rare side effects include priapism and cardiac arrhythmias.

Venlafaxine and duloxetine work as a reuptake inhibitor of serotonin and norepinephrine (SNRI). They are generally well tolerated, with a benign side effect profile similar to SSRIs. However, norepinephrine reuptake inhibition may result in palpitations, and hypertension. Therefore, blood pressure monitoring is recommended for patients on an SNRI. Venlafaxine mostly inhibits serotonin reuptake at low doses; its effect on norepinephrine reuptake inhibition is seen at doses higher than 150 mg a day. Venlafaxine should be slowly titrated up to prevent side effects. The extended release form of venlafaxine allows it to be dosed once or twice daily *(49)*. Duloxetine shows serotonin and norepinephrine reuptake inhibition at starting doses. Both medications have low P450 inhibition and moderate plasma protein binding *(50)*. Venlafaxine and duloxetine are preferably used for patients with comorbid depression and neuropathic pain.

Mirtazapine acts by blocking the 5-HT$_2$, 5-HT$_3$, and α2 adrenergic receptor sites. Its side effects of sedation and weight gain are beneficial for many cancer patients with insomnia and weight loss. It also has antiemetic properties *(51)*. At lower doses, the sedating effect is greater and at doses higher than 30 mg a day the sedating effect is less pronounced and the antidepressant effect becomes more prominent. It is also available in a dissolvable tablet form, which is particularly useful for patients who cannot swallow or who have difficulty with nausea and vomiting. Interactions with the P450 system are minimal *(51)*.

Psychostimulants and wakefulness-promoting agents are helpful to treat depressed cancer patients' symptoms of fatigue, and poor concentration. Psychostimulants exert dopaminergic effects. Psychostimulants used in cancer patients include dextroamphetamine and methylphenidate. They have a major advantage over antidepressants due to their fast onset of action, decreasing fatigue, promoting wakefulness and countering opioid-related sedation. Side effects may be anorexia, anxiety, insomnia, euphoria, irritability, and mood lability. However, side effects are not common at low doses and can be avoided by slow titration. Hypertension and cardiac complications can occur; thus, it is advisable to monitor cardiac function *(52, 53)*. For depressed cancer patients with short survival expectancy, psychostimulants provide rapid relief from distressing depressive symptoms. However, initiating antidepressants at low doses and titration upward as tolerated provides similar benefits over a longer period of time *(16)*. Modafinil is known as a wakefulness-promoting agent with unknown mechanism of action. It produces increased alertness, wakefulness, and energy. It is better tolerated than the psychostimulants, but may also cause anxiety, restlessness, and insomnia. It should be used with caution in patients with poorly controlled hypertension *(54, 55)*.

Psychotherapy

Several different psychotherapeutic techniques have been successfully employed with depressed cancer patients, and psychotherapy is often combined with a pharmacologic intervention. The most commonly utilized forms of psychotherapy are supportive psychotherapy and cognitive-behavioral therapy. In supportive psychotherapy, the clinician adopts an empathic approach, offers emotional support, provides information to help the patient focus on adaptive coping strategies, emphasizing past strengths and supporting previously successful ways of coping. Cognitive-behavioral therapy aims to alter patients' thoughts and behaviors that adversely impact mood. Cognitive-behavioral interventions encourage the patient to reframe their problems more constructively to reduce overwhelming distress.

Group therapy can be helpful to improve social networks, connecting the patient with others who have the same diagnosis and/or treatment, decreasing the patient's sense of isolation. Supportive-expressive and cognitive-existential group psychotherapies have been used successfully for cancer patients *(56, 57)*.

An important aspect of the treatment of depressed cancer patients is social support provided by family, friends, and community or religious groups. Vulnerable family members are also identified and encouraged to seek individual or group support.

Electroconvulsive Therapy

Electroconvulsive therapy (ECT) is an effective treatment modality for depressed patients. ECT should be considered in patients who are refractory to psychopharmacologic treatment, have severe weight loss secondary to depression, exhibit acute psychosis, or have a high suicide risk *(58)*. Although there are no absolute contraindications to ECT, it is used with caution among individuals with central nervous system tumors or cardiac problems.

CONCLUSION

Depression is a common psychiatric complication of cancer, and is an important risk factor for suicide. Diagnosis of depression in the context of cancer is challenging. Recognizing the risk factors for depression, with careful attention to the signs and symptoms of depression, leads to improved recognition and treatment of depressive disorders, thus increasing adherence to cancer treatment, improving quality of life, and reducing serious consequences such as desire for hastened death and suicide.

REFERENCES

1. Bukberg J, Penman D, Holland JC. Depression in hospitalized cancer patients. Psychosom Med 1984;46:199–212.
2. Massie MJ. Prevalence of depression in patients with cancer. J of National Cancer Inst Monogr 2004;32:57–71.
3. McDaniel JS, Musselman DL, Porter MR, Reed DA, Nemeroff CB. Depression in patients with cancer: diagnosis, biology, and treatment. Arch Gen Psychiatry 1995;52:89–99.
4. Blazer DG, Kessler KC, McGonagle KA, Swartz MS. The prevalence and distribution of major depression in a national community sample: The National Comorbidity Survey. Am J Psychiatry 1994;151:979–986.
5. Chochinov HM, Wilson KG, Enns M, Lander S. Prevalence of depression in the terminally ill: Effects of diagnostic criteria and symptom threshold judgments. Am J Psychiatry 1994;151:537–540.
6. Coups EJ, Winell J, Holland JC. Depression in the context of cancer. In: Licinio J, Ma-Le Wong, eds. Biology of Depression: From Novel Insights to Therapeutic Strategies, Vol. 1. Weinheim, Germany: Wiley, 2005:365–385.
7. Roth AJ, Holland JC. Treatment of depression in cancer patients. Prim Care Cancer 1994;14:23–29.
8. Cohen-Cole SA, Brown FW, McDanile JS. Diagnostic assessment of depression in the medically ill. In: Stoudemire A, Fogel BS, eds. Psychiatric Care of the Medical Patient. New York: Oxford University Press, 1993:53–70.
9. Spitzer RL, Endicott J, Robins E. Research diagnostic criteria: rationale and reliability. Arch Gen Psychiatry 1978;35:773–782.
10. American Psychiatric Association. Diagnostic and Statistical Manual of Mental Disorders, 4th ed. Washington, DC: American Psychiatric Association, 1994.
11. Medical Letter. Drugs that cause psychiatric symptoms. Med Lett 1993;35:65–70.
12. Newport DJ, Nemeroff CB. Assessment and treatment of depression in the cancer patient. J Psychosom Res 1998;45:215–237.
13. Ebrahimi B, Tucker SL, Li D, et al. Cytokines in pancreatic carcinoma. Cancer 2004;101:2727–2736.
14. Lerner DM, Stoudemire A, Rosenstein DL. Cytokine-induced neuropsychiatric toxicity. In: Holland SM, ed. Cytokine Therapeutics in Infectious Diseases. Philadelphia, PA: Lippincott Williams & Wilkins, 2001:323–332.
15. Musselman DL, Lawson DH, Gumnick JF, Manatunga AK, Penna S, et al. Paroxetine for the prevention of depression induced by high-dose interferon alfa. N Engl J Med 2001;344:961–966.
16. Holland JH, Friedlander MM. Oncology. In: Blumenfield M, Strain JJ, eds. Psychosomatic Medicine. Philadelphia, PA: Lippincott Williams & Wilkins, 2006:121–144.
17. Plumb MM, Holland JC. Comparative studies of psychological function in patients with advanced cancer – II. Interviewer-rated current and past psychological symptoms. Psychosom Med 1981;43:243–254.
18. Spiegel D, Sand S, Koopman C. Pain and depression in patients with cancer. Cancer 1994;74:2570–2578.
19. Kathol RG, Mutgi A, Williams J, Clamon G, Noyes R Jr. Diagnosis of major depression in cancer patients according to four sets of criteria. Am J Psychiatry 1990;147:1021–1024.
20. Schroevers MJ, Ranchor AV, Sanderman R. The role of social support and self-esteem in the presence and course of depressive symptoms: a comparison of cancer patients and individuals from the general population. Soc Sci Med 2003;57:375–385.
21. Kessler RC, McGonagle KA, Swartz M, Blazer DG, Nelson CB. Sex and depression in the National Comorbidity Survey. I: Lifetime prevalence, chronicity and recurrence. J Affect Disord 1993;29:85–96.
22. DeFlorio ML, Massie MJ. Review of depression in cancer: gender differences. Depression 1995;3:66–80.
23. Bolund C. Suicide and cancer. II: Medical and care factors in suicide by cancer patients in Sweden. 1973–1976. J Psychosoc Oncol 1985;3:17–30.
24. Farberow NL, Ganzler S, Cuter F, Reynolds D. An eight-year survey of hospital suicides. Suicide Life Threat Behav 1971;1:198–201.
25. Louhivuori KA, Hakama J. Risk of suicide among cancer patients. Am J Epidemiol 1979;109:59–65.
26. Weisman AD. Coping behavior and suicide in cancer. In: Cullen JW, Fox BH, Ison RN, eds. Cancer: The Behavioral Dimensions. New York: Raven press, 1976.
27. Conwell Y, Caine ED. Rational suicide and the right to die: reliability and myth. N Engl J Med 1991;325:1100.
28. Chochinov HM, Wilson KG, Ennis M, et al. Desire for death in the terminally ill. Am J Psychiatry 1995;152:1185–1191.
29. Chochinov HM, Wilson KG, Ennis M, Lander S. Depression, hopelessness, and suicidal ideation in the terminally ill. Psychosomatics 1998;39:336–370.

30. Rosenfeld B, Krevo S, Breitbart W, et al. Suicide, assisted suicide, and euthanasia in the terminally ill. In: Chochinov H, Breitbart W, eds. Handbook of Psychiatry in Palliative Medicine. New York, NY: Oxford University Press, 2000:51–63.

31. Achte KA, Vanhkouen ML. Cancer and the psyche. Omega 1971;2:46–56.

32. Breitbart W. Suicide risk and pain in cancer and AIDS patients. In: Chapman CR, Foley KM, eds. Current and Emerging Issues in Cancer Pain: Research and Practice. New York, NY: Raven press, 1993:49–65.

33. Kendal WS. Suicide and cancer: a gender-comparative study. Ann Oncol 2006 Oct 19; epub ahead of print.

34. Schairer C, Brown LM, Chen BE, et al. Suicide after breast cancer: an international population-based study of 723 810 women. J Natl Cancer Inst 2006;98:1416–1419.

35. Holland JC, Gooen-Piels J: Psycho-oncology. In: Holland JC, Frei E, eds. Cancer Medicine, 6th ed. Hamilton, Ontario: B.C. Decker Inc, 2003:1039–1053.

36. Hietanen P, Lonnqvist J. Cancer and suicide. Ann Oncol 1991;2:19.

37. Breitbart W, Cohen K. Delirium. In: Holland JC, ed. Psycho-Oncology. New York, NY: Oxford University Press, 1998:564–575.

38. Recklitis CJ, Lockwood RA, Rothwell MA, Diller LR. Suicidal ideation and attempts in adult survivors of childhood cancer. J Clin Oncol 2006;24:3852–3857.

39. Dubovsky SL. Averting suicide in terminally ill patients. Psychosomatics 1978;19:113–115.

40. Potash M, Breitbart W. Affective disorders in advanced cancer. Hematol/Oncol Clin North Am 2002;16:671–700.

41. American Psychiatric Association. Practice Guidelines for the Treatment of Patients with Major Depressive Disorder, 2nd ed. Arlington, VA: American Psychiatric Publishing, Inc., 2000.

42. The National Comprehensive Cancer Network. Distress Management Clinical Practice Guidelines in Oncology, version 1.2007.

43. Frazer A, Benmansour S. Delayed pharmacological effects of antidepressants. Mol Psychiatry 2002;7(Suppl 1):S23–S28.

44. Hemaryeck A, Belpaire FM. Selective serotonin reuptake inhibitors and cytochrome P-450 mediated drug–drug interactions: an update. Curr Drug Metab 2002;3:13–37.

45. Joshi N, Breitbart WS. Psychopharmacologic management during cancer treatment. Semin Clin Neuropsychiatry 2003;8:241–252.

46. DeVane CL. Differential pharmacology of newer antidepressants. J Clin Psychiatry 1998;59(Suppl 20):85–93.

47. Burke WJ. Escitalopram. Expert Opin Investig Drugs 2002;11:1477–1486.

48. Masand PS, Gupta S. Selective serotonin-reuptake inhibitors: an update. Harv Rev Psychiatry 1999;7:69–84.

49. Horst WD, Preskorn SH. Mechanisms of action and clinical characteristics of three atypical antidepressants: venlafaxine, nefazodone, bupropion. J Affect Disord 1998;51:237–254.

50. Dugan SE, Fuller MA. Duloxetine: a dual reuptake inhibitor. Ann Pharmacother 2004;38:2078–2085.

51. Nutt DJ. Tolerability and safety aspects of mirtazaoine. Hum Psychopharmacol 2002;17(Suppl 1):S37–S41.

52. DeMarchi R, Bansal V, Hung A, et al. Review of awakening agents. Can J Neurol Sci 2005;32:4–17.

53. Morrow GR, Shelke AR, Roscoe JA, et al. Management of cancer-related fatigue. Cancer Invest 2005;23:229–239.

54. Robertson P Jr., Hellrigel ET. Clinical pharmacokinetic profile of Modafinil. Clin Pharmacokinet 2003;42:123–137.

55. Wisor JP, Eriksson KS. Dopaminergic–adrenergic interactions in the wake promoting mechanism of Modafinil. Neuroscience 2005;132:1027–1034.

56. Classen C, Butler LD, Koopman C, Miller E, DiMiceli S, Giese-Davis J, Fobair P, Carlson RW, Kraemer HC, Spiegel D. Supportive-expressive group therapy and distress in patient with metastatic cancer: a randomized clinical intervention trial. Arch Gen Psychiatry 2001;58:494–501.

57. Kissane DW, Bloch S, Smith GC et al. Cognitive-existential group psychotherapy for women with primary breast cancer: a randomized controlled trial. Psychooncology 2003;12:532–546.

58. Beale MD, Kellner CH, Parsons PJ. ECT for the treatment of mood disorders in cancer patients. Convuls Ther 1997;13:222–226.

8 Anemia

George M. Rodgers

ABSTRACT

Anemia management is an important aspect of comprehensive care of the cancer patient. Many cancer patients receive suboptimal care in terms of anemia treatment. These patients should have an initial laboratory evaluation to exclude conditions such as iron or vitamin deficiency, and hemolysis. If these diagnoses are excluded, a diagnosis of anemia of cancer or chemotherapy is suggested. This condition results in functional iron deficiency and erythropoietin deficiency, and can be treated successfully in most patients with erythropoietic drugs and parenteral iron. This chapter summarizes appropriate use of these drugs and reviews their recommended doses, benefits, and risks.

From: *Cancer and Drug Discovery Development: Supportive Care in Cancer Therapy*
DOI: 10.1007/978-1-59745-291-5_8, Edited by: D. S. Ettinger © Humana Press, Totowa, NJ

Key Words: Erythropoietin, Darbepoetin, Epoetin, Parenteral iron, Anemia, Chemotherapy.

INTRODUCTION

While anemia is commonly associated with cancer and its treatment, many cancer patients receive no supportive therapy for their anemia. For example, a survey published in 2002 reported that the annual number of cancer patients receiving chemotherapy was ~800,000; of these, only ~200,000 or 25% received anemia treatment *(1)*. Although the number of cancer patients receiving supportive care for anemia has probably improved over the past few years, anemia management remains an important aspect of quality cancer care, and the Centers for Medicare and Medicaid Services has established a 2005 Demonstration Project focused on measuring patient outcomes in supportive care of cancer patients, including anemia management.

This chapter will review strategies for evaluating the anemic cancer patient and suggest one approach to managing these patients. The treatment approach is based on recent guideline recommendations issued by the National Comprehensive Cancer Network (NCCN) Anemia Panel *(2)*. The role of parenteral iron therapy will be discussed, as well as potential adverse effects of anemia therapies.

INITIAL LABORATORY EVALUATION

For purposes of this discussion, anemia is defined as a hemoglobin (Hb) <11 g/dL. Anemia in cancer patients may result from numerous causes, including bleeding associated with thrombocytopenia related to the tumor or its treatment, nutritional deficiency of vitamin B_{12} or folic acid, hemolysis as seen in some lymphoproliferative disorders, or as a result of the "chronic disease" or chemotherapy state. Before it is assumed that anemia in a cancer patient is due to chemotherapy or "chronic disease," it is prudent to exclude other treatable causes as mentioned above. Otherwise, patients with iron or vitamin deficiency, or hemolysis *(2)* will have a suboptimal response to erythropoietic drugs until correction of the underlying problem. An appropriate initial laboratory evaluation would include iron studies (serum iron, total iron binding capacity, ferritin), vitamin B_{12} and folic acid levels, a chemistry panel to include lactate dehydrogenase and bilirubin, and a Coombs test to exclude hemolysis. Evaluation of the peripheral blood smear may also be helpful.

If the baseline evaluation does not suggest another etiology, then a diagnosis of "anemia of cancer or chemotherapy" is suggested.

PATHOPHYSIOLOGY OF THE ANEMIA OF CANCER OR CHEMOTHERAPY

Figure 1 illustrates mechanisms contributing to the anemia of cancer or chemotherapy. Similar mechanisms are seen in the "anemia of chronic disease" associated with renal failure, inflammation, etc. In all of these anemias, inflammatory cytokines such as interleukin-1 or tumor necrosis factor elaborated from activated mononuclear cells suppress erythropoiesis and inhibit endogenous erythropoietin production. Red blood cell survival is usually shortened in these patients. Although serum iron levels in these patients are low, bone marrow iron stores are adequate or increased, indicating a defect in iron utilization. This state has been termed "functional iron deficiency."

TREATMENT OPTIONS FOR THE ANEMIA OF CANCER
OR CHEMOTHERAPY

The reasons to treat anemia in this setting include reducing complications of severe anemia (ischemia), and improving quality of life (QOL). Standard treatment in the past consisted of packed red cell transfusions for symptomatic relief of anemic symptoms. While efficacious in promptly relieving symptoms, chronic red cell transfusion may lead to problems, including iron overload, alloimmunization leading to diminished transfusion response, as well as potential viral infection risks.

Appreciation of the mechanisms contributing to the anemia of cancer or chemotherapy (Fig. 1) suggests alternative treatment options, specifically erythropoietic drugs and iron therapy. The positive results of clinical studies using erythropoietic drugs that

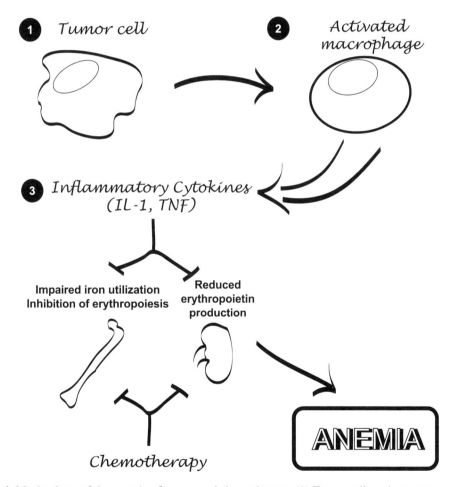

Fig. 1. Mechanisms of the anemia of cancer and chemotherapy. (1) Tumor cells activate mononuclear cells (T-cells, macrophages). (2) Activated mononuclear cells secrete inflammatory cytokines. (3) Cytokines inhibit red cell production by impairing iron utilization and suppressing growth of erythroid progenitors. Cytokines also reduce renal erythropoietin production. Chemotherapeutic agents also contribute to anemia by suppression of erythropoiesis and by reducing renal erythropoietin production. Red blood cell survival is also shortened in this condition (not shown).

took into consideration QOL issues as an endpoint have dramatically changed the supportive care of cancer patients with anemia. Cancer or treatment-related fatigue is underrecognized and suboptimally managed (1); one study reported that cancer patient fatigue occurred on at least a few days of each month in 76% of chemotherapy patients (3).

The first trial reporting the effects of an erythropoietic agent (epoetin alfa) on both reducing red cell transfusion requirements and improving anemia-specific QOL in cancer patients receiving chemotherapy was published by Littlewood et al. (4). Similar results have been demonstrated with darbepoetin alfa (5). Numerous studies have subsequently confirmed beneficial effects of erythropoietic drug therapy (2), and the treating physician has several treatment options to manage anemia in the cancer patient (discussed below).

THE TARGET HEMOGLOBIN FOR ERYTHROPOIETIC DRUG THERAPY

The erythropoietic drugs are very active in increasing hemoglobin, hematocrit, and red cell mass in cancer patients. Excessive improvement or normalization of hemoglobin levels may lead to hypertension, thrombosis, and even death. Consequently, recommendations for use of these drugs strongly suggest that physicians target hemoglobin levels less than that considered typically normal. The data on which the recommended target hemoglobin level is based is from an analysis of two large community oncology trials in which epoetin alfa was the erythropoietic drug used (6).

Results of this analysis indicated that there was a positive correlation between improving hemoglobin levels and improving QOL scores. Maximum QOL gain occurred at a hemoglobin level of 12 g/dL. The greatest incremental gain in QOL occurred when hemoglobin levels increased from 11 g/dL to 12 g/dL (6). Thus, previous guidelines for erythropoietic drug therapy recommended initiating treatment at a hemoglobin level <11 g/dL and targeting a level of 12 g/dL (7). More recently, based on safety concerns (discussed below), guidelines now recommend initiating therapy at a hemoglobin level <10 g/dL and targeting a level of 10 to <12 g/dL (2).

FDA-APPROVED REGIMENS FOR ERYTHROPOIETIC DRUGS IN CANCER- AND TREATMENT-RELATED ANEMIA

Table 1 summarizes the recommended regimens for darbepoetin alfa and epoetin alfa as of July 2008. Epoetin alfa is approved for weekly subcutaneous dosing both in a weight-based and standard dosage format (150 U/kg tiw or 40,000 U/week). If there is no hemoglobin response after four weeks, dose escalation is recommended (300 U/kg tiw or 60,000 U/week). Clinical trials supporting the epoetin alfa regimens have been published (reviewed in (2)).

Darbepoetin alfa is approved for both weekly and every 3-week dosing regimens: 2.25 µg/kg/week and 500 µg q3 week, respectively (5, 8). Dose escalation for the weekly regimen is approved for 4.5 mg/kg/week if there is no hemoglobin response by four weeks.

Table 1
Recommended doses and regimens for erythropoietic drugs in cancer patients receiving chemotherapy

Epoetin alfa	
	150 U/kg tiw (300 U/kg tiw if no response after 4 weeks)
	Or
	40,000 U/week (60,000 U/week if no response after 4 weeks)
Darbepoetin alfa	
	2.25 µg/kg/week (4.5 µg/kg/week if no response after 6 weeks)
	Or
	500 µg q3 week

tiw three times weekly, *q3 week* every 3 weeks

COMMONLY USED, OFF-LABEL ERYTHROPOIETIC DRUG REGIMENS

Both epoetin alfa and darbepoetin alfa have been studied in cancer patients treated every two weeks *(9, 10)*. An every-3-week epoetin alfa regimen has also been investigated *(11)*.

INITIATION OF ERYTHROPOIETIC THERAPY

The revised ASCO/ASH anemia guideline was published in 2008; recommendations were based on the literature through 2007. This guideline recommended a Hb value <10 g/dL to initiate treatment with erythropoietic drugs *(12)*. The NCCN guideline recommends a threshold Hb <11 g/dL for treatment initiation *(2)*. This higher threshold Hb value is supported by a meta-analysis that included data from 1999–2004 *(13)*. Results of this analysis suggested a clinical benefit associated with initiating treatment at a Hb >10 g/dL; such intervention significantly reduced the relative risk of red cell transfusion and a subsequent Hb decline below 10 g/dL. Significant QOL benefits were also identified with early intervention *(13)*.

DOSE MODIFICATION OF ERYTHROPOIETIC DRUGS

To avoid complications of overly rapid correction of red cell mass (hypertension, thrombosis), the NCCN guideline recommends that if the Hb increase is more than 1 g/dL in a 2-week period, that dose should be reduced by 25–50%. If the Hb value exceeds 12 g/dL, erythropoietic drug, therapy should be held and then restarted when the Hb falls below 12 g/dL with a 25–50% dose reduction.

MONITORING OF IRON STORES

Current recommendations of the NCCN Anemia Panel are to check serum ferritin levels as well as serum iron/total iron binding capacity prior to initiation of erythropoietic therapy *(2)*. If the serum ferritin is <300 ng/mL, or if the transferrin saturation is <20%, functional iron deficiency likely exists and the patient will probably benefit from parenteral iron therapy in combination with an erythropoietic drug (discussed below). The Auerbach study that investigated the effectiveness of oral versus i.v. iron therapy in anemic cancer patients receiving chemotherapy had treatment iron value criteria of ferritin ≤200 ng/mL, or ferritin ≤300 ng/mL with a transferrin saturation ≤19% *(14)*.

While the patient continues to receive erythropoietic drug therapy, iron studies should be monitored on a regular basis to ensure that functional iron deficiency will not occur and diminish the patient's response.

ADVERSE EVENTS ASSOCIATED WITH ERYTHROPOIETIC THERAPY

Use of epoetin alfa and darbepoetin alfa in cancer patients is associated with potential risks. Compared to placebo-treated patients, cancer patients who received either erythropoietic drug were more likely to experience the following adverse events: edema, diarrhea, hypertension, and thrombosis. In terms of the thrombosis risk, the largest clinical trial comparing the two drugs head to head in cancer patients found that 6% of darbepoetin alfa and 7% of epoetin alfa patients experienced cardiovascular/thromboembolic events *(15)*. There were no cases of neutralizing antibodies to erythropoietin found nor cases of pure red cell aplasia *(15)*.

CONTROVERSIAL ISSUES WITH ERYTHROPOIETIC DRUG THERAPY

Are Epoetin Alfa and Darbepoetin Alfa Equivalent?

The clinical equivalence of the two erythropoietic agents in cancer patients has been investigated in both retrospective studies (medication use evaluations, chart audits) as well as prospective trials. Endpoints of these studies have included red cell transfusion rates, change in hemoglobin level, time to target hemoglobin, necessity for dose escalation, and drug safety.

Four prospective comparison studies of epoetin alfa versus darbepoetin alfa in cancer patients receiving chemotherapy have been published *(15– 18)*. Three of the four trials found that the two drugs were similar in terms of efficacy and safety *(15–17)*; all three of these trials studied the every-2-week time interval for darbepoetin treatment. The statistical term used in many of these studies to imply equivalence was "noninferiority." One trial found that therapy with epoetin alfa resulted in a higher response rate *(18)*; this study compared weekly epoetin alfa (40,000 U) versus darbepoetin alfa (200 µg every 2 weeks).

Two recent reviews surveyed the medical literature on the subject of comparative trials of the two erythropoietic drugs in chemotherapy-related anemia *(19, 20)*. Both trials concluded that the drugs have equivalent efficacy and safety *(19, 20)*. One study calculated the odds ratio (OR) for transfusions; for epoetin alfa, the OR for transfusion was 0.44 (95% CI 0.35–0.55), and for darbepoetin alfa, the OR for transfusion was 0.41 (95% CI 0.31–0.55) *(16)*. Thus, the preponderance of the data at this time indicates that the two erythropoietic drugs are equivalent. The decision as to which drug to use is based on patient and physician preference (dose schedules) and cost.

Do Erythropoietic Drugs Affect Cancer Patient Survival?

This provocative question was raised by the results of two trials, one in breast cancer patients *(21)* and the other in head and neck cancer patients *(22)*. The breast cancer trial had as its primary objective measuring survival and QOL in breast cancer patients who received either placebo or epoetin alfa to maintain hemoglobin levels in the 12–14 g/dL range. The study was prematurely terminated because of higher mortality in the epoetin alfa group from vascular events (arterial and venous thrombosis). Although the time to disease progression was similar in both the placebo and epoetin alfa groups, an effect of the drug on tumor progression could not be excluded *(21)*. The major conclusion from this breast cancer study was that normalization of hemoglobin levels should not be achieved, and that tight control of hemoglobin levels is desirable.

The second trial in head and neck cancer patients receiving radiation therapy (no chemotherapy) randomized patients to receive either epoetin beta or placebo *(22)*. Patients who received epoetin beta had increased tumor progression and decreased survival. However, post hoc trial analysis indicated methodologic concerns that may have confounded the trial results, including lack of prognostic factor balance that would favor the placebo group, protocol variations, and excessive Hb correction in the epoetin beta group *(23)*.

In contrast to these two individual studies, a meta-analysis of 57 clinical trials in which epoetin or darbepoetin therapy were compared with placebo was reported *(24)*. The authors concluded that (a) erythropoietic drugs reduce the relative risk for red cell transfusion; (b) there is suggestive evidence that these drugs improve QOL; (c) erythropoietic drugs increase the relative risk of thromboembolism (RR 1.67); and (d) no definitive effect of erythropoietic drugs on cancer patient survival can be demonstrated, favorably or unfavorably *(24)*. A more recent meta-analysis by Bennett et al. of phase III trials between 1985–2008 found that erythropoietic drug therapy was associated with a significantly higher risk for death *(25)*. However, when the data was analyzed based on anemia of cancer trials vs. anemia of cancer and chemotherapy trials, the mortality effect was restricted to the anemia of cancer subgroup *(25)*.

At this time, the preponderance of the data indicates no definite effect of erythropoietic drugs on survival of cancer patients receiving chemotherapy. Several prospective clinical trials are ongoing to directly address this question, and they will have sufficient power individually to detect an absolute difference in survival between 7–11%; collectively, a meta-analysis of these trials will have an 80% power to detect a hazard ratio for survival as low as 1.15 *(26)*. Additionally, an updated Cochrane group meta-analysis of patient-level data is pending *(27)*. Until this data is available it would be prudent to use erythropoietic drugs in a manner that minimizes possible risk by not exceeding a target Hb level of 12 g/dL. The NCCN guideline suggests that patients be counseled about the risks and benefits of erythropoietic drug therapy vs. red cell transfusion *(2)*.

What is the Role of Parenteral Iron Therapy?

The discussion above has focused on the role of erythropoietic drugs to improve the anemia of cancer or chemotherapy. However, as shown in Fig. 1, there is another potential treatment strategy — iron therapy. Even though many cancer patients will have improvement in Hb levels with erythropoietic therapy alone, ~30% of these patients will have a suboptimal response (failure to achieve the target Hb or a Hb rise <2 g/dL (28); adding iron therapy to a patient's erythropoietic drug therapy would be expected to enhance their erythropoietic response.

When erythropoietic drugs are used to treat anemia in other "chronic disease" settings, such as the hemodialysis setting, large amounts of iron are necessary to keep up with the demands of erythropoietic agent-induced erythropoiesis. In the hemodialysis setting, oral iron supplementation is inadequate, and intravenous iron replacement is required (29). The first study to suggest that parenteral iron therapy is important in managing patients with anemia of cancer or chemotherapy was reported by Auerbach et al. (30). This study randomized nonmyeloid cancer patients with anemia into four groups: no iron therapy, oral iron therapy (325 mg twice daily), i.v. iron dextran bolus (100 mg weekly), and i.v. iron dextran (total dose infusion at the initial visit). All patients received epoetin alfa 40,000 U weekly, so the major variable was whether iron supplementation was received, and, if so, whether oral or i.v. iron was used. Major endpoints in this trial were Hb increase and QOL measures.

Although all groups demonstrated a Hb increase from baseline (all patients received epoetin alfa), the Hb increase in patients receiving either i.v. bolus iron or i.v. total dose infusion was statistically greater than the Hb increase seen in the no iron and oral iron patient groups. Similarly, both i.v. iron groups demonstrated increased QOL scores compared to the groups receiving no iron or oral iron (30). These results clearly indicate that intravenous iron optimizes the response to erythropoietic drugs.

How Should This Information Be Translated into Routine Clinical Practice?

Many physicians are wary of iron dextran, whose use has been associated with anaphylaxis and death. Therefore, it is important to note that not all iron dextran products are equivalent. The older iron dextran products (Imferon®, DexFerrum®) are high-molecular-weight (HMW) products with a higher incidence of adverse events (31). In contrast, InFed® is a low-molecular-weight (LMW) iron dextran product with a better safety profile (31). The Auerbach et al. study primarily used InFed® (30).

If iron dextran is used to treat functional iron deficiency of cancer or chemotherapy, patients should be treated with methylprednisolone before and after the infusion (30), or with diphenhydramine and acetaminophen before infusion (32). Alternatively, other parenteral iron products are available to treat functional iron deficiency, including iron gluconate (Ferrlecit®) and iron sucrose (Venofer®) (33). Table 2 summarizes parenteral iron therapy options currently available, as well as their advantages and disadvantages, recommended dosing of each drug, and cost. DexFerrum® is not listed because of its unfavorable safety profile; clinicians who desire to use an iron dextran product are urged to consider InFed®. The safest parenteral iron product is probably iron sucrose (Venofer®) (34); however, it is more expensive and repeated doses are necessary to fully

Table 2
Parenteral iron products and their use

Product	Trade names	Dosage	Test dose	Life-threatening adverse events[a] (per million)	Cost[b]
Iron dextran	InFed®	100 mg over 2–5 min or total dose infusion	Required on first infusion	3.3	$377
Iron gluconate	Ferrlecit®	125 mg over 10 min 1–3 times/week	Not required	0.9	$689
Iron sucrose	Venofer®	100 mg over 5 min 1–3 times/week	Not required	0.6	$688

[a]Data obtained from Chertow et al. (31)
[b]As of September 2006, University of Utah Pharmacy. Cost is listed per gram of iron

replete patients' iron stores. Trials in cancer patients receiving iron gluconate *(35)* and iron sucrose *(36)* have been reported. Despite the lack of a requirement for a test dose with iron gluconate and iron sucrose, it is the author's recommendation to give patients who receive any parenteral iron product an initial test dose and routine premedication, since life-threatening adverse events have been associated with all parenteral iron products *(34)*.

For physicians who remain uncertain as to whether the use of parenteral iron products up front is necessary in their patients with anemia of cancer and chemotherapy, one option would be to consider using parenteral iron therapy only in those patients who have had a suboptimal erythropoietic response despite dose escalation. Many of these "nonresponders" will likely be salvaged with the addition of parenteral iron therapy, as has been seen in hemodialysis patients with functional iron deficiency *(29)*. An argument for using parenteral iron therapy "up front" is that iron will enhance the effectiveness of erythropoietic drugs, likely reducing the amount and cost of erythropoietic agent used, as has been seen in the hemodialysis setting *(29)*. Such a strategy will also reduce patient exposure to unnecessarily high doses of erythropoietic drugs.

FUTURE DIRECTIONS

Even under optimal circumstances when erythropoietic drugs are used in combination with parenteral iron, a significant number of patients may not respond *(30)*, and these patients may require red cell transfusion. Whether novel erythropoietic molecules currently under development will be more effective or safer than current therapy in managing the anemia of cancer or chemotherapy remains to be seen. Trials of these agents are ongoing *(37, 38)*.

REFERENCES

1. Tchekmedyian NS. Anemia in cancer patients: significance, epidemiology, and current therapy. Oncology 2002;16(9 Suppl 10):17–24.

2. Rodgers GM, Becker PS, Bennett CL, et al. Cancer- and treatment-related anemia. J Natl Compr Canc Netw 2008;6:536–64.

3. Curt GA, Breitbart W, Cella D, et al. Impact of cancer-related fatigue on the lives of patients: new findings from the Fatigue Coalition. Oncologist 2000;5:353–60.

4. Littlewood TJ, Bajetta E, Nortier JW, et al. Effects of epoetin alfa on hematologic parameters and quality of life in cancer patients receiving nonplatinum chemotherapy: results of a randomized, double-blind, placebo-controlled trial. J Clin Oncol 2001;19:2865–74.

5. Vansteenkiste J, Pirker R, Massuti B, et al. Double-blind, placebo-controlled, randomized phase III trial of darbepoetin alfa in lung cancer patients receiving chemotherapy. J Natl Cancer Inst 2002;94:1211–20.

6. Crawford J, Cella D, Cleeland CS, et al. Relationship between changes in hemoglobin level and quality of life during chemotherapy in anemic cancer patients receiving epoetin alfa therapy. Cancer 2002;95:888–95.

7. Rodgers GM. Guidelines for the use of erythropoietic growth factors in patients with chemotherapy-induced anemia. Oncology 2006;20(Suppl 6):12–15.

8. Canon JL, Vansteenkiste J, Bodoky G, et al. Randomized, double-blind, active-controlled trial of every-3-week darbepoetin alfa for the treatment of chemotherapy-induced anemia. J Natl Cancer Inst 2006;98:273–84.

9. Thames WA, Smith SL, Scheifele AC, et al. Evaluation of the US Oncology Network's recommended guidelines for therapeutic substitution with darbepoetin alfa 200 microg every 2 weeks in both naive patients and patients switched from epoetin alfa. Pharmacotherapy 2004;24:313–23.

10. Henry DH, Gordan LN, Charu V, et al. Randomized, open-label comparison of epoetin alfa extended dosing (80 000 U Q2W) vs weekly dosing (40 000 U QW) in patients with chemotherapy-induced anemia. Curr Med Res Opin 2006;22:1403–13.

11. Patton J, Kuzur M, Liggett W, et al. Epoetin alfa 60,000 U once weekly followed by 120,000 U every 3 weeks increases and maintains hemoglobin levels in anemic cancer patients undergoing chemotherapy. Oncologist 2004;9:90–6. Erratum in: Oncologist 2004;9:240.

12. Rizzo JD, Somerfield MR, Hagerty KL, et al. Use of epoetin and darbepoetin in patients with cancer: 2007 American Society of Hematology/American Society of Clinical Oncology clinical practice guideline update. Blood 2008;111:25–41.

13. Lyman GH, Glaspy J. Are there clinical benefits with early erythropoietic intervention for chemotherapy-induced anemia? A systematic review. Cancer 2006;106:223–33.

14. Auerbach M, Barker L, Bahrain H, et al. Intravenous iron optimizes the response to erythropoietin in patients with anemia of cancer and chemotherapy: results of a multicenter, open-label, randomized trial. Blood 2001;98:799a (abstract).

15. Glaspy J, Vadhan-Raj S, Patel R, et al. Randomized comparison of every-2-week darbepoetin alfa and weekly epoetin alfa for the treatment of chemotherapy-induced anemia: the 20030125 Study Group Trial. J Clin Oncol 2006;24:2290–7.

16. Schwartzberg LS, Yee LK, Senecal FM, et al. A randomized comparison of every-2-week darbepoetin alfa and weekly epoetin alfa for the treatment of chemotherapy-induced anemia in patients with breast, lung, or gynecologic cancer. Oncologist 2004;9:696–707.

17. Senecal FM, Yee L, Gabrail N, et al. Treatment of chemotherapy-induced anemia in breast cancer: results of a randomized controlled trial of darbepoetin alfa 200 microg every 2 weeks versus epoetin alfa 40,000 U weekly. Clin Breast Cancer 2005;6:446–54.

18. Waltzman R, Croot C, Justice GR, et al. Randomized comparison of epoetin alfa (40,000 U weekly) and darbepoetin alfa (200 microg every 2 weeks) in anemic patients with cancer receiving chemotherapy. Oncologist 2005;10:642–50.

19. Ross SD, Allen IE, Henry DH, et al. Clinical benefits and risks associated with epoetin and darbepoetin in patients with chemotherapy-induced anemia: a systematic review of the literature. Clin Ther 2006;28:801–31.

20. Cersosimo RJ, Jacobson DR. Epoetin alfa versus darbepoetin alfa in chemotherapy-related anemia. Ann Pharmacother 2006;40:58–65.

21. Leyland-Jones B, Semiglazov V, Pawlicki M, et al. Maintaining normal hemoglobin levels with epoetin alfa in mainly nonanemic patients with metastatic breast cancer receiving first-line chemotherapy: a survival study. J Clin Oncol 2005;23:5960–72.

22. Henke M, Laszig R, Rube C, et al. Erythropoietin to treat head and neck cancer patients with anaemia undergoing radiotherapy: randomised, double-blind, placebo-controlled trial. Lancet 2003;362:1255–60.

23. Glaspy JA. Cancer patient survival and erythropoietin. J Natl Compr Canc Netw 2005;3:796–804.

24. Bohlius J, Wilson J, Seidenfeld J, et al. Erythropoietin or darbepoetin for patients with cancer. Cochrane Database Syst Rev 2006;3:CD003407.

25. Bennett CL, Silver SM, Djulbegovic B, et al. Venous thromboembolism and mortality associated with recombinant erythropoietin and darbepoetin administration for the treatment of cancer-associated anemia. JAMA 2008;299:914–24.

26. Crawford J. Erythropoiesis-stimulating protein support and survival. Oncology 2006;20(Suppl 6):39–43.

27. Glaspy JA. Erythropoiesis-Stimulating Agents in Oncology. J Natl Compr Canc Netw 2008;6:565–575.

28. Steensma DP, Loprinzi CL. Epoetin alfa and darbepoetin alfa go head to head. J Clin Oncol 2006;24:2233–6.

29. Fishbane S, Frei GL, Maesaka J. Reduction in recombinant human erythropoietin doses by the use of chronic intravenous iron supplementation. Am J Kidney Dis 1995;26:41–6.

30. Auerbach M, Ballard H, Trout JR, et al. Intravenous iron optimizes the response to recombinant human erythropoietin in cancer patients with chemotherapy-related anemia: a multicenter, open-label, randomized trial. J Clin Oncol 2004;22:1301–7.

31. Chertow GM, Mason PD, Vaage-Nilsen O, Ahlmen J. On the relative safety of parenteral iron formulations. Nephrol Dial Transplant 2004;19:1571–5.

32. Laman CA, Silverstein SB, Rodgers GM. Parenteral iron therapy: a single institution's experience over a 5-year period. J Natl Compr Canc Netw 2005;3:791–5.

33. Silverstein SB, Rodgers GM. Parenteral iron therapy options. Am J Hematol 2004;76:74–8.

34. Chertow GM, Mason PD, Vaage-Nilsen O, Ahlmen J. Update on adverse drug events associated with parenteral iron. Nephrol Dial Transplant 2006;21:378–82.

35. Henry DH, Dahl NV, Auerbach M, et al. Intravenous ferric gluconate significantly improves response to epoetin alfa versus oral iron or no iron in anemic patients with cancer receiving chemotherapy. Oncologist 2007;12:231–42.

36. Hedenus M, Birgegård G, Näsman P, et al. Addition of intravenous iron to epoetin beta increases hemoglobin response and decreases epoetin dose requirement in anemic patients with lymphoproliferative malignancies: a randomized multicenter study. Leukemia 2007;21:627–32.

37. Stead RB, Lambert J, Wessels D, et al. Evaluation of the safety and pharmacodynamics of Hematide, a novel erythropoietic agent, in a phase 1, double-blind, placebo-controlled, dose-escalation study in healthy volunteers. Blood 2006;108:1830–4.

38. Macdougall IC, Eckardt KU. Novel strategies for stimulating erythropoiesis and potential new treatments for anaemia. Lancet 2006;368:947–53.

9   Neutropenia

Jeffrey Crawford

ABSTRACT

The development and use of myeloid growth factors in support of cancer patients receiving chemotherapy has had a huge impact on the practice of oncology. While there are several areas of importance, this chapter will focus on the problem of chemotherapy-induced neutropenia and its impact on patient outcomes and potential strategies for management, including dose reduction, prophylactic antibiotics, and myeloid growth factors. In this context, the biology, pharmacology, and pharmacodynamics of myeloid growth factors will be reviewed, as well as the clinical evidence of benefit that have led to the current guidelines for use. Lastly, while the focus will be predominantly around support for chemotherapy-induced neutropenia, the impact of myeloid growth factors in other settings, including high-dose chemotherapy and the management of chronic neutropenia will also be briefly addressed.

Key Words: Neutropenia, Myeloid growth factors, Prophylactic antibiotics.

THE PROBLEM OF NEUTROPENIA IN THE CANCER PATIENT

Since the initial development of cancer chemotherapy, the primary dose-limiting toxicity of chemotherapy has been neutropenia *(1)*. Severe or grade 3 neutropenia is defined as <1,000 neutrophils/MM^3 while grade 4 life-threatening neutropenia is <500 neutrophils/MM^3. While definitions of febrile neutropenia have varied with studies, they generally include a temperature of ≥38.2°C along with either grade 3 or grade 4

From: *Cancer and Drug Discovery Development: Supportive Care in Cancer Therapy*
DOI: 10.1007/978-1-59745-291-5_9, Edited by: D. S. Ettinger © Humana Press, Totowa, NJ

neutropenia, most commonly the latter. While fever and infection can develop at any of these levels of neutropenia, it is most commonly associated with neutropenia <500 cells/ MM^3, the highest risk subgroup of patients with neutrophil count <100 neutrophils/ MM^3. While the depth of neutropenia is a risk factor, the best established relationship of neutropenia to the risk of developing fever and infection relates to the duration of neutropenia. This is well established in early studies of patients with leukemia *(1)*, but also has been well described in the setting of chemotherapy-induced neutropenia in patients with solid tumors *(2)*. In these studies, the risk of fever and infection is roughly linear over the first week to ten days of grade 4 neutropenia; for example, the risk of developing febrile neutropenia is approximately 10% per day. Therefore, for patients with five days of grade 4 neutropenia, a 50% risk of febrile neutropenia can be expected and even 1–2 days of grade 4 neutropenia can be associated with 10–20% risk.

The development of febrile neutropenia should be considered an oncologic emergency. Patients should undergo thorough history, physical examination, and laboratory evaluation, including blood and urine cultures, chest X-ray and other studies as dictated by the clinical presentation. With detailed evaluation, a clinically or microbiologically documented source of infection will be determined in approximately half of patients. While most patients will recover uneventfully, chemotherapy-induced neutropenia still carries substantial risk of both morbidity and mortality. The mortality risk varies with the patient population, disease setting, and type of chemotherapy, but in general is <5% for the majority of solid tumors other than lung cancer, where the risk approaches that of lymphoma and hematologic malignancies. The latter groups have a higher risk of mortality because of the more prolonged duration of neutropenia associated with regimens. For the lung cancer population, the higher mortality may relate to the increased comorbidity that exists in this population and the higher risk for development of life-threatening and fatal pneumonia in the setting of neutropenia. Recent paradigms have attempted to develop risk stratification models to identify patients at low risk for complications of febrile neutropenia that might be managed by treatment and careful follow-up in the outpatient setting. However, in the absence of a well-structured support system to accomplish this, standard care for the majority of patients with febrile neutropenia remains hospitalization and intravenous broad spectrum empiric antibiotics pending laboratory imaging and culture results to help direct therapy. The duration of therapy is based both on the initial and ongoing evaluation in the hospital and is most often dictated by recovery of the neutrophil count to >500 or 1,000 neutrophils/MM^3. Continued use of antibiotics after neutrophil recovery is not necessary in the patient who has been afebrile and had no source of infection identified. On the other hand, patients who have an infection in this setting should continue on appropriate antibiotic therapy after neutrophil recovery as appropriate to that infection. However, several critical clinical points are the early recognition of fever in the setting of neutropenia, prompt evaluation, and urgent administration of appropriate antibiotics and medical management. For patients whose fever is an indicator of Gram negative bacteremia, for example, a delay in treatment, even hours can literally mean a difference between life and death.

In addition to the major clinical consequences of febrile neutropenia, even mild to moderate neutropenia can pose a problem. While neutrophil counts between 1,000 and 1,500 neutrophils/MM^3 are not known to be associated with increased likelihood of infection in the absence of other risk factors, neutrophil counts in this range on the day of planned treatment do generally lead to chemotherapy dose delays or reductions depending on the regimen. The impact of these dose reductions and delays on ultimate treatment outcome has not been well studied and will be discussed further under treatment strategies in the next section. However, at a minimum, these alterations in treatment plan do result in patient concern about not receiving the planned treatments and logistical difficulties in time lost from work for both patients and their care providers, and complicates scheduling for both patients and practitioners. Thus, in addition to the potential physical consequences of neutropenia and increasing risk of infection, there is a psychological impact in increasing anxiety for patients around alterations in treatment planning and general concern that the neutropenia may worsen leading to a risk for infection. Furthermore, health care providers continue to provide varied information to patients about special diets, avoiding crowds, etc. that can lead to social isolation. Much of this advice is unwarranted in most patients receiving outpatient chemotherapy in which the likelihood of prolonged neutropenia is relatively low, but it continues to be a factor that impacts quality of life for these patients. Formal studies of quality of life related to symptoms of both anxiety and fatigue that may occur as a result of neutropenia per se have been studied by Cella and colleagues *(3)* in the development of the FACT neutropenia scale and other instruments, but it has been difficult to fully assess the relationship of quality of life measures to neutropenia per se, since patients who experience neutropenia are also often more likely to have other chemotherapy-related side effects, including anemia, mucositis, etc., that may also complicate such analyses. The economic impact of neutropenia in patients receiving cancer chemotherapy is substantial, in terms of the direct expenses associated with hospitalization, IV antibiotics, and follow-up care; in the altered treatment plans associated with lesser degrees of neutropenia; and the indirect costs of care *(4)*. The costs of myeloid growth factors must also be considered but when used by current practice guidelines they can minimize or actually reduce overall healthcare costs.

STRATEGIES FOR MANAGEMENT OF CHEMOTHERAPY-INDUCED NEUTROPENIA

Dose Reduction Delay

Because of the major clinical consequences of chemotherapy-induced neutropenia, the primary strategy for management should be that of prevention. However, because we haven't fully identified patient risk models, even with application of appropriate practice guidelines, neutropenia and febrile neutropenia will continue to be a common complication of chemotherapy. In the area of prevention, there are three basic strategies that can be considered alone or in combination and they include chemotherapy dose reduction and/or delay, the use of prophylactic antibiotics, and/or the use of myeloid growth factors.

Chemotherapy dose reduction and delay have been the time-honored approaches to reduce toxicities of chemotherapy. Prior to the advent of myeloid growth factors, these were literally the only fully effective approaches for this, but with unclear impact on potential reduction in treatment benefit. As we are all aware, the dose and schedule of chemotherapy regimens that we use have largely been developed to deliver treatment at the maximum tolerated dose (MTD). With the vast majority of cytotoxic chemotherapy agents alone, and in combination, the MTD is generally determined by neutropenia. Furthermore, the patient population generally treated on clinical trials defining the MTD of these regimens is in general younger and healthier patients with less comorbid disease than seen in clinical practice. Thus, the oncologist is often faced with administering full standard dose chemotherapy, using a planned dose reduction, if necessary, in treatment to reduce the potential risks of the chemotherapy. In addition, regardless of whether the patient is treated at full or reduced dose initially, unplanned dose reductions may occur as a result of consequences of chemotherapy, again commonly due to neutropenia, as well as other chemotherapy complications.

The evidence that maintenance of full dose chemotherapy across all cycles of treatment is essential to optimal treatment outcome is limited by a lack of studies that directly address this question. The two areas that have been studied better than others include the adjuvant treatment of early stage breast cancer, as well as chemotherapy in the setting of patients with lymphoma. These studies have looked at the relative dose intensity (RDI) of the chemotherapy planned. The RDI can be determined by measuring the actual amount of chemotherapy delivered per unit time, such as milligrams/week divided by the reference standard, full dose, on time, resulting in a percentage. In a retrospective analysis by Bonadonna of women with breast cancer receiving adjuvant chemotherapy, those who received less than 85% of full dose therapy had virtually no benefit of treatment with outcomes similar to the controls *(5)*. Similar prospective data from CALGB have also shown an important dose threshold *(6)*. Similarly, in lymphoma studies that have looked at planned reduced dose of chemotherapy at 50%, RDI results in poor outcomes for these patients, compared to those treated at full standard doses *(7)*. Despite the potential impact of delivering reduced chemotherapy doses in these populations, large surveys of community practice in the United States have shown a high frequency of both planned and unplanned chemotherapy dose reductions in breast cancer *(8)*, as well as lymphoma *(9)*. The full reasons for these dose reductions and delays are likely multifactorial and prospective survival data is not available, but is much needed in this area. At present, what can be said is that in the practice of medical oncology, delivery of reduced dose intensity chemotherapy rather than the evidence-based dosing from clinical trials is a common practice. Prospective studies are clearly needed in this area to understand the impact of delivery of full dose chemotherapy with appropriate supportive care versus dose reduction in optimizing treatment outcomes and quality of care for patients across the range of curative, adjuvant, and palliative settings in oncology.

Prophylactic Antibiotics

In addition to or instead of chemotherapy dose reduction, a second strategy to try to reduce febrile neutropenia involves the use of prophylactic antibiotics. Initial attempts that utilize either trimethoprim/sulfamethoxazole and/or incompletely absorbed antibiotics result in very inconsistent results *(10)*. More consistent results have been seen in the era of fluoroquinolone prophylaxis, resulting in a significant reduction in Gram negative infections, but no reduction in Gram positive infections. Subsequent strategies involving fluoroquinolone prophylaxis in combination with antibiotics against Gram positive organisms have resulted in reduction in both Gram negative and Gram positive infections, but have had limited application due to increase in adverse events from these antibiotic combinations.

A full discussion of antibiotic prophylaxis in neutropenic patients is beyond the scope of this chapter, but will be briefly summarized here. A meta-analysis of 96 randomized controlled trials between 1973 and 2004 was reported and included more than 9,000 patients. Seventy-nine studies were focused on inpatients with hematologic malignancies and/or patients receiving peripheral progenitor stem cell support, thus representing patients with more prolonged neutropenia. Fifty-two of these trials involved quinolone prophylaxis. Only seven trials included myeloid growth factors also, limiting any comparisons *(11)*. In these trials comparing antibiotic prophylaxis versus placebo or no intervention, there was a reduction in both causes of mortality and infection-related mortality with the results most positive in the setting of fluoroquinolones. For patients receiving fluoroquinolones, the relative risk of fever was 0.67 (0.56–0.81), documented infection was 0.50 (0.35–0.70), infection-related death was 0.38 (0.21–0.69), and all cause mortality was 0.52 (0.35–0.77). The adverse events were numerically greater in the fluoroquinolone group at 1.30 (0.61–2.76), as well as the development of resistant bacteria at 1.69 (0.73–3.92).

The advantages of fluoroquinolones in neutropenic patients include a broad antimicrobial spectrum, preservation of the anaerobic flora of the alimentary tract, a high fecal concentration, systemic bacterial activity, good tolerability, and the lack of myelosuppression. However, the limitations of this approach are that there were an insufficient number of outpatient solid tumor chemotherapy patients to be applicable to this setting. Furthermore, prophylactic antibiotics are not recommended by the Infectious Disease Society of America (IDSA) guidelines, because of concerns regarding the increase in antibiotic resistance if these approaches were widely used. However, routine application can certainly be considered in high-risk patients with prolonged neutropenia in the setting of hematologic malignancies and stem cell transplants.

Subsequent to this meta-analysis, there have been two important trials that further explore the role of prophylactic antibiotics in the prevention of infection after chemotherapy. The first is the GIMEMA trial which was focused again on patients with hematologic malignancy or solid tumor transplant patients who had grade 3 or 4 neutropenia lasting more than 7 days. Unlike the majority of the prior studies, this was a large prospective randomized trial using levofloxacin versus placebo in a total of 760 patients *(12)*. The levofloxacin group had a 24% reduction in fever along with a reduction in Gram negative bacteremia. No difference in overall mortality could be seen in this one study. Again noted was an increase in levofloxacin-resistant Gram negative oraganisms.

The other trial of note is the SIGNIFICANT trial which explored the role of prophylactic antibiotics in solid tumor and lymphoma patients receiving standard dose multicycle chemotherapy. This was again a very large trial, with over 1,500 patients randomized to receive levofloxacin at 500 mg daily for 7 days versus placebo. The primary endpoint was reduction in febrile episodes, attributed to infection *(13)*. In this study, in the first cycle of treatment, febrile episodes were noted in 7.9% of placebo patients compared to 3.5% of levofloxacin patients. Febrile episodes across all cycles of treatment were reduced from 15% in the placebo group to 11% in the levofloxacin group. The problem of infection was reduced from 19% in the placebo group to 14% in the levofloxacin group in the first cycle and 41% versus 34% across all cycles. The hospitalization rate was also decreased in the levofloxacin group, but there was no significant difference in overall mortality, with 2% overall mortality in the placebo group and 1% in the levofloxacin group. Because of the relative low risk of febrile episodes in this population, it would be necessary to treat 23 patients in order to benefit one patient. This suggests that while this strategy of prophylactic antibiotics can result in a significantly lower rate of fever and infection in standard dose chemotherapy patients, the number of patients requiring antibiotics is large and therefore concerns about side effects particularly the emergence of antibiotic resistance.

The evidence comparing the strategy of using prophylactic antibiotics versus myeloid growth factors is limited. However, there are some trials that are instructive from the population of patients with small-cell lung cancer. In this population, patients are randomized to receive a standard combination of cyclophosphamide, doxorubicin, and etoposide (CDE), along with either placebo or prophylactic antibiotics with ciprofloxacin and roxithromycin *(14)*. In addition, a second group of patients was randomized to receive a more dose-intensive CDE chemotherapy regimen with granulocyte colony-stimulating-factor support. In a combined analysis, the placebo patients had a 43% rate of febrile neutropenia, compared to 24% in the group that received antibiotics ($p = 0.007$). In a subset analysis, most of the reduction in the risk of febrile neutropenia occurred in the dose-intense CDE group with granulocyte colony-stimulating-factor and antibiotic support. A subsequent trial using standard dose CDE randomized patients to prophylactic antibiotics alone or prophylactic antibiotics plus granulocyte colony-stimulating factor *(15)*. In this trial, the investigators believed that the prophylactic antibiotics alone would be as effective as the combination. However, as expected, there was significantly less neutropenia in the group receiving myeloid growth factor and despite the prophylactic antibiotics in all patients, the myeloid growth factor group had a lower rate of febrile neutropenia and there was a trend toward a lower rate of febrile neutropenia-related mortality. While these two studies certainly cannot be considered definitive, it would appear that myeloid growth factors along with prophylactic antibiotics are more effective than antibiotics alone. Since there was no group of patients receiving myeloid growth factors alone, it is difficult to know what the additional benefit of the prophylactic antibiotics are; an extrapolation from other standard dose chemotherapy settings indicates that the additional benefit of prophylactic antibiotics is likely to be small. On the other hand, in settings where patients have prolonged neutropenia, there may be additional benefit of this combination approach, warranting further study.

Use of Myeloid Growth Factors

The third preventive strategy for the management of chemotherapy-induced neutropenia became available in the early 1990s with the approval of the myeloid growth factors. These include granulocyte colony-stimulating factor (G-CSF) or filgrastim and granulocyte monocyte colony-stimulating factor (GM-CSF) or sargramostim. Outside the United States, G-CSF is also available as lenograstim, a glycosylated form of a protein and GM-CSF as molgramastim. Both filgrastim and sargramostim were initially approved by the FDA in 1991. Subsequently, a long-acting form of filgrastim was developed, pegfilgrastim, with a polyethylene glycol moiety attached to the protein backbone of filgrastim. This agent was approved in 2002. The current FDA-approved indications for these

Table 1
FDA-approved indications for myeloid growth factors

Growth factor/cytokine	Generic name	Trade name(s)	Distributor(s)/manufacturer(s)	Indication(s)
G-CSF	Filgrastim Pegfilgrastim	Neupogen Neulasta	Amgen	Cancer patients receiving myelosuppressive chemotherapy Patients with nonmyeloid malignancy following BMT Patients with severe chronic neutropenia Following induction chemotherapy in AML
GM-CSF	Sargramostim	Leukine Prokine	Berlex	Following autologous BMT BMT engraftment delay or failure Following induction chemotherapy in older patients with AML Allogeneic BMT for mobilization of PBPCs and for use after PBPC transplantation

myeloid growth factors are outlined in Table 1. Pegfilgrastim and filgrastim are both approved for use in reducing neutropenia in cancer patients receiving myelosuppressive chemotherapy. GM-CSF or sargramostim does not have this indication. Both filgrastim and sargramostim are approved for mobilization of peripheral blood stem cells and in the settings of bone marrow transplantation and acute leukemia. In addition, filgrastim is indicated for management of patients with severe or chronic neutropenia.

While G-CSF and GM-CSF both share the property of being able to stimulate neutrophil production, they are biologically distinct. G-CSF is the endogenous cytokine that regulates neutrophil production in the setting of infection and stress and is lineage specific for neutrophils, while also acting synergistically with early-acting cytokines, including stem cell factor, for broader effects on the myeloid compartment. By contrast, GM-CSF is a broader acting cytokine, affecting neutrophils, monocytes, and eosinophils and appears to be very important for generating an inflammatory response at the local site of infection. Specifically, GM-CSF has chemo-attractant properties which lead to neutrophil migration toward the site of the cytokine release. While perhaps somewhat of an oversimplification, endogenous G-CSF can be thought of as a systemic biologic response modifier in generating increased neutrophil numbers and enhanced neutrophil function, while endogenous GM-CSF, which shows some of these functions, can be thought of as a more locally acting cytokine in response to infection and inflammation.

The recombinant forms of both of these proteins are outlined in Table 1 and have documented clinical utility. G-CSF, either filgrastim or pegfilgrastim, are approved agents for clinical use in decreasing the risk of infection as manifested by febrile neutropenia, along with reduction in duration of hospitalization and IV antibiotic use in patients receiving myelosuppressive chemotherapy. These effects on marrow hematopoiesis are achieved by expansion of the neutrophil progenitor precursor cell population and also by shortening the time of maturation of the postmitotic compartment from 5–6 days to 1 day, to greatly enhance the number of circulating neutrophils. When cytotoxic chemotherapy is administered, the precursor cells and the myeloid compartment are reduced, resulting in a decreased production of neutrophils over several days. Endogenous granulocyte colony-stimulating hormone does not increase until neutropenia develops. At that point, G-CSF acts to enhance neutrophil production and release, but this process requires several days. By the use of colony-stimulating factors after chemotherapy, but prior to the development of neutropenia, neutrophil production can be accelerated so that neutropenia can either be avoided or reduced in magnitude.

The initial randomized phase III trials that led to the approval of filgrastim included two studies in small-cell lung cancer *(16, 17)* and one study in non-Hodgkin's lymphoma *(18)*. All of these trials showed approximately a 50% reduction in the duration of neutropenia in the patients receiving filgrastim, compared to the placebo group. Associated with this 50% reduction in duration of neutropenia was an approximately 50% reduction in the rate of febrile neutropenia, with associated reductions in IV antibiotic use and the incidence of hospitalization. From these data, the relationship between duration of neutropenia and risk of febrile neutropenia was redefined, and as outlined in Table 1 demonstrates the general relationship between days of neutropenia and risk of febrile neutropenia; while the relationship is not entirely linear, the risk of febrile neutropenia was approximately 10% for every day of grade 4 neutropenia.

To achieve the benefit of reduction of neutropenia, filgrastim must be administered daily because of its relatively short half-life of 4–6 h. This half-life is determined predominantly by renal clearance and secondarily by neutrophil mediated clearance by G-CSF receptors. To provide a more sustained duration molecule, pegfilgrastim was developed. In this case, a 20-kDa polyethylene glycol molecule was added to the interminous of recombinant human G-CSF. This changed the molecular weight of the molecule such that renal clearance was essentially eliminated *(19)*. The dose of pegfilgrastim administered saturates all of the binding sites on existing neutrophils resulting in a steady state of plasma levels that require production of new neutrophils in order to clear the molecule; the half-life is prolonged to several days depending upon the rate of neutrophil production. In the setting of chemotherapy-induced neutropenia, there is virtually no clearance of the molecule until neutrophil recovery occurs after the neutrophil nadir. With neutrophil recovery, the molecule is rapidly cleared from the circulation. Thus, a single injection of pegfilgrastim in this setting is self-regulating. By administering pegfilgrastim after chemotherapy, a steady state of plasma level is achieved, driving production of neutrophil progenitors and neutrophils and as those neutrophils recover post chemotherapy, the molecule is cleared from the circulation. Importantly, the process of pegylation was shown not to alter the biologic properties of filgrastim in proliferation assays, receptor binding, neutrophil response, and neutrophil function studies.

In the registrational trials of pegfilgrastim *(20, 21)*, a single dose of pegfilgrastim, 24 hours after chemotherapy with doxorubicin and docetaxel was compared to daily administration of filgrastim in women with breast cancer. One study dosed the pegfilgrastim by weight and the other used a fixed 6-mg dose of pegfilgrastim. Filgrastim was administered at 5 mcg/kg. With either dosing schedule, comparable neutrophil recovery occurred with either pegfilgrastim or filgrastim. The incidence of bone pain was similar with both agents and the fixed dose of 6 mg was effective across a broad range of body weights. Interestingly, there was a trend toward a lower rate of febrile neutropenia in the pegfilgrastim compared to filgrastim arms, but this was a secondary endpoint of the study. Based on these data, pegfilgrastim was approved for use to be administered 24 h after chemotherapy for myelosuppressive chemotherapy regimens that had a period of at least 14 days between chemotherapy dosing. Since that time, a number of q2week dosing regimens have been developed with pegfilgrastim showing comparable safety and efficacy as the every-3-week chemotherapy schedule in the registration trials.

It is clear from the biology of these agents that use of myeloid growth factors is most effective when used in a prevention strategy, rather than a treatment strategy. This is born out by the clinical trial results using these agents at the time of neutropenia or febrile neutropenia. Those studies clearly show a lesser effect on neutrophil recovery and other clinical endpoints likely related to delayed time of initiation of treatment. As outlined by ASCO guidelines *(22)*, the colony-stimulating factors are recommended for use in prevention of febrile neutropenia as will be discussed in the subsequent section, but not for routine use in treatment of either asymptomatic neutropenia or in the routine use in patients with febrile neutropenia. In the latter setting, colony-stimulating factors can be considered in the high-risk patient with tissue infection, suspected bacteremia, or in patients who are likely to have prolonged neutropenia.

PRACTICE GUIDELINES FOR THE MYELOID GROWTH FACTORS

Shortly after the initial approval of filgrastim and sargramostim, ASCO convened an expert panel guidelines committee to help develop parameters for use of these agents in the clinical practice of oncology. In the initial registrational trials mentioned above, the risk of febrile neutropenia was quite high in the small-cell lung cancer and lymphoma trials, with a rate of 44–77% in the control group of the three studies. Based on the lack of data demonstrating benefit at lower rates of febrile neutropenia, the panel recommended that the use of these agents be limited to high-risk settings. Since most standard chemotherapy regimens are not associated with a 40% or greater risk of neutropenia, most of the use of CSFs prior to recent guideline updates were in a reactive rather than proactive mode. For patients who developed febrile neutropenia or other neutropenic complications delaying therapy in a cycle of treatment, in the absence of myeloid growth factor, the myeloid growth factor was then introduced in subsequent cycles of chemotherapy. By this reactive use, the benefits of these agents were reduced by exposing patients to the risks and complications of myelosuppressive chemotherapy.

Subsequent studies clearly demonstrated benefits of colony-stimulating factors at lower rates of febrile neutropenia. In the registrational trials for pegfilgrastim, the expected rate of febrile neutropenia with the doxorubicin/docetaxel regimen was 38%. In the subsequent randomized trials, the rates of febrile neutropenia were 18–20% in the filgrastim group and 9–13% in the pegfilgrastim groups (20, 21).

Subsequently, a study in small-cell lung cancer, using a lower dose of chemotherapy with prophylactic antibiotics previously discussed (15), demonstrated a reduction in the rate of febrile neutropenia from 30% in the control group to 18% in the group receiving filgrastim. The study that most influenced current guidelines of use attempted to define the benefit of myeloid growth factors in patients receiving chemotherapy with approximately a 20% risk of febrile neutropenia. In this large trial of over 900 patients, single agent docetaxel at 100 mg/m2 was administered to women with breast cancer. The placebo group had a 17% rate of febrile neutropenia and, surprisingly, this was reduced to 1% in the pegfilgrastim group. The assumption had been that the myeloid growth factor would be less effective at low rates of febrile neutropenia, but the opposite was observed. From studies of the associated neutrophil profile of these patients, it appears that this may likely be due to the fact that when neutropenia duration is brief, this can be largely abolished by the use of myeloid growth factor. A meta-analysis of prophylactic use of G-CSF in febrile neutropenia has demonstrated benefit in reducing the risk of febrile neutropenia across the whole range of risks (23).

PRACTICE GUIDELINES

From all of the randomized trials noted above, the highest risk of febrile neutropenia occurs in the first cycle of treatment, therefore emphasizing the importance of identifying patients at risk for prophylactic strategies at the time of the first cycle of treatment. In 2005, the National Comprehensive Cancer Network formed a myeloid growth factors panel to address the emerging clinical trial data and develop clinical practice guidelines. In their assessment of the available data, they felt that evaluation for risk for chemotherapy-induced neutropenia and febrile neutropenia must include the disease itself, the chemotherapy regimen, patient risk factors, and whether the treatment intent was curative or palliative. The primary interventions to be considered were the use of a colony-stimulating factor including filgrastim, sargramostim, or pegfilgrastim versus dose reduction or alternative treatment strategies. In the refinement of risks, high risk was considered risk of 20% or greater for the development of febrile neutropenia or other neutropenic events that would compromise treatment. Ten to twenty percent was considered an immediate risk and <10% a low risk subgroup. Furthermore, the NCCN group felt that it was important to define treatment goals in terms of whether the planned therapy was curative or adjuvant treatment, whether the intent was prolonged survival and improved quality of life, or whether the main goal of treatment was mainly symptom management. In this decision analysis, myeloid growth factors were routinely recommended for first cycle use in all three settings if the risk was 20% or greater. However, in the population receiving treatment predominantly for symptom management, the caveat was that other alternatives, such as the use of a less myelosuppressive chemotherapy regimen or dose reduction providing comparable benefit, should also be considered. In the intermediate category of 10–20% risk, in the curative and adjuvant setting, use of myeloid growth factors could be considered. At this same intermediate risk in the more palliative setting, the same caveat as previously mentioned would apply. In the low-risk group, below 10%, no colony-stimulating factor use was recommended *(24)*.

Subsequent to the NCCN guidelines, the ASCO expert panel reconvened and also agreed that 20% marked a high-risk population that should be considered for first cycle prophylaxis. The EORTC reached a similar conclusion for the greater-than-20% group. All three groups differ somewhat in the wording indicating when they would recommend or consider usage in patients at less than 20% risk, but most of this had to do with developing patient-specific algorithms around specific risk factors.

With the new threshold of 20% risk, several chemotherapy regimens now qualify for first cycle use of myeloid growth factors, including several regimens used in bladder cancer, breast cancer, lymphoma, small-cell lung cancer, sarcoma and testicular cancer, as well as ovarian cancer. However, it is critical to evaluate not only the chemotherapy regimen, but also the specific patient risk factors *(25)*. Some of the individual treatment risk factors to be considered are whether patients had a prior chemotherapy and/or radiation treatment to bone marrow-containing areas, whether there is a history of previous severe neutropenia, whether the planned dose and relative dose intensity is greater than 80%. The patient risk factors to be considered are age, with most studies showing patients older than age 65 are at increased risk for neutropenia. In addition, female gender seems to be a risk factor. There are multiple possible explanations for this, including smaller body surface area (BSA) which could lead to a higher relative dosing of chemotherapy. Poor performance status, comorbid disease, poor nutritional status, and decreased immune function have all been associated with increased risk of developing febrile neutropenia. In terms of cancer-related factors, bone marrow involvement with tumor, advanced or uncontrolled cancer, hematologic malignancies, and lung cancer have all been associated with increased risk of febrile neutropenia. In addition, conditions associated with an increased risk of severe or serious infection in the setting of neutropenia would include open wounds or other active tissue infection at the time neutropenia occurs. Specific comorbidities that need to be considered include chronic obstructive pulmonary disease, cardiovascular disease, liver disease, diabetes, and anemia.

What is needed to help the clinician sort through all the potential factors that might alter an individual patient's risk with a given chemotherapy regimen is a readily available risk model that can be applied. The ANC study group has performed a large prospective nationwide study of the incidence of severe neutropenia and febrile neutropenia in patients receiving chemotherapy in the settings of breast cancer, lymphoma, ovarian cancer, lung cancer, colon cancer, and other assorted malignancies. This prospective observational database again documented the presence of severe neutropenia in 20–50% of patients with 50–70% of that neutropenia occurring in the first cycle of treatment. The overall rate of febrile neutropenia among this heterogeneous population of patients, diseases, and treatment regimens was approximately 13%. The plan is to use this database to develop a refined risk model to identify patients at higher and lower risk of febrile neutropenia that can then be prospectively tested to best develop strategies for the rational and patient-specific use of myeloid growth factors versus alterations of treatment regimen or chemotherapy dose depending on the goals of therapy.

In conclusion, the last fifteen years have seen a tremendous explosion of our biological understanding of cytokines and hematopoiesis and specifically in our ability to modify neutropenia and its complications through the use of myeloid growth factors in a variety of clinical settings. This chapter has focused on the specific problem of chemotherapy-induced neutropenia, but these same myeloid growth factors have had a substantial impact on the technology and development of peripheral blood progenitor cell support and transplantation in the field of high-dose chemotherapy. Likewise, the myeloid growth factors have been found to be safe and effective in shortening the duration of neutropenia in the setting of acute myeloid leukemia. In children with severe chronic neutropenia, the long-term use of filgrastim has lessened the degree of neutropenia in these patients reducing the number of infections and promoting mucosal integrity. The second generation molecules such as pegfilgrastim provide convenience and safety and may ultimately be shown to be more effective than daily dosing. In addition, a number of small molecules that stimulate the G-CSF receptor are also in development and will add both to our understanding of this field as well as options for our patients. In current clinical practice, the NCCN, ASCO, and EORTC guidelines have reached similar conclusions in regard to the optimum use of these agents based on risk. Thus, defining patient-specific risks and risk factors, and incorporating them in a simple tool that can be studied prospectively, will be critical to the optimal use of these supportive care approaches in the years ahead.

REFERENCES

1. Bodey G, Buckley M, Sathe Y, Freireich E. Quantitative relationships between circulating leukocytes and infection in patients with acute leukemia. *Ann Intern Med* 1966;64:328–340.
2. Crawford J, Blackwell S. Hematopoietic growth factors. In: The Chemotherapy Source Book, 3rd Edition. Perry MC (Ed.), Philadelphia: Lippincott Williams & Wilkins, 2001. 94–103.
3. Anderson N, Cella D, Calhoun E, et al. Rationale for the development of the FACT-N: a neutropenia-specific quality-of-life tool. Proceedings from the 2003 annual congress of the Oncology Nursing Society. Abstract 117.
4. Lyman G, Kuderer N, Green J, Balducci. The economics of febrile neutropenia: implications for the use of colony-stimulating factors. *Eur J Cancer* 1998;34:1857–1864.
5. Bonadonna G, Valagussa B, Moliterni A, Zambetti M, Brambilla C. Adjuvant Cyclophosphamide, methotrexate, and fluorouracil in node-positive breast cancer — The results of 20 years of follow-up. *N Engl J Med* 1995;332:901–906.
6. Budman D, Berry D, Cirrincione C, Henderson IC, Wood W, Weiss R, Rerree C, Muss H, Green M, Norton L, Frei E. Dose and dose intensity as determinants of outcome in the adjuvant treatment of breast cancer. *J Natl Cancer Inst* 1998;90:1205–1211.
7. Kwak L, Halpern J, Olshen R, Horning S. Prognostic significance of actual dose intensity in diffuse large-cell lymphoma: results of a tree-structured survival analysis. *J Clin Oncol* 1990;8:963–977.
8. Lyman G, Dale D, Crawford J. Incidence and predictors of low dose-intensity in adjuvant breast cancer chemotherapy: a nationwide study of community practices. *J Clin Oncol* 2003;21: 4524–4531.
9. Lyman G, Dale D, Friedberg J, Crawford J, Risher R. Incidence and predictors of low chemotherapy dose-intensity in aggressive non-Hodgkin's lymphoma: a nationwide study. *J Clin Oncol* 2004;22:4302–4311.
10. Moon S, Williams S, Cullen M. Role of prophylactic antibiotics in the prevention of infection after chemotherapy: a literature review. *Support Cancer Ther* 2006;3:207–213.
11. Gafter-Gvili A, Fraser A, Mical P, Leibovici L. Meta-analysis: antibiotic prophylaxis reduces mortality in neutropenic patients. *Ann Intern Med* 2005;142:979–995.
12. Bucaneve G, Micozzi A, Menichetti F, Martino P, Dionisi M, Martinelli G, Allione B, D'Antonio D, Buelli M, Nosari M, Cilloni D, Zuffa E, Cantaffa R, Specchia G, Amadori S, Fabbiano F, Deliliers G, Lauria F, Foa R, Del Favero A, the Gruppo Italiano Malattie Ematologiche dell'Adulto (GIMEMA) Infection Program. Levofloxacin to prevent bacterial infection in patients with cancer and neutropenia. *N Engl J Med* 2005;353:977–987.
13. Cullen M, Steven N, Billingham L, Gaunt C, Hastings M, Simmonds P, Stuart N, Rea D, Bower M, Fernando I, Hudddart R, Gollins S, Stanley A. Simple investigation in neutropenic individuals of the frequency of infection

after chemotherapy +/– antibiotic in a number of tumours (SIGNIFICANT) Trial Group. N *Engl J Med* 2005;353:988–998.

14. Tjan-Heijnen VCG, Postmus P, Ardizzoni A, Manegold C, Burghouts J, van Meerbeeck J, Gans S, Mollers M, Buccholz E, Biesma B, Legrand C, Debruyne C, Giaccone G. Reduction of chemotherapy-induced febrile leucopenia by prophylactic use of ciprofloxacin and roxithromycin in small-cell lung cancer patients: an EORTC double-blind placebo-controlled phase III study. *Ann Oncol* 2001;12:1359–1368.

15. Timmer-Bonte J, de Boo T, Smit H, Biesma B, Wischut F, Cheragwandi S, Termeer A, Hensing C, Akkermans J, Adang E, Bootsma G, Tjan-Heijnen V. Prevention of chemotherapy-induced febrile neutropenia by prophylactic antibiotics plus or minus granulocyte colony-stimulating factor in small-cell lung cancer: a Dutch randomized phase III study. *J Clin Oncol* 2005;23:7974–7984.

16. Crawford J, Ozer H, Stoller R, Johnson D, Lyman G, Tabbara I, Kris M, Grous V, Picozzi V, Rausch G, et al. Reduction by granulocyte colony-stimulating factor of fever and neutropenia induced by chemotherapy in patients with small-cell lung cancer. *N Engl J Med* 1991;325:164–170.

17. Trillet-Lenoir V, Green J, Manegold C, Von Pawel J, Gatzemeier U, Lebeau B, Depierre A, Johnson P, Decaster G, Tomita D, et al. Recombinant granulocyte colony-stimulating factor reduces the infectious complications of cytotoxic chemotherapy. *Eur J Cancer* 1993;16A:319–324.

18. Pettengell R, Gurney H, Radford JA, Deakin DP, James R, Wilkinson PM, Kane K, Bentley J, Crowther D. Granulocyte colony-stimulating factor to prevent dose-limiting neutropenia in non-Hodgkin's lymphoma: a randomized controlled trial. *Blood* 1992;80:1430–1436.

19. Blackwell S, Crawford J. G-CSF in the chemotherapy setting. In: Granulocyte Colony-Stimulating Factor in the Clinical. Morstyn, G. (Ed.), New York: Marcel Dekker, 1994; 103–116.

20. Holmes FA, O'Shaughnessy JA, Vukelja S, Jones SE, Shgan J, Savin M, Glaspy J, Moore M, Meza L, Wiznitzer I, Neumann TA, Hill LR, Liang BC. Blinded, randomized, multicenter study to evaluate single administration pegfilgrastim once per cycle versus daily filgrastim as an adjunct to chemotherapy in patients with high-risk stage II or stage III/IV breast cancer. *J Clin Oncol* 2002;20:727–731.

21. Green MD, Koelbl H, Baselga J, Galid A, Guillem V, Gascon P, Siena S, Lalisang RI, Samonigg H, Clemens MR, Zani V, Liang BC, Renwick J, Piccart MJ. A randomized double-blind multicenter phase III study of fixed-dose single-administration pegfilgrastim versus daily filgrastim in patients receiving myelosuppressive chemotherapy. *Ann Oncol* 2003;14:29–35.

22. ASCO 2006 Update of recommendations for the use of white blood cell growth factors: an evidence-based clinical practice guideline.

23. Lyman G, Kuderer N, Djulbegovic B. Prophylactic granulocyte colony-stimulating factor in patients receiving dose-intensive cancer chemotherapy: a meta-analysis. *American Journal of Medicine* 2002; 112:406–411.

24. National Comprehensive Cancer Network, Clinical Practice Guidelines in Oncology. Myeloid Growth Factors. V.1.2007.

25. Lyman G, Risk assessment in oncology clinical practice: from risk factors to risk models. *Oncology* 2003;17:8–13.

Words: Chemotherapy side effects, Nausea, Antiemetics, Emesis.

INTRODUCTION

Historically, approximately 70–80% of all cancer patients receiving chemotherapy experienced emesis *(3)*; fortunately, there have been dramatic improvements since the introduction of effective antiemetic therapy *(1)*. In the last 20 years, several studies have attempted to quantify the burden of chemotherapy side effects on cancer patients. Repeatedly, nausea and vomiting are mentioned as "major physical side effects" *(4)* and "most troublesome" *(5)*. Although there have been recent advancements in pharmacologic prevention of CINV, a 1997 study by de Boer-Dennert and colleagues revealed that nausea and vomiting, respectively, ranked as the first and third most distressing side effects of chemotherapy, despite decrease in overall incidence and severity with the introduction of 5-hydroxytryptamine-3 (5-HT3) antagonists *(6)*. Grunberg and colleagues surveyed patients, medical oncologists, and oncology nurses in 2001–2002 to assess the frequency and provider perception of CINV. Though improvements in the prevention of acute nausea and vomiting were seen (acute nausea in approximately 35% and acute emesis in 13%), delayed symptoms were seen more frequently (50–60% with nausea and 30–50% with emesis, depending on the chemotherapy used). Strikingly, more than 75% of physicians and nurses underestimated the occurrence of delayed nausea and vomiting *(1)*. Progress in relieving the symptoms of CINV will come only with further education of oncology physicians and nurses, more aggressive use of current medications, and continued development of pharmacologic and alternative therapies.

PATHOPHYSIOLOGY OF NAUSEA AND VOMITING

Vomiting is controlled by the central nervous system via a complex pathway of varied afferent inputs and neurotransmitters. Borison and Wang were the first to describe two areas of the brainstem involved in nausea and vomiting: the chemoreceptor trigger zone (CTZ) and the emetic center (EC) *(7)*. The CTZ, located in the area postrema in the floor of the fourth ventricle, lies outside of the blood–brain barrier and is, therefore, susceptible to emetogenic stimuli from the bloodstream, such as chemotherapy or, more likely, its metabolites *(8)*. Several receptors have been identified in the CTZ including muscarinic, dopamine D2, serotonin (5-HT3), neurokinin-1, and histamine H-1 receptors.

In addition to receiving impulses from the CTZ, the EC coordinates afferent pathways from the gastrointestinal tract and pharynx via the vagus and splanchnic nerves that are coordinated in the emetic center *(9)*. The phenomenon of anticipatory emesis suggests that inputs from the cerebral cortex, in particular, may also be involved. The EC also receives afferent impulses and coordinates the efferent activities of the salivation center, abdominal muscles, respiratory center, and autonomic nerves that result in vomiting. The emetic center, composed of these indistinct receptor and effector nuclei, is located in the nucleus tractus solitarius of the brainstem *(8)*.

Current findings suggest that the most critical neuroreceptors involved in these pathways are serotonin, dopamine, and substance P. Others include acetylcholine, corticosteroid, histamine, cannabinoid, opiate, and neurokinin-1 receptors *(10)*. Receptors for dopamine, serotonin (5-HT3), and substance P have demonstrated clinical relevance. The most

10 Nausea and Vomiting

Tara L. Lin and David S. Etti

ABSTRACT

Chemotherapy-induced nausea and vomiting (CINV) remains a sig
for many cancer patients despite recent advances in pharmacologic th
et al. Cancer 2004;100(10):2261–8). In addition to significant physic
including dehydration, nutritional compromise, and metabolic alteratic
a dramatic impact on a patient's quality of life (Mitchell EP Semin Oncol 1
79). Despite the dissemination of detailed guidelines for preventive a
mens, some patients continue to receive suboptimal prophylaxis
Symptoms of nausea and vomiting after chemotherapy are often more di
age than if the symptoms had been prevented initially with appropriate
intervention. Notably, some patients actually develop a psychological
their nausea and vomiting as a result of inadequate management in the pa:
physiology of CINV, principles of antiemetic prophylaxis, the emetogeni
common chemotherapeutics, classes of antiemetic therapy, and guideline:
tion and acute management of CINV will be discussed.

From: Cancer and Drug Discovery Development: Supportive Care in Cancer Ther.
DOI: 10.1007/978-1-59745-291-5_10, Edited by: D. S. Ettinger © Humana Press, Toto

significant advancement in antiemetic therapy came in the early 1990s when the 5-HT3 receptor antagonists became available *(6)*. Substance P, which binds to the neurokinin-1 receptor, is an emerging target in antiemetic therapy *(11)*, and one approved NK-1 receptor antagonist has shown clinical utility *(12, 13, 14, 15)*.

The exact mechanism by which chemotherapy and its metabolites have emetic effects remains unclear. Metabolites may stimulate the CTZ directly. Serotonin and other neurotransmitters may be released from intestinal cells damaged by chemotherapy. Sensory neurons release substance P, and numerous NK-1 receptors have been identified in both the CTZ and nucleus tractus solitarius. Given that this mechanism is not defined and the fact that no single common pathway controlling the emetic response has been uncovered, it is unlikely that any single agent will be able to provide complete antiemetic protection from chemotherapy.

TYPES OF EMESIS

Three distinct types of chemotherapy-induced emesis have been identified: acute, delayed, and anticipatory. *Acute emesis* is defined as nausea and vomiting within 24 h of chemotherapy. It has its onset within 1–2 h of chemotherapy and peaks in 4–6 h without adequate prophylaxis. *Delayed emesis* refers to symptoms that start more than 24 h after chemotherapy. It typically peaks at 48–72 h and may last for 6–7 days. Although delayed emesis may be less frequent and less severe than acute emesis, it is less well-controlled than acute emesis. Cisplatin is most frequently associated with delayed emesis, although it is also seen with carboplatin, cyclophosphamide, and anthracyclines. *Anticipatory emesis* is seen in patients who have previously experienced significant nausea and vomiting following chemotherapy. In these patients, symptoms develop as a conditioned response before the chemotherapy is administered. It may be triggered by sights and activities associated with the chemotherapy (e.g., driving to the treatment center). As control of CINV has improved, the incidence of anticipatory emesis has declined *(16)*.

Despite the prevalence of CINV, it is important to remember that there are other potential causes of nausea and vomiting in cancer patients including partial or complete bowel obstruction, brain metastases, uremia, electrolyte disturbances (i.e., hyperglycemia, hypercalcemia, hyponatremia), and gastroparesis. Medications commonly prescribed in cancer patients, such as opiates, may cause emesis as well.

PRINCIPLES OF PREVENTION AND CONTROL OF CHEMOTHERAPY-INDUCED NAUSEA AND VOMITING IN THE CANCER PATIENT

The most important principle in managing CINV is that prevention of symptoms, rather than treatment of symptoms, be the ultimate goal. Symptoms may persist for days following the administration of chemotherapy and prophylactic therapy should be given over all days of potential symptoms. Individual patient characteristics may influence the risk of CINV independent of the chemotherapy given. Additionally, antiemetics should be given at the lowest efficacious dose with consideration of their side effect profiles. Chemotherapeutic agents and their likelihood of causing acute or delayed emesis, followed by a review of the currently available pharmacologic and nonpharmacologic interventions to prevent and treat CINV will be discussed.

EMETOGENIC CHEMOTHERAPY (TABLE 1)

The severity and frequency of CINV are affected by variables of both the patient and the chemotherapy. The most predictive factor is the specific chemotherapy agent used, although the route and rate of administration and drug dosage may play a role (17). There are also patient-related factors predicting a higher incidence of CINV such as a history of prior chemotherapy, history of prior CINV, female sex, younger age, history of motion sickness, and no or minimal history of alcohol use.

There is no universally accepted classification system of chemotherapy agents by emetogenic potential. The most widely accepted, devised by Hesketh and colleagues, divides chemotherapy into five levels of emetogenicity based on the percentage of patients who experience nausea and vomiting following each without any antiemetic prophylaxis. Level 1 drugs result in emesis in less than 10% without antiemetic therapy; Level 2, 10–30%; Level 3, 30–60%; Level 4, 60–90%; and Level 5, more than 90% of patients experiencing emesis without prophylaxis (18). A recently proposed modification would classify chemotherapy into four risk categories: high risk (level 5, more than 90%); moderate risk (levels 3 and 4, 30–90%); low risk (level 2, 10–30%); and minimal risk (level 1, less than 10%) (19).

These classification systems were developed with a focus on acute emesis. It is clear from recent data that the frequency and severity of delayed symptoms are often underestimated and remain a significant problem for many patients (1). To optimally manage both acute and delayed symptoms, adequate antiemetic prophylaxis is required for the duration of days that symptoms are anticipated.

CLASSES OF ANTIEMETICS (TABLE 2)

Our understanding of the neurotransmitters involved in the central nervous system pathways that regulate the vomiting response provides potential targets for antiemetic therapy. In return, successful clinical application of these agents confirms the importance of these neurotransmitters and receptors in the vomiting pathway. Neuroreceptors involved in the control of emesis include: muscarinic (M1), dopamine (D2), histamine (H1), 5-HT3 (receptor site for serotonin), and neurokinin-1 (receptor site for substance P) (20, 21). The most effective and most commonly used classes of agents are the 5-HT3 receptor antagonists, the dopamine antagonists, and corticosteroids. An emerging class of agents, the neurokinin-1 receptor antagonists, further expands the repertoire of antiemetic agents.

5-HT3 Receptor Antagonists

Four 5-HT3 receptor antagonists have been approved in the United States: ondansetron, granisetron, dolasetron, and, most recently, palonosetron. When first approved in the early 1990s, these agents revolutionized the antiemetic prophylaxis of highly and moderately emetogenic chemotherapy. Studies of 5-HT3 receptor

Table 1
Emetogenic potential of single chemotherapy agents

Level	*Agent*	
High risk, Level 5 (>90% predicted frequency of emesis without prophylaxis)	Carmustine > 250 mg/m^2	Dacarbazine
	Cisplatin ≥ 50 mg/m^2	Mechlorethamine
	Cyclophosphamide > 1,500 mg/m^2	Procarbazine (oral dosing)
		Streptozocin
Moderate risk, Level 4 (60–90% predicted frequency of emesis without prophylaxis)	Amifostine > 500 mg/m^2	Cytarabine > 1g/m^2
	Busulfan > 4 mg/day	Dactinomycin
	Carboplatin	Doxorubicin > 60 mg/m^2
	Cisplatin < 50 mg/m^2	Epirubicin > 90 mg/m^2
	Cyclophosphamide > 750 mg/m^2 and ≤1,500 mg/m^2	Melphalan > 50 mg/m^2
		Methotrexate > 1,000 mg/m^2
Moderate risk, Level 3 (30–60% predicted frequency of emesis without prophylaxis)	Amifostine > 300 mg/m^2 and ≤500 mg/m^2	Ifosfamide
	Arsenic trioxide	Interleukin-2 > 12–15 million units/m^2
	Cyclophosphamide ≤ 750 mg/m^2	Irinotecan
	Cyclophosphamide (oral dosing)	Lomustine
	Doxorubicin 20 mg/m2 and <60 mg/m^2	Methotrexate 250–1,000 mg/m^2
	Epirubicin ≤ 90 mg/m^2	Mitoxantrone < 15 mg/m^2
		Oxaliplatin > 75 mg/m^2
Low risk, Level 2 (10–30% predicted frequency of emesis without prophylaxis)	Amifostine ≤ 300 mg/m^2	Gemcitabine
	Bexarotene	Laybepilope
	Cytarabine 100–200 mg/m^2	Methotrexate > 50 mg/m^2 and <250 mg/m^2
	Capecitabine	Mitomycin
	Docetaxel	Paclitaxel
	Doxorubicin (liposomal formulation)	Paclitaxel-albumin
	Etoposide	Pemetrexed
	5-FU < 1,000 mg/m^2	Temozolomide
		Topotecan
Minimal risk, Level 1 (<10% predicted frequency of emesis without prophylaxis)	Alemtuzumab	Lenalidomide
	Asparaginase	Melphalan (low-dose, oral dosing)
	Alpha interferon	Methotrexate ≤ 50 mg/m^2
	Beracizumab	Nelarabine
	Bleomycin	Pentostatin
	Bortezomib	Rituximab
	Chlorambucil (oral dosing)	Sorafenib
	Cladribine	Sunitinib
	Dasatinib	Thalidomide
	Decitabine	Thioguanine (oral dosing)
	Dexrazoxane	Trastuzumab
	Denileukin diftitox	Valrubicin
	Fludarabine	Vinblastine
	Gefitinib	Vincristine
	Gemtuzumab ozogamicin	Vinorelbine
	Hydroxyurea	
	Imatinib mesylate	
	Lapatinib	

Table 2
Classes and recommended doses of selected antiemetics

Agent	Class	Route	Dose
Ondansetron	5HT$_3$ receptor antagonist	IV	8–12 mg
		PO	12–24 mg
Granisetron	5HT$_3$ receptor antagonist	IV	1 mg or 0.01 mg/kg
		PO	2 mg
Dolasetron	5HT$_3$ receptor antagonist	IV	100 mg or 1.8 mg/kg
		PO	100 mg
Palonosetron	5HT$_3$ receptor antagonist	IV	0.25 mg
Aprepitant	NK-1 receptor antagonist	PO	125 mg day 1
Fasoapropitant	NK-1 receptor antagonist	IV	115 mg day 1
			80 mg day 2, 3
Dexamethasone	Steroid	IV	8–20 mg
		PO	8–20 mg
Prochlorperazine	Dopamine receptor antagonist	IV	10 mg
		PO	10 mg
		Spansule	15 mg
		Suppository	25 mg
Metoclopramide	Dopamine receptor antagonist	IV	1–2 mg/kg
		PO	20–40 mg
Haloperidol	Dopamine receptor antagonist	IV	1–3 mg
		PO	1–2 mg
Dronabinol	Cannabinoid	PO	5–10 mg
Nabilone	Cannabinoid	PO	1–2 mg

antagonists used alone demonstrated superior efficacy compared to high-dose metoclopramide alone (22) and equivalence to the combination of high-dose metoclopramide and dexamethasone, the previous standard of care (23). However, the combination
of 5-HT3 receptor antagonist and dexamethasone was the most effective combination
tested (24). Importantly, the 5-HT3 receptor antagonists were well tolerated with few
adverse effects.

Before 2003, there were three FDA-approved 5-HT3 receptor antagonists: ondansetron, granisetron, and dolasetron. Numerous clinical trials demonstrated their clinical
equivalence, despite differences seen in preclinical models (24–30). A single dose
prechemotherapy was shown to be as effective as repeat dosing (31–33), and there was
no significant difference whether given orally or intravenously (34, 35).

In July 2003, a new 5-HT3 receptor antagonist, palonosetron, was approved by the
Food and Drug Administration (FDA) for antiemetic prophylaxis. Palonosetron may
have advantages over the other serotonin antagonists because of its higher binding
affinity to the 5-HT3 receptor and its longer half-life. Two Phase III randomized clinical trials demonstrated the superiority of palonosetron compared to ondansetron and
dolasetron, particularly in preventing delayed nausea and vomiting. In the first, 592
patients were randomized to receive palonosetron at either 0.25 mg or 0.75 mg or
dolasetron at 100 mg, 30 min prior to moderately emetogenic chemotherapy. Less
than 5% of patients received concomitant corticosteroids. A statistically significant

difference was observed between the palonosetron 0.25 mg and dolasetron arms in complete response (CR, defined as absence of emesis and no rescue medication in the first 24 h). CR rates were 63% in the palonosetron 0.25-mg arm versus 52.9% in the dolasetron arm ($p = 0.049$), and 57% for the palonosetron 0.75-mg arm ($p = 0.412$). For complete control (CC, defined as no emesis, no need for rescue medication and no symptoms other than mild nausea) of delayed nausea and vomiting (24–120 h), palonosetron 0.25 mg and 0.75 mg demonstrated statistically significant improvements compared to dolasetron 100 mg (48.1% for palonosetron 0.25 mg compared to 36.1% for dolasetron, $p = 0.027$; 51.9% for palonosetron 0.75 mg, $p = 0.016$). There was no difference among the groups in observed adverse effects including headache, constipation, and fatigue (36).

In the second study, palonosetron was compared to ondansetron 32 mg. Five-hundred seventy patients receiving moderately emetogenic chemotherapy were randomized to one of two doses of palonosetron (0.25 mg or 0.75 mg) or ondansetron 32 mg on day 1 of chemotherapy. No patients received corticosteroids. CR rates were superior for the palonosetron 0.25-mg arm compared to the ondansetron group in prevention of both acute (81% vs. 68.6%, $p = 0.009$) and delayed (74.1% vs. 55.1%, $p < 0.001$) symptoms. Although palonosetron 0.75 mg demonstrated numeric improvement over ondansetron, the results were not statistically significant. Side effects were similar in all groups and included headache, diarrhea, constipation, and fatigue (37).

The 5-HT3 antagonists remain the cornerstone of prophylaxis for both highly and moderately emetogenic chemotherapy. Initial data shows the superiority of palonosetron over the others, particularly in the prevention of delayed symptoms. Further studies are needed to define the differences between palonosetron and the other 5-HT3 antagonists. All of the 5-HT3 antagonists are well tolerated; the most common adverse effect is headache, occurring in 15–20% of patients. Less commonly seen side effects include constipation and dizziness.

Dopamine Receptor Antagonists

There are three classes of dopamine receptor antagonists effective in the prevention and treatment of nausea and vomiting: phenothiazines, butyrophenones, and benzamides. In the 1960s, the phenothiazines were the first drugs proven to have efficacy in prevention of CINV. Prochlorperazine is the most commonly used in this class and has efficacy in all classes except the most highly emetogenic chemotherapy (38). Extrapyramidal effects including dystonia may be seen; treatment is diphenhydramine and cessation of the drug. The butyrophenones, including haloperidol, are less frequently used for CINV and have adverse effects similar to the phenothiazines. They may be effective in the treatment of breakthrough nausea and vomiting when the addition of a drug from another class is required.

Of the benzamides, metoclopramide is the best studied and most widely used in CINV. It blocks central and peripheral D2 receptors at low doses and exhibits weak 5-HT3 inhibition at high doses. Besides its effects in the central nervous system, there are gastrointestinal effects as well; it speeds gastric emptying and increases sphincter tone at the gastroesophageal junction. Prior to the introduction of the 5-HT3 antagonists, a combination of high-dose intravenous metoclopramide and dexamethasone was the most effective antiemetic prophylaxis for highly emetogenic chemotherapy (39).

Because metoclopramide crosses the blood–brain barrier, side effects including dystonia and tardive dyskinesia may be seen, particularly at high doses and in elderly patients. Diphenhydramine was commonly given as part of the combination regimen to prevent these adverse effects. This previous standard of care has generally been replaced by a combination containing a 5-HT3 receptor antagonist because of its improved efficacy and safety profile *(22–24)*. The regimen of metoclopramide, dexamethasone, and diphenhydramine may be useful in patients intolerant of 5-HT3 receptor antagonists or those who have failed first-line treatment.

Corticosteroids

Corticosteroids, most commonly dexamethasone, are effective in preventing nausea and vomiting when used alone or in combination for all emetogenic classes of chemotherapy. For moderately and highly emetogenic chemotherapy, a regimen containing dexamethasone plus a 5-HT3 receptor antagonist is used. A meta-analysis of 32 randomized clinical trials including 5,613 patients from 1984–1998 demonstrated the efficacy of dexamethasone in both moderately and highly emetogenic chemotherapy either alone or in combination with other agents *(40)*. Later studies revealed the superiority of a combination of 5-HT3 receptor antagonist and dexamethasone compared to either agent alone in highly emetogenic chemotherapy *(41)*. The site of action of corticosteroids along the vomiting reflex pathway is unknown. Side effects including insomnia, increased energy, and mood disturbances may be seen.

Neurokinin-1 Receptor Antagonists

Neurokinin-1 (NK-1) receptors are found in the nucleus tractus solitarius and the area postrema, and they are activated by substance P *(11)*. Inhibitors of the NK-1 receptor have demonstrated antiemetic effects and represent a new target for antiemetic therapy. The first approved medication in this class, aprepitant, has been shown to prevent both acute and delayed emesis resulting from highly and moderately emetogenic chemotherapy *(13–15)*.

Following promising preliminary data, two randomized Phase III multicenter trials demonstrated the efficacy of aprepitant for prevention of both acute and delayed nausea and vomiting. Five-hundred twenty-three patients receiving highly emetogenic chemotherapy (cisplatin > 70 mg/m^2) received as emetic prophylaxis either aprepitant in combination with 5-HT3 receptor antagonists and dexamethasone (aprepitant 125 mg PO, ondansetron 32 mg IV, and dexamethasone 12 mg PO on day 1, followed by aprepitant 80 mg PO and dexamethasone 8 mg PO on days 2–3, and dexamethasone 8 mg PO on day 4) or a regimen of a 5-HT3 receptor antagonist and dexamethasone alone (ondansetron 32 mg IV plus dexamethasone 20 mg PO on day 1, followed by dexamethasone 8 mg PO BID on days 2–4). In the first study, overall complete response (absence of emesis and no need for rescue medication in the first 24 h) was 62.7% in the aprepitant arm versus 43.3% in the standard therapy arm ($p < 0.001$). CR rates for the aprepitant arm and the standard therapy arm, respectively, for acute (82.8% vs. 68.4%, $p < 0.001$)

and delayed (67.7% as compared to 46.8%, $p < 0.001$) symptoms demonstrated the superiority of the aprepitant arm *(13)*. The second study, which evaluated the same regimens in 521 patients receiving high-dose cisplatin chemotherapy, confirmed these results. Overall CR rates were 72.7% in the aprepitant group versus 52.3% in the standard arm ($p < 0.001$). CR rates in both acute and delayed emesis were also superior in the aprepitant arm (89.2% vs. 78.1%, respectively, $p < 0.001$ and 75.4% vs. 55.8%, respectively, $p < 0.001$) *(14)*. These data led to the FDA approval of aprepitant as prophylaxis for highly emetogenic chemotherapy in 2003.

In 2006, FDA approval for aprepitant in the prophylaxis of moderately emetogenic chemotherapy was granted following a study of 866 breast cancer patients evaluating symptoms of CINV during their first cycle of cyclophosphamide plus anthracycline chemotherapy. Patients were randomized to a control regimen of ondansetron 8 mg BID plus dexamethasone 20 mg on day 1, followed by ondansetron 8 mg BID on days 2–3 or to the aprepitant-containing regimen consisting of aprepitant 125 mg PO, ondansetron 8 mg BID, and dexamethasone 12 mg on day 1, followed by aprepitant 80 mg qd on days 2–3. With a primary endpoint of absence of emesis, the aprepitant containing regimen had a superior CR rate (51% vs. 41%, $p = 0.015$). Analysis of acute and delayed emesis separately showed some advantage for the aprepitant arm, but this difference was not statistically significant (15).

Aprepitant is a substrate, moderate inducer and moderate inhibitor of the cytochrome P450 enzyme 3A4 (CYP3A4) *(42)*. Chemotherapy and other drugs are metabolized by this enzyme, and caution must be used when adding aprepitant in these patients. Docetaxel, paclitaxel, etoposide, irinotecan, ifosfamide, imatinib, vinorelbine, vinblastine, and vincristine are metabolized by CYP3A4. Although in its clinical trials, aprepitant was given to patients receiving these agents without any alteration in dose, observed adverse effects, or decreased efficacy, caution is urged. In addition, aprepitant may interact with nonchemotherapy agents; for example, it may induce metabolism of warfarin, leading to reduced levels. Aprepitant appears to increase the active levels of oral dexamethasone and methylprednisolone, and reduced dosing of prophylactic dexamethasone is recommended when used in combination with aprepitant. Other drugs with interactions include oral contraceptives, midazolam, ketoconazole, erythromycin, carbamazepine, rifampin, and phenytoin.

Other Classes of Antiemetics

Additional classes of antiemetic agents that may be useful in patients include the benzodiazepines, anticholinergics, and cannabinoids. The most commonly used benzodiazepines, lorazepam and alprazolam, although not antiemetics, have their greatest utility in the treatment of anticipatory nausea and reduction in the anxiety associated with chemotherapy when used in addition to the classic antiemetics *(43)*. The anticholinergic promethazine, and less frequently, transdermal scopolamine, may be used for treatment of breakthrough CINV. There is less randomized clinical trial data to recommend the use of cannabinoids such as marijuana or its synthetic versions, nabilone and dronabinol *(44)*. A meta-analysis of 30 studies including cannabinoids by Tramer et al., suggests that dronabinol and nabilone are more effective antiemetics than prochlorperazine, metoclopramide, chlorpromazine, and haldol. However, these findings were not consistent in patients receiving very low or very high emetogenic potential chemotherapy *(45)*. Additionally, the authors found that the side effects of cannabinoids (such as euphoria, sedation, dysphoria, depression, and hallucinations) would limit more widespread use. A recently published study of 64 patients receiving moderately to highly emetogenic chemotherapy randomized patients to receive antiemetic prophylaxis consisting of dexamethasone and ondansetron, with or without dronabinol on day 1, followed by placebo, dronabinol, ondansetron or the combination of dronabinol and ondansetron on days 2–5. The authors concluded that dronabinol and ondansetron were similarly effective at prevention of CINV and that the combination of dronabinol and ondansetron was no more effective than either agent alone *(46)*. Further randomized studies to evaluate cannabinoids when used with or compared to optimal antiemtic prophylaxis (regimens containing $5HT_3$ antagonists, NK-1 receptor antagonists) are needed to clarify their role.

RECOMMENDATIONS FOR PREVENTION AND TREATMENT OF CHEMOTHERAPY-INDUCED EMESIS (TABLE 3)

The goal of antiemetic therapy is complete prevention of chemotherapy-induced nausea and vomiting. In patients receiving highly and moderately emetogenic chemotherapy, the period of risk for nausea and vomiting lasts at least 4 days following chemotherapy, and protection with antiemetics is needed daily throughout this period of risk. The choice of antiemetic prophylaxis is driven by the emetogenic potential of the specific chemotherapy agents and patient risk factors.

Table 3
Guidelines for prevention of acute and delayed nausea and vomiting in patients depending on emetic risk

Emetic risk	Acute	Delayed
High (>90%)	Aprepitant +$5HT_3$ Antagonist +Dexamethasone +/–Lorazepam	Aprepitant +Dexamethasone
Moderate (30–90%)	$5HT_3$ Antagonist +Dexamethasone +Aprepitant in select patients +/–Lorazepam	Aprepitant if used on day 1 + Dexamethasone or Dexamethasone or $5HT_3$ Antagonist +/–Lorazepam
Low (10–30%)	Dexamethasone or Phenothiazine or Metoclopramide +/–Lorazepam	None
Minimal (<10%)	None	None

Highly Emetogenic Chemotherapy

Cisplatin and cyclophosphamide are the most frequently used highly emetogenic chemotherapy agents. Nausea and vomiting are virtually assured without adequate prophylaxis. Prior to the approval of the NK-1 receptor antagonist aprepitant, the previous recommendation was a combination of a 5-HT3 antagonist and dexamethasone. A regimen of a 5-HT3 receptor antagonist, aprepitant (125 mg PO) and dexamethasone (12 mg PO or IV) on day 1, followed by aprepitant (80 mg PO) and dexamethasone (8 mg PO or IV) on days 2–4 is recommended in all patients receiving highly emetogenic chemotherapy. All prophylaxis should begin prior to the administration of chemotherapy. Faso-aprepitant (115 mg IV) can be substituted for the 125 mg PO dose one day.

Moderately Emetogenic Chemotherapy

A combination of a 5-HT3 receptor antagonist and dexamethasone is recommended in all patients receiving moderately emetogenic chemotherapy. Given recent data and its superior efficacy in preventing delayed symptoms, palonosetron (0.25 mg on day 1 only) is the preferred 5-HT3 receptor antagonist. If others are used, they should be given on day 1 prior to chemotherapy and then repeated daily on days 2–4. Dexamethasone is given as 12 mg IV or PO on day 1 and then at a daily dose of 8 mg on days 2–4 (either 8 mg daily or 4 mg in divided doses BID). In select patients (those with breakthrough nausea and vomiting despite adequate prophylaxis or those with other patient variables which suggest higher risk of symptoms), aprepitant (125 mg PO on day 1, followed by 80 mg PO on days 2–3) should be considered.

Low-Risk Chemotherapy

Options for antiemetic prophylaxis in patients receiving chemotherapy of low emetogenic potential include dexamethasone (12 mg PO or IV) or prochlorperazine (10 mg PO or IV q4–6 h) or metoclopramide (20–40 mg PO q4–6 h or 1–2 mg/kg UV q3–4 h with diphenhydramine to prevent extrapyramidal symptoms). All prophylaxis should be given prior to the administration of chemotherapy.

Minimally Emetogenic Chemotherapy

No routine prophylaxis is recommended. Should nausea and vomiting occur, the use of dexamethasone, prochlorperazine, or metoclopramide is recommended. Prophylactic use of these medications should be considered prior to the next cycle of therapy.

SPECIAL SITUATIONS

Breakthrough Nausea and Vomiting

Of course, the best treatment for breakthrough nausea and vomiting is to prevent it from occurring at all with optimal use of antiemetic prophylaxis. At times, despite aggressive prophylaxis, symptoms still occur. The best management of breakthrough symptoms is to add an agent from another class of antiemetics. In addition, an alternative route other than oral, such as intravenous or rectal, may be useful. These medications are most effective if taken on a schedule rather than on an as-needed basis. When breakthrough nausea and vomiting occur, the prophylactic regimen should be reevaluated and enhanced prior to the next cycle of chemotherapy.

Anticipatory Nausea and Vomiting

Prevention of anticipatory nausea and vomiting is achieved through the use of optimal antiemetic prophylaxis with each cycle of chemotherapy. Once symptoms have developed, agents such as the benzodiazepines may be added to the prophylactic regimen, in large part due to their antianxiety effects (43). Other strategies which have proven useful for some patients include behavioral therapy, systemic desensitization, and hypnosis (47, 48).

Radiation-Induced Nausea and Vomiting

Radiation-induced nausea and vomiting (RINV) is seen in nearly all patients receiving total body irradiation prior to bone marrow transplantation and in more than 80% of those receiving radiation to the upper abdomen (49). Studies have demonstrated the efficacy of prophylactic 5-HT3 receptor antagonists to placebo (50) and the superiority of prophylaxis with 5-HT3 receptor antagonists as compared to combinations with metoclopramide and prochlorperazine (51, 52). The recommendation is for all patients undergoing either upper abdominal radiation therapy or total body irradiation to receive prophylaxis with an oral 5-HT3 receptor antagonist dosed either BID or TID with or without oral dexamethasone (53).

CONCLUSIONS

Dramatic progress has been made in the prevention and treatment of chemotherapy-induced emesis, especially since the introduction of the 5-HT3 receptor antagonists in the early 1990s and the 2003 introduction of the NK1 receptor antagonist, aprepitant. Recent surveys indicate the need for heightened awareness of the frequency and severity of acute and, particularly, delayed nausea and vomiting from chemotherapy. Fortunately, new agents have been added to the antiemetic arsenal to further enhance the efficacy of antiemetic prophylaxis. Appropriate implementation of guidelines for prophylaxis based on the specific chemotherapy agents used will ensure that fewer patients experience these most distressing of side effects.

REFERENCES

1. Grunberg SM, Deuson RR, Mavros P, . Incidence of chemotherapy-induced nausea and emesis after modern antiemetics. *Cancer* 2004;100(10):2261–8.
2. Mitchell EP. Gastrointestinal toxicity of chemotherapeutic agents. *Semin Oncol* 1992;19(5):566–79.
3. Morran C, Smith DC, Anderson DA, McArdle CS. Incidence of nausea and vomiting with cytotoxic chemotherapy: a prospective randomised trial of antiemetics. *Br Med J* 1979;1(6174):1323–4.
4. Coates A, Abraham S, Kaye SB, . On the receiving end – patient perception of the side-effects of cancer chemotherapy. *Eur J Cancer Clin Oncol* 1983;19(2):203–8.
5. Lindley C, McCune JS, Thomason TE, . Perception of chemotherapy side effects cancer versus noncancer patients. *Cancer Pract* 1999;7(2):59–65.

6. de Boer-Dennert M, de Wit R, Schmitz PI, . Patient perceptions of the side-effects of chemotherapy: the influence of 5HT3 antagonists. *Br J Cancer* 1997;76(8):1055–61.

7. Borison HL, Wang SC. Physiology and pharmacology of vomiting. *Pharmacol Rev* 1953;5(2):193–230.

8. Miller AD, Leslie RA. The area postrema and vomiting. *Front Neuroendocrinol* 1994;15(4):301–20.

9. Carpenter DO. Neural mechanisms of emesis. *Can J Physiol Pharmacol* 1990;68(2):230–6.

10. Dodds LJ. The control of cancer chemotherapy-induced nausea and vomiting. *J Clin Hosp Pharm* 1985;10(2):143–66.

11. Saito R, Takano Y, Kamiya HO. Roles of substance P and NK(1) receptor in the brainstem in the development of emesis. *J Pharmacol Sci* 2003;91(2):87–94.

12. de Wit R, Herrstedt J, Rapoport B, . Addition of the oral NK1 antagonist aprepitant to standard antiemetics provides protection against nausea and vomiting during multiple cycles of cisplatin-based chemotherapy. *J Clin Oncol* 2003;21(22):4105–11.

13. Poli-Bigelli S, Rodrigues-Pereira J, Carides AD, . Addition of the neurokinin 1 receptor antagonist aprepitant to standard antiemetic therapy improves control of chemotherapy-induced nausea and vomiting Results from a randomized, double-blind, placebo-controlled trial in Latin America. *Cancer* 2003;97(12):3090–8.

14. Hesketh PJ, Grunberg SM, Gralla RJ, . The oral neurokinin-1 antagonist aprepitant for the prevention of chemotherapy-induced nausea and vomiting: a multinational, randomized, double-blind, placebo-controlled trial in patients receiving high-dose cisplatin – the Aprepitant Protocol 052 Study Group. *J Clin Oncol* 2003;21(22):4112–19.

15. Warr DG, Hesketh PJ,Gralla RJ, . Efficacy and tolerability of aprepitant for the prevention of chemotherapy-induced nausea and vomiting in patients with breast cancer after moderately emetogenic chemotherapy. *J Clin Oncol* 2005;23(12):2822–30.

16. Moher D, Arthur AZ, Pater JL. Anticipatory nausea and/or vomiting. *Cancer Treat Rev* 1984;11(3):257–64.

17. Pollera CF, Giannarelli D. Prognostic factors influencing cisplatin-induced emesis Definition and validation of a predictive logistic model. *Cancer* 1989;64(5):1117–22.

18. Hesketh PJ, Kris MG, Grunberg SM, . Proposal for classifying the acute emetogenicity of cancer chemotherapy. *J Clin Oncol* 1997;15(1):103–9.

19. Koeller JM, Aapro MS, Gralla RJ, . Antiemetic guidelines: creating a more practical treatment approach. *Support Care Cancer* 2002;10(7):519–22.

20. Mitchelson F. Pharmacological agents affecting emesis A review (Part I). *Drugs* 1992;43(3):295–315.

21. Bountra C, Gale JD, Gardner CJ, . Towards understanding the aetiology and pathophysiology of the emetic reflex: novel approaches to antiemetic drugs. *Oncology* 1996;53(Suppl 1):102–9.

22. Chevallier B, Cappelaere P, Splinter T, . A double-blind, multicentre comparison of intravenous dolasetron mesilate and metoclopramide in the prevention of nausea and vomiting in cancer patients receiving high-dose cisplatin chemotherapy. *Support Care Cancer* 1997;5(1):22–30.

23. Warr D, Wilan A, Venner P, . A randomised, double-blind comparison of granisetron with high-dose metoclopramide, dexamethasone and diphenhydramine for cisplatin-induced emesis An NCI Canada Clinical Trials Group Phase III Trial. *Eur J Cancer* 1992;29A(1):33–6.

24. Heron JF, Goedhals L, Jordaan JP, Cunningham J, Cedar E. Oral granisetron alone and in combination with dexamethasone: a double-blind randomized comparison against high-dose metoclopramide plus dexamethasone in prevention of cisplatin-induced emesis The Granisetron Study Group. *Ann Oncol* 1994;5(7):579–84.

25. Bonneterre J, Hecquet B. Granisetron (IV) compared with ondansetron (IV plus oral) in the prevention of nausea and vomiting induced by moderately emetogenic chemotherapy A cross-over study. *Bull Cancer* 1995;82(12):1038–43.

26. Stewart A, McQuade B, Cronje JD, . Ondansetron compared with granisetron in the prophylaxis of cyclophosphamide-induced emesis in out-patients: a multicentre, double-blind, double-dummy, randomised, parallel-group study Emesis Study Group for Ondansetron and Granisetron in Breast Cancer Patients. *Oncology* 1995;52(3):202–10.

27. Martoni A, Angelelli B, Guaraldi M, Strocchi E, Pannuti F. An open randomised cross-over study on granisetron versus ondansetron in the prevention of acute emesis induced by moderate dose cisplatin-containing regimens. *Eur J Cancer* 1996;32A(1):82–5.

28. Hesketh P, Navari R, Grote T, . Double-blind, randomized comparison of the antiemetic efficacy of intravenous dolasetron mesylate and intravenous ondansetron in the prevention of acute cisplatin-induced emesis in patients with cancer Dolasetron Comparative Chemotherapy-induced Emesis Prevention Group. *J Clin Oncol* 1996;14(8):2242–9.

29. Audhuy B, Cappelaere P, Martin M, . A double-blind, randomised comparison of the anti-emetic efficacy of two intravenous doses of dolasetron mesilate and granisetron in patients receiving high dose cisplatin chemotherapy. *Eur J Cancer* 1996;32A(5):807–13.

30. Lofters WS, Pater JL, Zee B, . Phase III double-blind comparison of dolasetron mesylate and ondansetron and an evaluation of the additive role of dexamethasone in the prevention of acute and delayed nausea and vomiting due to moderately emetogenic chemotherapy. *J Clin Oncol* 1997;15(8):2966–73.

31. Seynaeve C, Schuller J, Buser K, Comparison of the anti-emetic efficacy of different doses of ondansetron, given as either a continuous infusion or a single intravenous dose, in acute cisplatin-induced emesis A multi-centre, double-blind, randomised, parallel group study. Ondansetron Study Group. *Br J Cancer* 1992;66(1):192–7.

32. Ettinger DS, Eisenberg PD, Fitts D, Friedman C, Wilson-Lynch K, Yocom K. A double-blind comparison of the efficacy of two dose regimens of oral granisetron in preventing acute emesis in patients receiving moderately emetogenic chemotherapy. *Cancer* 1996;78(1):144–51.

33. Harman GS, Omura GA, Ryan K, Hainsworth JD, Cramer MB, Hahne WF. A randomized, double-blind comparison of single-dose and divided multiple-dose dolasetron for cisplatin-induced emesis. *Cancer Chemother Pharmacol* 1996;38(4):323–8.

34. Perez EA, Hesketh P, Sandbach J, . Comparison of single-dose oral granisetron versus intravenous ondansetron in the prevention of nausea and vomiting induced by moderately emetogenic chemotherapy: a multi-center, double-blind, randomized parallel study. *J Clin Oncol* 1998;16(2):754–60.

35. Gralla RJ, Navari RM, Hesketh PJ, . Single-dose oral granisetron has equivalent antiemetic efficacy to intravenous ondansetron for highly emetogenic cisplatin-based chemotherapy. *J Clin Oncol* 1998;16(4): 1568–73.

36. Eisenberg P, Figueroa-Vadillo J, Zamora R, . Improved prevention of moderately emetogenic chemotherapy-induced nausea and vomiting with palonosetron, a pharmacologically novel 5-HT3 receptor antagonist: results of a phase III, single-dose trial versus dolasetron. *Cancer* 2003;98(11):2473–82.

37. Gralla R, Lichinitser M, Van Der Vegt S, . Palonosetron improves prevention of chemotherapy-induced nausea and vomiting following moderately emetogenic chemotherapy: results of a double-blind randomized phase III trial comparing single doses of palonosetron with ondansetron. *Ann Oncol* 2003;14(10):1570–7.

38. Moertel CG, Reitemeier RJ, Gage RP. A controlled clinical evaluation of antiemetic drugs. *JAMA* 1963;186:116–18.

39. Kris MG, Gralla RJ, Tyson LB, . Improved control of cisplatin-induced emesis with high-dose metoclopramide and with combinations of metoclopramide, dexamethasone, and diphenhydramine Results of consecutive trials in 255 patients. *Cancer* 1985;55(3):527–34.

40. Ioannidis JP, Hesketh PJ, Lau J. Contribution of dexamethasone to control of chemotherapy-induced nausea and vomiting: a meta-analysis of randomized evidence. *J Clin Oncol* 2000;18(19):3409–22.

41. Dexamethasone, granisetron, or both for the prevention of nausea and vomiting during chemotherapy for cancer The Italian Group for Antiemetic Research. *N Engl J Med* 1995;332(1):1–5.

42. Shadle CR, Lee Y, Majumdar AK, . Evaluation of potential inductive effects of aprepitant on cytochrome P450 3A4 and 2C9 activity. *J Clin Pharmacol* 2004;44(3):215–23.

43. Razavi D, Delvaux N, Farvacques C, . Prevention of adjustment disorders and anticipatory nausea secondary to adjuvant chemotherapy: a double-blind, placebo-controlled study assessing the usefulness of alprazolam. *J Clin Oncol* 1993;11(7):1384–90.

44. Sallan SE, Zinberg NE, Frei E, 3rd. Antiemetic effect of delta-9-tetrahydrocannabinol in patients receiving cancer chemotherapy. *N Engl J Med* 1975;293(16):795–7.

45. Tramer MR, Carroll D, Campbell FA, Reynolds DJ, Moore RA, McQuay HJ. Cannabinoids for control of chemotherapy-induced nausea and vomiting: quantitative systematic review. *BMJ* 2001;323(7303):16–21.

46. Meiri E, Jhangiani H, Vredenburgh JJ, . Efficacy of dronabinol alone and in combination with ondansetron versus ondansetron alone for delayed chemotherapy-induced nausea and vomiting. *Curr Med Res Opin* 2007;23(3):533–43.

47. Morrow GR, Morrell C. Behavioral treatment for the anticipatory nausea and vomiting induced by cancer chemotherapy. *N Engl J Med* 1982;307(24):1476–80.

48. Redd WH, Andrykowski MA. Behavioral intervention in cancer treatment: controlling aversion reactions to chemotherapy. *J Consult Clin Psychol* 1982;50(6):1018–29.

49. Horiot JC. *Prophylaxis versus treatment: is there a better way to manage radiotherapy-induced nausea and vomiting? Int J Radiat Oncol Biol Phys* 2004;60(4):1018–25.

50. Franzen L, Nyman J, Hagberg H, . A randomised placebo controlled study with ondansetron in patients undergoing fractionated radiotherapy. *Ann Oncol* 1996;7(6):587–92.

51. Okamoto S, Takahashi S, Tanosaki R, . Granisetron in the prevention of vomiting induced by conditioning for stem cell transplantation: a prospective randomized study. *Bone Marrow Transplant* 1996;17(5):679–83.

52. Priestman TJ, Roberts JT, Upadhyaya BK. A prospective randomized double-blind trial comparing ondansetron versus prochlorperazine for the prevention of nausea and vomiting in patients undergoing fractionated radiotherapy. *Clin Oncol (R Coll Radiol)* 1993;5(6):358–63.

53. Feyer P, Maranzano E, Molassiotis A, . Radiotherapy-induced nausea and vomiting (RINV): antiemetic guidelines. *Support Care Cancer* 2005;13(2):122–8.

11 Oral Mucositis

Nathaniel Treister and Stephen Sonis

ABSTRACT

Mucositis is a common, painful, treatment-disrupting toxicity of both radiotherapy and chemotherapy. Patients with cancers of the head and neck receiving radiation therapy with and without induction or concomitant chemotherapy, and individuals being treated with high-dose chemotherapy regimens are at particularly high risk. Importantly, even patients receiving conventional dosing schemes for other forms of cancer have a meaningful chance of developing painful lesions of the mouth and throat during their treatment. The fact that the pathobiology of mucositis is complex and multifaceted provides opportunities for mechanistically based interventions. While palifermin is the only agent currently approved for treatment, it also represents an example of other agents in development for which efficacy is based on disruption of the biological pathways leading to mucositis. This chapter discusses the clinical characteristics of mucositis, how it is evaluated and scored, its pathogenesis, and current and evolving prevention and treatment strategies.

Key Words: Oral complications, Mucosal injury, Radiation therapy, Cancer chemotherapy, Oral disease, Head and neck cancer, Hematopoietic cell transplantation.

From: *Cancer and Drug Discovery Development: Supportive Care in Cancer Therapy*
DOI: 10.1007/978-1-59745-291-5_11, Edited by: D. S. Ettinger © Humana Press, Totowa, NJ

INTRODUCTION

Mucosal injury is a common side effect of many forms of drug and radiation therapy that are used to treat cancer. While mucositis of the oral cavity and oropharynx has been best studied, virtually every component of the gastrointestinal tract is susceptible. For example, esophagitis is a frequent consequence of radiation therapy used to treat lung cancers, and proctitis is an unfortunate and very bothersome side effect among men treated for prostate cancer. The widespread application and success of growth factors for management of hematological toxicities associated with cancer therapies (e.g., anemia, infections) has brought control of mucositis to the forefront of objectives in oncological supportive care. This review will focus on oral mucositis as its clinical impact, features, and pathobiology serve as a paradigm for other forms of the condition.

CLINICAL FEATURES AND COURSE OF MUCOSITIS

Clinically, oral mucositis generally occurs in sequential stages. For patients receiving stomatotoxic chemotherapy, early mucosal changes and symptoms are noted for about 4–5 days following drug infusion. At this time, patients may complain of soreness and a reduced ability to tolerate spicy or acidic foods. The tissue may appear red and smooth (Fig. 1). Within the next few days, pain intensifies as the integrity of the mucosa breaks down and ulceration occurs. Ulceration associated with mucositis may be discrete or, as it worsens, become confluent involving extensive areas of mucosa (Fig. 2). The pain associated with ulcerative mucositis is significant, often requiring opioid analgesics and diet modification. Ulcerative mucositis lasts for upward of 1 week and then most cases

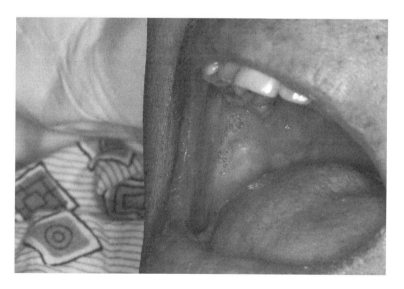

Fig. 1. Moderate mucositis of the right buccal mucosa. The tissue is erythematous and atrophic, with whitish-grey leukoedemetous changes. There is a small well-defined central zone of ulceration due to the presence of a fibrin pseudomembrane.

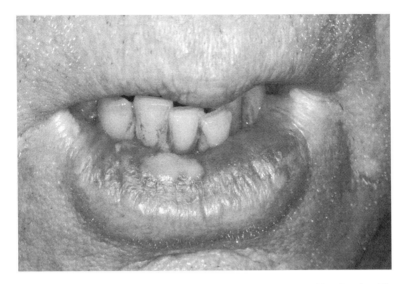

Fig. 2. Ulcerative mucositis of the labial mucosa extending to the vermillion border. There is patchy ulceration of the nonkeratinized mucosa with generalized erythema. The lips are particularly sensitive and mucositis in this location makes eating especially difficult.

resolve spontaneously. Lesions in myelosuppressed patients may be prolonged, especially if they become secondarily infected. Ulcers vary in size, but usually have a whitish, yellowish necrotic center. Unlike aphthous ulcers (canker sores), the lesions may have an irregular form and no peripheral border of erythema. Bleeding is not uncommon, especially in thrombocytopenic patients.

Radiation-induced mucositis begins at cumulative doses of 10 Gy with symptoms of pain and subtle tissue changes consisting of superficial epithelial sloughing and erythema. Mild mucosal sensitivity can usually be controlled with NSAIDs. However, as radiation continues, mucosal damage increases resulting in frank ulceration by 30 Gy. As the esophagus is often within the field of radiation, throat pain and dysphagia are common. These exquisitely painful lesions persist for the remainder of the patient's radiation course and often necessitate aggressive analgesic management with opioids. Patients' ability to eat is compromised and a relatively large number of patients require the placement of feeding tubes. Indeed, severe mucositis is so prevalent in this group that prophylactic gastrostomy-tube (g-tube) placement is common practice at many centers. In most cases, lesions last until at least 2–3 weeks after the cessation of radiation treatment. Since patients may have ulcerative mucositis for 6–7 weeks, it is not unusual for some to request breaks in treatment to better cope with this toxicity.

There is no sentinel anatomic site for oral mucositis. Chemotherapy-induced lesions may affect any part of the movable, nonkeratinized oral mucosa. Although mucositis is most common on the buccal mucosa, ventral lingual mucosa, and the soft palate, it also occurs on the labial mucosa (inner aspects of the lips) and the floor of the mouth. Chemotherapy mucositis does not occur on the dorsal surface of the tongue, the gingival, or the hard palate (i.e., those areas of oral mucosa that are most keratinized). Lesions in these locations are most commonly infectious in nature (i.e., recrudescent

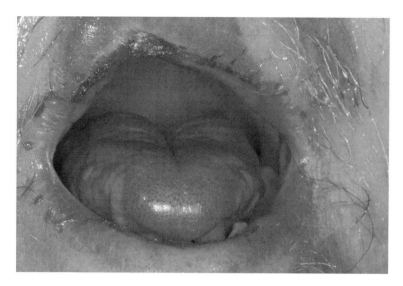

Fig. 3. Severe mucositis secondary to chemoradiation. There are extensive ulcerations on the ventrolateral tongue bilaterally that extend to involve the lateral aspects of the tongue dorsum. There is minimal saliva due to radiation-induced acute salivary gland necrosis which exacerbates the friction and pain.

HSV). Radiation-induced mucositis may occur in the same areas as that induced by chemotherapy except that the hard palate may also be affected. The mucosa of the dorsum of the tongue is rarely affected, but when it is, it is almost always the consequence of the extension of established lesions from the lateral tongue border (Fig. 3).

MUCOSITIS ASSESSMENT AND SCORING

It is likely that the lack of a consistent and uniformly accepted scoring scheme for grading mucositis severity has contributed to inconsistencies in reported toxicities, as well as insufficient clinical efficacy studies. There are more than a dozen different mucositis grading scales. Some are institutional, others more global. In general, mucositis scales can be grouped into three different functional categories:

- Those designed for toxicity assessment and reporting. The NCI-CTC v.3 scale and the WHO scale are the most common examples, although collaborative oncology group scales (i.e., RTOG) also fall into this category.
- Those scales designed primarily as research tools. The OMAS (1) and OMI (2) scales are the most frequently cited examples.
- Scales designed to assist in the nursing management of oncology patients. The Walsh (3) and Eiler's scales (4) are examples.

For any scale to be of value it must be consistently administered, easy to use, and validated for interobserver and intersite consistency. The following criteria summarize the characteristics of an ideal mucositis scale:

- Accurately reflects severity and course of objective and subjective clinical changes
- Easy to teach and use, with minimal interobserver variability

- Does not require lesion measurement
- Sensitive enough to discriminate treatment efficacy
- Clinically meaningful and easily interpretable end points for clinicians, patients, and FDA (labeling)

Toxicity Scales

The two most commonly used toxicity scales are the NCI-CTC scale and the WHO scale (Tables 1 and 2). They have similarities, but their differences are important. The NCI-CTC provides mucositis assessment in two ways (two separate scales): first, a clinical, descriptive score in which the criteria include the presence or absence of objective findings of mucositis (erythema and ulceration) and a description of the extent of ulceration; and second, an assessment of a patient's ability to function as influenced by mucositis (scored as ability to eat). However, in common usage the objective score is the only one that is usually reported. The criteria for clinical scoring include the presence or absence of erythema, and the extent of ulceration – single or "patchy" ulcers vs.

Table 1
National Cancer Institute Common Toxicity Criteria version 3 scoring criteria for oral mucositis

Mucositis functional/symptomatic score

Grade 0	No mucositis
Grade 1	Able to eat solids
Grade 2	Requires liquid diet
Grade 3	Alimentation not possible
Grade 4	Symptoms associated with life-threatening consequences

Mucositis/stomatitis clinical score

Grade 0	No mucositis
Grade 1	Erythema of the mucosa
Grade 2	Patchy ulceration or pseudomembranes
Grade 3	Confluent ulcerations or pseudomembranes
Grade 4	Tissue necrosis

Table 2
World Health Organization scoring criteria for oral mucositis

Grade 0	Normal
Grade 1	Soreness with or without erythema; no ulceration
Grade 2	Ulceration and erythema; patient can swallow a solid diet
Grade 3	Ulceration and erythema; patient can not swallow a solid diet
Grade 4	Ulceration or pseudomembrane formation of such severity that alimentation not possible

"confluent" lesions. This differentiation may be arbitrarily decided by the grader as the criteria are not specifically defined. Consequently, the extent of mucositis is determined by its clinical manifestations, rather than its clinical impact, and the NCI score may thereby underestimate the symptomatic impact of mucosal injury.

The WHO score combines objective and subjective findings into a single number. Like the NCI-CTC clinical criteria, the objective elements of the WHO score include erythema and ulceration. Unlike the NCI score, there is no attempt to assess the amount of ulceration; it is simply either present or absent. The WHO score relies on the impact of the ulcer on function within a particular grade to reflect extent. Thus, a patient who has an ulcer, but is able to eat normally, has a grade of 2, whereas a patient who has an ulcer of such severity as to necessitate a liquid diet has a grade of 3. Because of this incorporation of function and objective findings into a single score, the WHO scale tends to be more globally sensitive.

Research Scales

A number of unique scales have been validated for mucositis studies. While some of these scales have very quantitative endpoints that rely on ulcer size, severity of erythema, and impact on pain and function, others evaluate a broad range of outcomes. The Oral Mucositis Assessment Scale (OMAS) and Oral Mucositis Index (OMI) scales are examples. The OMI scale and its modified version explore a wide range of fields thought to have value in assessing mucositis severity. While very descriptive, the scale's intensity is a barrier to its routine use. A significant drawback of many research scales, including those noted here, is that they are not easily interpretable by clinicians. Hence, their applicability is largely limited to efficacy screening for interventional trials.

Nursing Management Scales

For the most part, nursing management scales are useful for assessing a patient's overall oral health during cancer treatment. These scales capture a broad range of outcomes, some unrelated to mucositis such as oral hygiene levels, lip cracking, saliva consistency, and voice quality. Since each outcome category is scored equally, it is quite possible that a patient with poor oral hygiene and chapped lips could have a worse score than a patient with severe ulcerative mucositis only. As a result, the lack of specificity of these scales can result in dangerously miscalculating the true extent of mucosal injury.

MUCOSITIS EPIDEMIOLOGY

Oral mucositis has an overall reported occurrence of approximately 40% among patients receiving chemotherapy and 70% in individuals being treated with radiation for cancers of the head and neck (5, 6). Obtaining an accurate assessment of mucositis risk by treatment regimen and cancer diagnosis has been challenging as, like many side effects of chemotherapy, mucositis tends to be underreported, and its impact on patients underappreciated. For example, the reported frequency of oral mucositis differs dramatically when toxicities are reported incidentally compared to studies in which a particular toxicity is

Table 3
The reported frequencies of oral mucositis when reported as a treatment-related
toxicity vs. a study endpoint

Disease	Toxicity (%)	End point (%)	Difference	% Difference
Head and neck cancer	63	85	22	35
Hematologic malignancies	31	48	17	57
Lung cancer	15	54	39	265

the primary endpoint (Table 3). This problem is further compounded when only severe toxicities (grades 3 or 4) are recorded. The lack of a universally accepted grading scale makes comparisons even more difficult. Nonetheless, oral mucositis occurs in virtually all patients who receive radiation to the mouth and contiguous structures as treatment for cancers of the mouth, oropharynx, nasopharynx, and major salivary glands. About two-thirds of patients who are treated for cancers of the larynx and hypopharynx develop significant oral mucositis. Patients receiving hematopoeitic stem cell transplants (HSCT) are also at high risk for oral mucositis, particularly if the conditioning regimen includes total body irradiation or high-dose melphalan.

Together, HSCT and head and neck cancers affect about 55,000 patients per year in the United States. Of the remaining million or so newly diagnosed cancer patients (excluding cancers of the skin), at least 20% develop symptoms of oral mucositis to some extent. For patients receiving multicycle therapy for solid tumors, mucositis risk increases with each cycle. The type of chemotherapy, its dose, and form of administration all influence mucositis risk. Use of anthracyclines, antimetabolites, taxanes, and alkylating agents are associated with mucositis risks of 30% or more. For example, a recent study reported that among patients being treated for node positive breast cancer, oral mucositis occurred in 69.4% who receive TAC, compared to 52.9% in patients who received FAC (7). In contrast, the reported risk of mucositis, while still present, is less for topoisomerase 1 inhibitors, monoclonal antibodies, and plant alkaloids.

Since many multiagent treatment regimens are now the standard of care, assignment of mucositis risk based on a single agent is misleading and often inaccurate. For example, mucositis frequency for patients being treated for breast cancers ranged from 17% in patients receiving a combination regimen of epirubicin, vinorelbine, and 5-fluorouracil compared to over 69% in patients who had received a course of docetaxel, doxorubicin, and cyclophosphamid (7–12). In general, toxicities induced by chemotherapy are dose related. Similarly, radiation-induced mucositis is dependent on the cumulative dose of radiation given. Virtually any mucosal surface included in a field of 30 Gy or more of cumulative radiation will ulcerate.

Aside from treatment-related factors associated with risk, patient-related variables such as gender and body mass appear to impact the incidence and severity of mucositis (13, 14). However, the extent to which these predict risk is poorly defined. It is becoming increasingly clear that there is a strong genetic component to oral mucositis risk. Patients deficient in genes that control enzymes that metabolize stomatotoxic drugs such as fluoruracil and methotrexate suffer more frequent and severe mucositis than the normal population. Fortunately, such deficiencies are relatively rare. In contrast, individual variations in the extent of expression of genes that regulate the signaling pathways and mediators of mucosal injury appear to be more common. Thus, it is likely that mucositis risk is largely determined by an individual's genetic makeup. Importantly, this finding offers the potential opportunity for directed genetic testing as a means to predict patient toxicity risk.

HEALTH AND ECONOMIC IMPACT OF ORAL MUCOSITIS

In addition to its physiologic cost, oral mucositis is associated with significant health and economic burdens. Among patients receiving hematopoietic stem cell transplants, patients with significant mucositis have more days of fever, antibiotic use, total parenteral nutrition and narcotic use than did patients with mild or no mucositis (15). Among 599 patients being treated for a variety of nonhead and neck solid tumors, Elting and her colleagues reported increased infection and duration of hospitalization associated with mucositis (16). Importantly, mucositis is consistently found to be associated with longer hospitalizations in this patient cohort (15–18). Taken together, this greater utilization of resources culminates in mucositis being a driver of increased charges associated with treatment (6, 18).

The overwhelming majority of patients being treated with radiation with or without chemotherapy for squamous cell carcinomas of the head and neck develop clinically significant mucositis. As with other patient populations, mucositis in this cohort is also a driver of health resource use and cost of care. A number of studies have reported increased frequencies of mucositis-related hospital admissions (18, 19). As might be expected, the frequency of gastrostomy tube placement is increased among patients with mucositis (19, 20). In addition, it appears that the presence of mucositis results in a higher likelihood of unscheduled office or emergency room visits (20).

Mucositis indirectly but profoundly influences patients' ability to tolerate optimum cancer therapy. The painful and debilitating sequelae of mucositis are often reasons for which patients require a break or delay in their course of radiation or a reduction in the dose of chemotherapy. As a result, treatment outcomes may be compromised.

PATHOPHYSIOLOGY OF ORAL MUCOSITIS

Mucositis was traditionally thought to be the direct, nonspecific result of radiation- and chemotherapy-induced damage to the rapidly dividing basal cells of the mucosa, culminating in epithelial injury. Such targeted, clonogenic cell death was thought to interrupt the normal sequence of epithelial renewal, leading initially to atrophy, and ultimately, frank ulceration. Critical research advances have generated a tremendous body of data on tissue and cellular responses to cancer therapies and mucosal injury specifically, which have subsequently proved the classic model to be oversimplified and in large part inaccurate. In its place, a far more complex and dynamic landscape has been painted that includes nearly all the cells and structures of the mucosa and submucosa, in addition to the basal epithelium (21).

This has expanded our understanding of the underlying pathobiological mechanisms that lead to mucositis and has facilitated the identification of a broad range of promising targets for therapy, with a number of mechanistically based interventional approaches now in preclinical and clinical development. The highly coordinated cellular events have been modeled into the following five stages (Fig. 4) (22):

1. Initiation
2. Primary damage response
3. Signal amplification
4. Ulceration
5. Healing

While in reality these stages are not entirely discrete, it is helpful to envision mucositis as a progression and succession of biological activities. Importantly, depending on the type of therapy, the length, duration, and specific mechanisms of these stages may vary considerably. For example, in the case of fractionated radiation regimens for

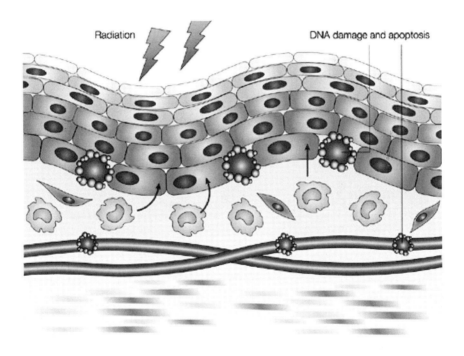

a

Fig. 4. The pathobiology of mucositis. (**a**) Radiation and chemotherapy generate reactive oxygen species that most importantly set in motion a biological cascade including multiple complementary damaging pathways. Mediators include proinflammatory cytokines, ceramide, and matrix metalloproteinases. These and other molecules cause direct cellular damage and also stimulate further upregulation through positive feedback loops. (**b**) The ulcerative phase of mucositis peaks approximately 10 days following the administration of stomatotoxic chemotherapy or at cumulative radiation doses of around 30 Gy. Bacterial colonization of ulcers follows, stimulating additional proinflammatory cytokine generation, and in severely myelosuppressed patients increasing the risk for sepsis. Healing takes place 3 weeks after chemotherapy infusion or 2–3 weeks following cessation of radiation therapy. ECM, extracellular matrix. Reproduced with permission (22).

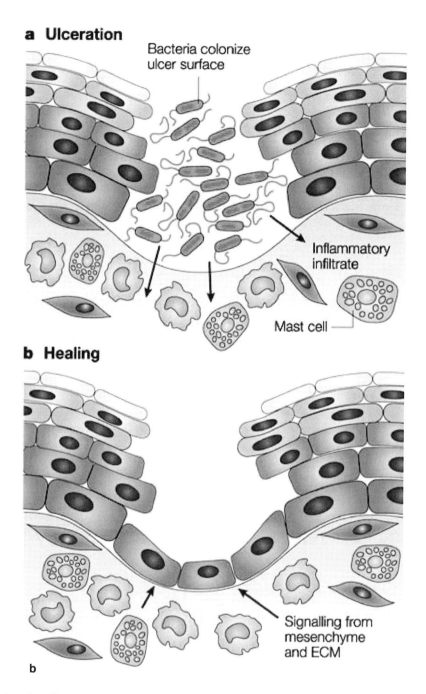

a Ulceration

Bacteria colonize
ulcer surface

Inflammatory
infiltrate

Mast cell

b Healing

Signalling from
mesenchyme
and ECM

b

Fig. 4. (continued)

head and neck cancers, damage is initiated in multiple, small daily doses over several weeks, whereas in the case of intensive conditioning regimens for hematopoietic cell transplantation, the chemotherapy and radiation doses are given in an intense, consolidated manner over a very short period of time.

Initiation

Chemotherapy and/or radiotherapy rapidly trigger the primary signals that ultimately result in mucosal injury by inducing DNA and non-DNA damage. Radiation is delivered from the "outside-in," affecting both the mucosa and the underlying submucosa, whereas chemotherapy, which enters via the endothelium within the submucosa, is delivered from the "inside-out," through the underlying connective tissue to the epithelium. While basal cell apoptosis develops at this early stage due to DNA strand breaks, these are insufficient to generate the level of tissue destruction observed clinically. More significant is the generation of free radicals, or reactive oxygen species (ROS), that have the ability not only to cause immediate direct epithelial damage, but also, importantly, to initiate a cascade of downstream events that culminate in mucosal damage and ulceration. These early activities occur almost immediately after exposure and well in advance of the development of any clinical signs or symptoms of mucositis.

Primary Damage Response

The initial response mechanisms activate a series of highly coordinated biochemical activities that lead to mucosal damage. Paramount to this is the early activation and upregulation of transcription factors that subsequently regulate the expression of numerous genes at the DNA level in the nucleus. Among those activated, nuclear factor-kappa B (NF-κB) has been identified as a key DNA transcription factor that acts as a master switch with the ability to affect the transcription of over 200 genes (23, 24). A number of the proteins influenced by NF-κB, such as tumor necrosis factor-alpha (TNF-α) and interleukins-1beta and 6, are proinflammatory cytokines that are known to be expressed at significantly elevated levels during mucositis and likely account for early damage to the connective tissue and endothelium (22, 25). Activation of sphingomyelinase and ceramide pathways also appears to play a significant role during this early phase (26).

Fibroblasts are a major structural component of the submucosa and the target of a number of pathogenic cellular pathways. It appears that NF-κB-regulated cytokines are effectors of both endothelial and fibroblast damage that precedes and initiates mesenchymal–epithelial crosstalk. It is this signaling that results in the select apoptosis of basal epithelial cells. Fibroblast injury is also mediated by AP1, a transcription factor which controls genes that regulate the production of matrix mellaloproteinases (MMPs). This diverse group of enzymes targets various structural components of the submucosa. For example, MMP1, an interstitial collagenase, facilitates degradation within the matrix of the submucosa, whereas MMP3 (stomelysin 1) targets and undermines the integrity of the basement membrane. This results in the exposure of additional molecular targets and receptors, which facilitates the diffusion and dissemination of additional pro-inflammatory signals and pathways (27).

The complexity of biological events was further illustrated by a recent study in which gene expression determined by microarray analysis was studied in patients undergoing chemoradiation for head and neck cancers. A comparison of samples taken prior to treatment with those taken 2 weeks after the start of therapy demonstrated that specific groups of genes were associated with the development of mucositis (the sentinenal toxicity) and that these could be grouped into 14 canonical pathways including those associated with signaling mediated by NF-κB, toll-like receptors, P13k/Akt, IL-6, p38, and MAPK. It is also apparent that apoptosis mediated by the ceramide pathway provides an additional conduit for tissue injury (28).

Signal Amplification

During this phase, a number of biologically capable proteins, such as the pro-inflammatory cytokines under the regulation of NF-κB, stimulate a number of positive feedback loops that result in amplification of the primary damage response described above (23). At the same time, initiation of further downstream pathways leads to the upregulation and activation of additional biologically active factors. For example TNF-α activates NF-κB, therefore further increasing TNF-α levels, while at the same time initiating mitogen-activated protein kinase (MAPK) signaling, which influences multiple pathways including programmed cell death signaling. The end result is a dramatic alteration of the mucosal environment with only minimal clinical signs and symptoms.

Ulceration

The ulcerative phase occurs when the mucosal integrity becomes so compromised that epithelium breaks down, leaving the submucosa raw and exposed to the oral cavity. Damage occurs secondary to normal physiologic oral functions, such as speaking, eating, and swallowing, due to normal movement of the oral tissues and low-grade trauma from the teeth and foods. These lesions are incredibly painful, in part due to exposed nerve endings, with secondary bacterial colonization by commensal oral organisms likely adding further insult to injury by activating infiltrating mononuclear cells that produce additional proinflammatory cytokines. In severely myelosuppressed patients, such as in the setting of hematopoietic cell transplantation, breaks in the mucosa may act as portals of entry leading to bacteremia and sepsis, and have been postulated to play a role in the development of acute graft-vs.-host disease (17, 29). In the case of fractionated radiation therapy protocols that may be given over 7–8 weeks, the ulcerative phase may persist for upward of 1–2 months.

Healing

Mucositis is a self-limiting condition that invariably resolves following the termination of cancer therapy. With the initiation and propagation mechanisms turned off, signaling from the extracellular matrix and mesenchyme promote the migration and proliferation of regenerative epithelial cells. As the duration of each phase is dependent on the type of cancer therapy (e.g., chemotherapy vs. radiation therapy), specific agents, and the dose and timing of therapy, healing may occur quickly or may take a more prolonged course. These five stages are dynamic and fluid, but follow a logical progression based on well-characterized changes. Strategies for intervention can be developed, which not only target specific mechanisms, but are also directed rationally at certain time points within the continuum of pathobiological activity (14).

PREVENTION AND TREATMENT OF ORAL MUCOSITIS

A large number of therapies have been evaluated with the goal of preventing and/or reducing the severity of mucosal toxicity associated with cancer therapies. The main challenge in developing such interventions has been to target and protect normal tissue without reducing or inhibiting the desired antineoplastic effects of the cancer treatment itself. In large part, the outcomes of these efforts have been disappointing for a number of reasons, including insufficient understanding of the underlying pathobiology, ineffective delivery strategies, and poor study design. In fact, recently conducted comprehensive evidence-based reviews of published mucositis studies by the Cochrane Collaboration and the Mucositis Study Group of the Multinational Association of Supportive Care in

Table 4
Summary of evidence-based clinical practice guidelines for care of patients with oral mucositis; adapted from the Mucositis Study Section of the Multinational Association of Supportive Care in Cancer and the International Society for Oral Oncology (MASCC/ISOO) (5)

Basic oral care and good clinical practices

- Multidisciplinary development and evaluation of oral care protocols, and patient and staff education in the use of such protocols to reduce the severity of oral mucositis from chemotherapy and/or radiation therapy
- Use of validated tools to regularly assess oral pain and oral cavity health; inclusion of oral health professionals is vital throughout the treatment and follow-up phases
- Patient-controlled analgesia with morphine as the treatment of choice for severe oral mucositis pain

Radiotherapy: Prevention

- Use of midline radiation blocks and three-dimensional radiation treatment to reduce mucosal injury
- Benzydamine rinses for prevention of radiation-induced mucositis in patients with head and neck cancer receiving moderate-dose radiation therapy

Standard-dose chemotherapy prevention

- Oral cryotherapy (30 min) to decrease oral mucositis in patients receiving bolus 5-FU or edatrexate chemotherapy

High-dose chemotherapy with or without total body irradiation plus HCST: Prevention

- Keratinocyte growth factor-1 (palifermin) in a dose of 60 lg kg^{-1} per day for 3 days prior to conditioning treatment and for 3 days posttransplantation in patients with hematologic malignancies receiving high-dose chemotherapy and total body irradiation with autologous stem cell transplantation
- Cryotherapy to prevent oral mucositis in patients receiving high-dose melphalan
- Low-level light therapy (LLLT) to reduce the incidence of oral mucositis and associated pain in patients receiving high-dose chemotherapy or chemoradiotherapy before HSCT if the treatment center is able to support the necessary technology and training

Cancer/International Society for Oral Oncology (MASCC/ISOO) concluded that for the most part findings were inconsistent, contradictory, and inconclusive, with few definitive clinical recommendations or guidelines (Table 4) (5–31).

Recently, however, we have seen advancements in the development of rational, mechanistically driven interventions, due to a greater understanding of the complex underlying pathobiology, the burgeoning field of biotechnology, and the recognized importance of well-designed clinical trials (Table 5) (30, 31). With its central role in the initiation of early events, ROS has been an obvious target for intervention. Amifostine (Ethyol, MedImmune, Gaithersburg, MD), an aminothiol and free-radical scavenger, is known to limit DNA injury following radiation exposure, and can be effective in reducing acute and long-term salivary gland damage. While recommended for prevention of radiation proctitis, results with respect to preventing oral mucositis have been mixed, although clinical studies are ongoing (5, 32). Palifermin (Kepivance, Amgen, Thousand Oaks, CA), recombinant human keratinocyte growth factor 1 (KGF1), has recently received FDA approval and has been incorporated into clinical practice for prevention of mucositis secondary to conditioning regimens for stem cell transplantation (33). KGF is a member of the fibroblast growth factor (FGF) superfamily, and while KGF1 has definite mitogenic effects on the mucosal epithelium resulting in increased thickness, it also appears to have a number of other biological activities that are likely as or more important with respect to mucositis prevention (34). For example, NRF2 is a transcription factor that mediates cellular responses to stress through the antioxidant-reponse element group of genes which encode proteins that limit the activities of ROS. KGF has been shown to induce NRF2 expression in keratinocytes, endothelial cells, and fibroblasts, thus offering another plausible mechanism of action other than its direct proliferative properties. The safety and efficacy of palifermin in a solid cancer population has been recently demonstrated in colorectal cancer patients on fluorouracil-containing protocols (35). Additional studies sponsored by both industry and cooperative groups are currently evaluating its efficacy in preventing mucositis in patients receiving chemoradiation for head and neck cancers, one of the most severely and most consistently affected patient populations (http://www.clinicaltrials.gov).

Another member of the FGF family, Valifermin (FGF-20), is also in clinical testing and likely has overlapping as well as unique activities compared to palifermin. With the recent growth in biotechnology, a number of other growth-factor-based, cytokine-based, and biologically based therapies are in various stages of clinical evaluation. These trials have moved forward with a certain degree of caution as growth factors have a theoretical risk of adversely affecting tumor behavior due to the presence of target receptors (34, 36). However, to date there is no data to support this hypothesis. N-acetylcysteine, an antioxidant that is also being clinically evaluated, has the ability to scavenge ROS but also, importantly, may suppress NF-κB activation. Benzydamine hydrochloride, while not approved for use in the United States, is a rinse with anti-inflammatory, analgesic, and antimicrobial properties, utilized in Europe and Canada for prevention of radiation-induced mucositis throughout Europe and other parts of the world (37). One of benzydamine's mechanisms of action appears to be down-regulation of TNF-α production and activity. This illustrates potential complementary mechanisms of action among multiple agents. A quite different approach, such as the one that takes place

Table 5
Biologically based treatments for the prevention or treatment of oral mucositis currently registered at http://www.clinicaltrials.gov

Product	Molecule	Sponsor(s)	Product category	State of development
Palifermin, FGF-7	Recombinant human fibroblast growth factor 7 (rhFGF-7)	Amgen (Thousand Oaks, CA), Radiation Therapy Oncology Group, National Cancer Institute	Growth factor	Clinical, Phase III, FDA approved for use in hematopoietic cell transplantation for hematologic malignancies
Valafermin, FGF-20CG 53135	Recombinant human fibroblast growth factor 20 (rhFGF-20)	CuraGen (Vernon, CT)	Growth factor	Clinical, Phase II
Sagramostin	GM-CSF	University of California San Francisco, National Cancer Institute	Growth factor	Clinical, Phase III
Traumeel-S	Homeopathic formulation of plant extracts	National Cancer Institute	Cytokine inhibitor	Clinical, Phase II
AES-14 (Saforis)	Glutamine	MGI Pharma (Bloomington, MN)	Amino acid	Clinical, Phase III
RK 0202	*N*-acetyl-l-cysteine	RxKinetix (Louisville, CO)	Antioxidant	Clinical, Phase II
ATL 104	Plant-derived growth factor	Alizyme (Cambridge, United Kingdom)	Growth factor	Clinical, Phase II
Tocopherol	Vitamin E	Hadassah Medical Organization (Jerusalem, Israel)	Vitamin	Clinical, Phase II
SNX-1012	Meclocycline sulfosalicylate	Serenex (Durhman, NC)	Anti-inflammatory	Clinical, Phase II
Amifostine	2-(3-aminopropylamino) ethylsulfanylphosphonic acid	Beth Israel Medical Center (New York, NY)	Antioxidant	Phase III
Light-emitting diode therapy	Light (LED array 670 nm 56 mW cm^{-2})	Medical College of Wisconsin (Milwaukee, WI)	Phototherapy	Clinical, phase II

during pathogenesis of mucositis, has focused attention on l-glutamine, a nonessential amino acid that is required to meet the metabolic cellular needs under intense catabolic periods of cellular activity. It is very likely that in the future we will find that multiple agents, used in various combinations, given in different ways (e.g., topical vs. systemic) and at different time-points (e.g., prior to vs. during therapy), will act synergistically through multiple pathways in preventing the untoward mucosal consequences of cancer therapies.

While there are tremendous ongoing advances in the pharmacologic management of mucosal injury, there are a number of nonpharmacologic approaches that can be quite effective in preventing and/or minimizing symptoms associated with mucositis. With head and neck cancer therapy, it is the cumulative dose of radiation that increases risk of mucositis; therefore, by reducing exposure to nontumor tissues while still delivering the full therapeutic dose to malignant cells, toxicity can be diminished. Use of intensity-modulated radiation therapy (IMRT) and three-dimensional treatment planning has been associated with decreased incidence and severity of mucosal as well as salivary gland toxicities (38). Although their utilization is not widespread or standardized, localized measures such as midline blocking shields (which must be custom-fabricated) (39) and physical separation of the oral mucosa from directly opposing metallic dental restorations using cotton rolls or custom stents can be quite effective in protecting areas inside the mouth (40, 41). Cryotherapy (i.e., ice chips), when applied intraorally during infusion of 5-fluorouracil and other stomatotoxic chemotherapy agents, has shown efficacy in reducing oral (but not gastrointestinal) mucositis, purportedly due to localized vasoconstriction therefore limiting diffusion of the cytotoxic agent into the oral mucosa (42). Low intensity light therapy, with laser or light-emitting diode technologies in the far-red to near-infrared range (630–1,000 nm), is an experimental treatment that has shown considerable promise in both the hematopoietic cell transplantation and head and neck cancer populations (43–45). While the exact mechanisms remain to be elucidated, there may be a combination of analgesic, anti-inflammatory, and wound healing effects, all of which may act to prevent or reduce the severity and duration of mucositis.

Palliative interventions continue to be the standard of care in managing oral symptoms and will likely always play an integral role in the treatment of mucosal barrier injury. Use of topical analgesics, including viscous lidocaine, "magic" or "miracle" mouthwash formulations (lidocaine, benzocaine, diphenhydramine, kaolin, milk of magnesia, and/or sucralfate, in various combinations and ratios), and morphine elixir are typically effective in reducing symptoms temporarily, which can be especially helpful prior to eating or performing oral hygiene. While opioid receptors are present within the oral mucosa, it is unclear to what extent topical morphine therapy may function via peripheral mechanisms rather than centrally through transmucosal absorption (46). Mucosal coating agents, such as Gelclair (Cambridge Laboratories, Dublin, Ireland) and Mucotrol (Cura Pharmaceutical Co., Eatontown, NJ), adhere to and block raw-exposed nerve endings in the ulcerated mucosa (47). Despite these measures, use of narcotic analgesics is typically required in severe cases, especially when mucositis extends beyond the oral cavity to the esophagus where topical therapy is ineffective. Even with narcotic pain medication, however, breakthrough pain and dose limiting toxicities are common (48).

While secondary colonization of ulcerations by the commensal oral microflora may play a minor role in pathogenesis, oral decontamination regimens have consistently been shown to be ineffective in reducing the incidence and severity of oral mucositis. Basic oral hygiene during cancer therapy, however, remains paramount to prevent infections, which may exacerbate mucositis and/or act as independent sources of pain (47). Erythematous and ulcerative lesions that may be misdiagnosed as mucositis, such as oral candidiasis and recrudescent herpes simplex virus, must be identified, cultured, and treated appropriately (49). Recognition and treatment of potential sources of local irritation, such as poorly fitting dentures, teeth or restorations with sharp edges, and orthodontic brackets may minimize development of mucositis lesions. All patients should be evaluated by an oral health care specialist prior to commencing cancer therapy to identify any areas of untreated dental and/or periodontal infections to minimize infectious complications.

CONCLUSIONS

Mucositis is a significant complication of chemotherapy- and radiotherapy-based cancer treatment protocols. Aside from pain and discomfort, patients with severe mucositis may require dose reductions and/or breaks in therapy resulting in potentially suboptimal outcomes. With a greater understanding of the underlying pathophysiology and mechanisms of mucositis, more targeted and biologically based approaches to treatment and prevention are now under investigation at preclinical and clinical levels. As has been demonstrated with successful application of growth factors for the management of treatment-associated hematological toxicities, prevention of mucositis will have a similar tremendous impact on oncological supportive care.

REFERENCES

1. Sonis ST, Eilers JP, Epstein JB, et al. Validation of a new scoring system for the assessment of clinical trial research of oral mucositis induced by radiation or chemotherapy. Mucositis Study Group. Cancer 1999; 85:2103–13
2. McGuire DB, Peterson DE, Muller S, Owen DC, Slemmons MF, Schubert MM. The 20 item oral mucositis index: Reliability and validity in bone marrow and stem cell transplant patients. Cancer Invest 2002; 20:893–903
3. Walsh LJ, Hill G, Seymour G, Roberts A. A scoring system for the quantitative evaluation of oral mucositis during bone marrow transplantation. Spec Care Dentist 1990; 10:190–5
4. Eilers J. Nursing interventions and supportive care for the prevention and treatment of oral mucositis associated with cancer treatment. Oncol Nurs Forum 2004; 31:13–23
5. Keefe DM, Schubert MM, Elting LS, et al. Updated clinical practice guidelines for the prevention and treatment of mucositis. Cancer 2007; 109:820–31
6. Elting LS, Cooksley CD, Chambers MS, Garden AS. Risk, outcomes, and costs of radiation-induced oral mucositis among patients with head-and-neck malignancies. Int J Radiat Oncol Biol Phys 2007; 68:1110–20
7. Martin M, Pienkowski T, Mackey J, et al. Adjuvant docetaxel for node-positive breast cancer. N Engl J Med 2005; 352:2302–13
8. Abu-Khalaf MM, Windsor S, Ebisu K, et al. Five-year update of an expanded phase II study of dose-dense and -intense doxorubicin, paclitaxel and cyclophosphamide (ATC) in high-risk breast cancer. Oncology 2005; 69:372–83
9. Berruti A, Bitossi R, Bottini A, et al. Combination regimen of epirubicin, vinorelbine and 5-fluorouracil continuous infusion as first-line chemotherapy in anthracycline-naive metastatic breast cancer patients. Eur J Cancer 2005; 41:249–55

10. Coleman RE, Biganzoli L, Canney P, et al. A randomised phase II study of two different schedules of pegylated liposomal doxorubicin in metastatic breast cancer (EORTC-10993). Eur J Cancer 2006; 42:882–7

11. Savio G, Laudani A, Leonardi V, et al. Treatment of metastatic breast cancer with vinorelbine and docetaxel. Am J Clin Oncol 2006; 29:276–80

12. Jones SE, Savin MA, Holmes FA, et al. Phase III trial comparing doxorubicin plus cyclophosphamide with docetaxel plus cyclophosphamide as adjuvant therapy for operable breast cancer. J Clin Oncol 2006; 24:5381–7

13. Barasch A, Peterson DE. Risk factors for ulcerative oral mucositis in cancer patients: Unanswered questions. Oral Oncol 2003; 39:91–100

14. Sonis ST, Elting LS, Keefe D, et al. Perspectives on cancer therapy-induced mucosal injury: Pathogenesis, measurement, epidemiology, and consequences for patients. Cancer 2004; 100:1995–2025

15. Sonis ST, Oster G, Fuchs H, et al. Oral mucositis and the clinical and economic outcomes of hematopoietic stem-cell transplantation. J Clin Oncol 2001; 19:2201–5

16. Elting LS, Cooksley C, Chambers M, Cantor SB, Manzullo E, Rubenstein EB. The burdens of cancer therapy. Clinical and economic outcomes of chemotherapy-induced mucositis. Cancer 2003; 98:1531–9

17. Ruescher TJ, Sodeifi A, Scrivani SJ, Kaban LB, Sonis ST. The impact of mucositis on alpha-hemolytic streptococcal infection in patients undergoing autologous bone marrow transplantation for hematologic malignancies. Cancer 1998; 82:2275–81

18. Vera-Llonch M, Oster G, Hagiwara M, Sonis S. Oral mucositis in patients undergoing radiation treatment for head and neck carcinoma. Cancer 2006; 106:329–36

19. Trotti A, Bellm LA, Epstein JB, et al. Mucositis incidence, severity and associated outcomes in patients with head and neck cancer receiving radiotherapy with or without chemotherapy: A systematic literature review. Radiother Oncol 2003; 66:253–62

20. Keefe DM, et al. Oral mucositis is associated with increased resource use among patients receiving treatment for cancers of the head and neck. ASCO abstract# 31629 2007; 25:6070

21. Sonis ST. Mucositis as a biological process: A new hypothesis for the development of chemotherapy-induced stomatotoxicity. Oral Oncol 1998; 34:39–43

22. Sonis ST. The pathobiology of mucositis. Nat Rev Cancer 2004; 4:277–84

23. Sonis ST. The biologic role for nuclear factor-kappaB in disease and its potential involvement in mucosal injury associated with anti-neoplastic therapy. Crit Rev Oral Biol Med 2002; 13:380–9

24. Logan RM, Gibson RJ, Sonis ST, Keefe DM. Nuclear factor-kappaB (NF-kappaB) and cyclooxygenase-2 (COX-2) expression in the oral mucosa following cancer chemotherapy. Oral Oncol 2007; 43:395–401

25. Lima V, Brito GA, Cunha FQ, et al. Effects of the tumour necrosis factor-alpha inhibitors pentoxifylline and thalidomide in short-term experimental oral mucositis in hamsters. Eur J Oral Sci 2005; 113:210–7

26. Hwang D, Popat R, Bragdon C, O'Donnell KE, Sonis ST. Effects of ceramide inhibition on experimental radiation-induced oral mucositis. Oral Surg Oral Med Oral Pathol Oral Radiol Endod 2005; 100:321–9

27. de Koning BA, Lindenbergh-Kortleve DJ, Pieters R, Buller HA, Renes IB, Einerhand AW. Alterations in epithelial and mesenchymal intestinal gene expression during doxorubicin-induced mucositis in mice. Dig Dis Sci 2007

28. Sonis S, Haddad R, Posner M, et al. Gene expression changes in peripheral blood cells provide insight into the biological mechanisms associated with regimen-related toxicities in patients being treated for head and neck cancers. Oral Oncol 2007; 43:289–300

29. Lark RL, McNeil SA, VanderHyde K, Noorani Z, Uberti J, Chenoweth C. Risk factors for anaerobic bloodstream infections in bone marrow transplant recipients. Clin Infect Dis 2001; 33:338–43

30. Keefe DM, Peterson DE, Schubert MM. Developing evidence-based guidelines for management of alimentary mucositis: Process and pitfalls. Support Care Cancer 2006; 14:492–8

31. Worthington HV, Clarkson JE, Eden OB. Interventions for preventing oral mucositis for patients with cancer receiving treatment. Cochrane Database Syst Rev 2006:CD000978

32. Bensadoun RJ, Schubert MM, Lalla RV, Keefe D. Amifostine in the management of radiation-induced and chemo-induced mucositis. Support Care Cancer 2006; 14:566–72

33. Spielberger R, Stiff P, Bensinger W, et al. Palifermin for oral mucositis after intensive therapy for hematologic cancers. N Engl J Med 2004; 351:2590–8

34. Blijlevens N, Sonis S. Palifermin (recombinant keratinocyte growth factor-1): A pleiotropic growth factor with multiple biological activities in preventing chemotherapy- and radiotherapy-induced mucositis. Ann Oncol 2007; 18:817–26

35. Rosen LS, Abdi E, Davis ID, et al. Palifermin reduces the incidence of oral mucositis in patients with metastatic colorectal cancer treated with fluorouracil-based chemotherapy. J Clin Oncol 2006; 24:5194–200

36. von Bultzingslowen I, Brennan MT, Spijkervet FK, et al. Growth factors and cytokines in the prevention and treatment of oral and gastrointestinal mucositis. Support Care Cancer 2006; 14:519–27

37. Epstein JB, Silverman S, Jr., Paggiarino DA, et al. Benzydamine HCl for prophylaxis of radiation-induced oral mucositis: Results from a multicenter, randomized, double-blind, placebo-controlled clinical trial. Cancer 2001; 92:875–85

38. Ship JA, Eisbruch A, D'Hondt E, Jones RE. Parotid sparing study in head and neck cancer patients receiving bilateral radiation therapy: One-year results. J Dent Res 1997; 76:807–13

39. Perch SJ, Machtay M, Markiewicz DA, Kligerman MM. Decreased acute toxicity by using midline mucosa-sparing blocks during radiation therapy for carcinoma of the oral cavity, oropharynx, and nasopharynx. Radiology 1995; 197:863–6

40. Farahani M, Eichmiller FC, McLaughlin WL. Measurement of absorbed doses near metal and dental material interfaces irradiated by X- and gamma-ray therapy beams. Phys Med Biol 1990; 35:369–85

41. Reitemeier B, Reitemeier G, Schmidt A, et al. Evaluation of a device for attenuation of electron release from dental restorations in a therapeutic radiation field. J Prosthet Dent 2002; 87:323–7

42. Rocke LK, Loprinzi CL, Lee JK, et al. A randomized clinical trial of two different durations of oral cryotherapy for prevention of 5-fluorouracil-related stomatitis. Cancer 1993; 72:2234–8

43. Bensadoun RJ. Low level laser therapy: A real hope in the management of chemo-induced and radiation-induced mucositis? Cancer J 2002; 8:236–8

44. Migliorati CA, Oberle-Edwards L, Schubert M. The role of alternative and natural agents, cryotherapy, and/or laser for management of alimentary mucositis. Support Care Cancer 2006; 14:533–40

45. Desmet KD, Paz DA, Corry JJ, et al. Clinical and experimental applications of NIR-LED photobiomodulation. Photomed Laser Surg 2006; 24:121–8

46. Cerchietti LC, Navigante AH, Bonomi MR, et al. Effect of topical morphine for mucositis-associated pain following concomitant chemoradiotherapy for head and neck carcinoma. Cancer 2002; 95:2230–6

47. Barasch A, Elad S, Altman A, Damato K, Epstein J. Antimicrobials, mucosal coating agents, anesthetics, analgesics, and nutritional supplements for alimentary tract mucositis. Support Care Cancer 2006; 14:528–32

48. Rubenstein EB, Peterson DE, Schubert M, et al. Clinical practice guidelines for the prevention and treatment of cancer therapy-induced oral and gastrointestinal mucositis. Cancer 2004; 100:2026–46

49. Scully C, Sonis S, Diz PD. Oral mucositis. Oral Dis 2006; 12:229–41

12

Diarrhea and Constipation: Supportive Oncology Management

Al B. Benson, III and Regina Stein

CONTENTS

    DIARRHEA
    CONSTIPATION
    SUMMARY
    REFERENCES

ABSTRACT

Gastrointestinal toxicity is often a complication of cancer and its treatment. It is a common complaint of patients being treated with tumor-directed therapy and requires appropriate supportive care. Approximately 148,600 cases of colorectal cancer are diagnosed annually. The sequelae of disease progression and the toxicity of treatment can result in significant gastrointestinal complications. Inadequate assessment and treatment can lead to debilitating symptoms and significantly impact quality of life. This chapter will review two common complaints encountered in patients with gastrointestinal malignancies: diarrhea and constipation. Strategies will be discussed for effective palliation and treatment of these common conditions.

Key Words: Chemotherapy-related toxicity, Diarrhea, Constipation, Treatment of gastrointestinal side effects, Supportive oncology.

DIARRHEA

Diarrhea is defined as the passage of more than three watery stools within a 24-h period (1). Normal physiology of the gastrointestinal tract is a fine balance between fluid secretion and absorption. On a daily basis, approximately 91 of fluid is ingested and secreted in the gastrointestinal tract. This includes oral intake, saliva which averages 11 a day, 21 of gastric secretions, 21 of pancreatic secretions, 11 of intestinal secretions, and 11 of bile. Following intestinal transit, on average 101 of fluid will be reabsorbed

From: *Cancer and Drug Discovery Development: Supportive Care in Cancer Therapy*
DOI: 10.1007/978-1-59745-291-5_12, Edited by: D. S. Ettinger © Humana Press, Totowa, NJ

yielding an average of 150–200 ml of fluid excreted in feces. Increased water content, total volume, or frequency of bowel movements are all typical symptoms of diarrhea.

Diarrhea can be classified into six major categories *(2)*. This includes secretory, exudative, dysmotility associated, osmotic, malabsorptive, and secondary causes of diarrhea which result from medications. Treatment aimed at curing various gastrointestinal malignancies will often lead to the development of diarrhea. Secretory diarrhea is characterized by an increased secretion of fluids and electrolytes and is associated with carcinoid syndrome and disorders of intestinal inflammation. Exudative diarrhea is characterized as a build-up of excess blood, serum proteins, and mucus in the intestinal lumen; it is associated with radiation colitis, infections, and malignancies of the colon. Dysmotility-associated diarrhea results from improper peristaltic movement throughout the intestines. This occurs following surgical procedures such as gastrectomy and ileocecal value resection. Chemotherapy-induced diarrhea is associated with specific chemotherapeutic agents and can be debilitating and have impact on therapy. Osmotic diarrhea results from the ingestion of oral solute that is not fully absorbed and often follows the ingestion of fruits, dietetic foods, medications sweetened with nonabsorbed carbohydrates, and pancreatic resection. Malabsorptive diarrhea results from malabsorption of solutes and is associated with lactase insufficiency, celiac sprue, Whipple's disease, and short-gut syndrome.

Diarrhea results from decreased absorption of fluid and electrolytes or increased secretion of fluid and electrolytes. It is a common complaint of patients in the hospital and outpatient cancer clinic. Since patients have many variable definitions for what constitutes diarrhea, it is important to have patients describe the consistency and frequency of their stools. Following a careful assessment, diarrhea can be classified as acute or chronic. Acute diarrhea is defined by symptoms that are less than 14 days in duration. Chronic diarrhea is characterized by symptoms that persist beyond 1 month *(1)*. The majority of diarrhea is acute, resulting from electrolyte imbalance, bacterial overgrowth, or as a side-effect of treatment (laxatives, antibiotics, chemotherapy, and radiation). A thorough list of common cause of diarrhea is found in Table 1.

Treatment-Induced Diarrhea

Diarrhea is a common side effect of chemotherapeutic drugs with an incidence identified up to 50–80% *(4)*. Dose limiting toxicity is often experienced with chemotherapy regimens which contain 5-flurouracil (5-FU), irinotecan, and cisplatin. Chemotherapy-induced diarrhea can result in significant morbidity and debilitation. Patients will often require hospitalization with aggressive hydration and electrolyte repletion. More importantly, the presence of refractory or severe diarrhea will require chemotherapy dose adjustments or the cessation of therapy altogether. This can have significant impact and lower the curative ability for certain malignancies. A study of 100 patients with colorectal cancer demonstrated that over 56% experienced diarrhea which resulted in treatment modifications *(5)*. Other causes of diarrhea should be ruled out, as other medications, radiation, infection, partial bowel obstruction, and fecal impaction can all result in acute diarrhea.

Irinotecan and fluorouracil containing chemotherapeutic regimens are often associated with diarrhea. The pathogenesis of chemotherapy-induced diarrhea results from damage to the epithelium of the intestinal mucosa *(6)*. An analysis conducted by Rothenberg et al.

Table 1
Causes of diarrhea

Dietary
  Lactose intolerance
  Sorbitol
  Alcohol intake
Malignancy
  Chemotherapy
  Radiation
  Medications
  Laxatives
  Antibiotics
HAART
  Blood pressure medications
  Digitalis
  Antacids containing magnesium
Infection
  Parasites
    Giardia lamblia
    Entamoeba histolytica
    Cryptosporidium.
  Fungal
    Candida
  Bacterial
    Clostridium difficile
    Shigella
    Salmonella
  Viral
    Rotavirus
    Cytomegalovirus
    Herpes simplex virus
    Hepatitis
    Norwalk virus
Traveler's Diarrhea
  E. coli
Intestinal disorders
  Ulcerative colitis
  Crohn's disease
  Irritable bowel disease
  Diverticulosis
  Celiac disease
  Graft vs. host disease
Pancreatic insufficiency
Fecal impaction
Intestinal/abdominal surgery
Psychiatric and emotional conditions

evaluated the deaths of 44 patients receiving irinotecan and 5FU and determined that the cause of death was largely the result of gastrointestinal toxicity and sudden thromboembolic events *(7)*. This study prompted the development of clinical guidelines which can be applied to all patients receiving chemotherapeutic regimens. In summary, all patients should be monitored closely with a history, physical examination, and laboratory evaluation. Patients who develop diarrhea should be started immediately on pharmacologic therapy including intravenous hydration and oral antibiotics. If the patient has concomitant neutropenia, antibiotics should be continued until the resolution of diarrhea. An infectious etiology should be ruled out as the cause of the diarrhea. The interruption or cessation of therapy must be implemented for severe or refractory cases.

The toxicity of diarrhea is categorized by severity and classified on a five-point scale (Table 2) *(8)*. Mild diarrhea can be managed with diet. Patients should attempt to increase their oral intake of fluids and limit lactulose and increased amounts of fiber. Mild to moderate diarrhea should be treated with pharmacologic therapy. Loperamide at an initial dose of 4 mg followed by 2 mg q4h is the first-line pharmacologic therapy for diarrhea following chemotherapy. Atropine-diphenoxylate 1–2 tablets every 6–8 h may be added to the loperamide for Grade I or II diarrhea. Refractory diarrhea or diarrhea classified as Grade III or IV should be treated with continuous hydration in conjunction with octreotide. Patients presenting with Grade III and Grade IV diarrhea should be hospitalized and treated with aggressive fluid and electrolyte repletion.

Carcinoid Syndrome

Carcinoid tumors are classified as neuroendocrine tumors and arise from hormone-producing cells of the gastrointestinal tract, respiratory tract, pancreas, and reproductive

Table 2
Common toxicity criteria (version 2.0) for diarrhea

Grade	0	1	2	3	4
Patients without a colostomy	None	Increase of<4 stools per day over pretreatment	Increase of 4–6 stools per day, or nocturnal stools	Increase of ≥7 stools per day or incontinence; or need for parenteal support for dehydration	Physiologic consequences requiring intensive care or hemodynamic collapse
Patients with a colostomy	None	Mild increase in loose watery colostomy output compared to pretreatment	Moderate increase in loose watery colostomy output compared with pretreatment, but not interfering with normal activity	Severe increase in loose watery colostomy output compared with pretreatment, interfering with normal activity	Physiologic consequences requiring intensive care or hemodynamic collapse

organs with the gastrointestinal tract being the most common site for the development
of these tumors *(9)*. These cells release bradykinin, serotonin, histamine, and prostaglandins. Excessive amounts of these hormones can result in the development of carcinoid syndrome. Approximately 20% of patients with midgut carcinoid tumors will
develop carcinoid syndrome *(10)*. Symptoms include flushing of the face, neck and
upper chest, abdominal pain, and diarrhea. Diarrhea can result from an obstructing
tumor in the intestinal cavity or from the over production of serotonin. When serotonin
excess is the cause, treatment is aimed at reducing the levels of circulating serotonin.
Octreotide has been demonstrated to slow the growth of carcinoid tumors. Approximately
50–70% of patients will have clinical improvement in their symptoms with the addition
of somatostatin analogs and interferon. Short- and long-acting preparations are available. When initiating therapy, the short-acting preparation should always be used first to
determine tolerability and assess for side effects *(11)*. Long-acting preparations can be
given every 2–4 weeks depending on response and control of symptoms. The initial
dose of octreotide LAR is usually 20 mg. Severe and refractory symptoms may need to
be treated with intravenous preparations

Clostridium Difficile Colitis (Antibiotic-Associated Colitis, Pseudomembranous Colitis)

Clostridium difficile colitis is a toxin-mediated infection of the colon resulting from
the overgrowth of the Gram positive organism *Clostridium difficile (12)*. It is often a
complication of antibiotic use (third generation cephalosporins, erythromycin, and clin-
damycin), chemotherapy, and intestinal radiation. It is the most common iatrogenic
infection acquired during hospitalization. Initial symptoms may include an elevated
white count, low grade fever, and mild watery or mucousy diarrhea. Symptoms may
progress to a high fever, abdominal cramping, dehydration, and severe watery and
bloody diarrhea. Rare complications include the development of toxic megacolon, peritonitis, and intestinal perforation *(13)*. Stool examination will often reveal an elevated
white count and the presence of clostridium toxin. A sigmoidoscopy may be necessary
to confirm the diagnosis. Clostridium difficile colitis has a distinctive endoscopic
appearance. Treatment includes the use of antibiotics – metronidazole and vancomycin.
Vancomycin should be reserved for refractory cases or patients with an intolerance to
metronidazole. Relapses are common, approximately 20% of cases, and often are the
result of inadequate eradication of the Clostridium organism.

General Treatment (Fig. 1)

Once an infectious etiology has been ruled out, the treatment for diarrhea includes
various nonspecific antidiarrheal agents. These medications are categorized into absorb-
ent agents, prostaglandin inhibitors, opioids, and somatostatin inhibitors.

Absorbent Agents

Methyl cellulose; Citrucel: 1–4 g per day.
Mechanism: Synthetic, orally administered, bulk forming laxative. This substance
acts to absorb liquid in the gastrointestinal tract to increase the bulk or stool. The
increased bulk will increase peristalsis.

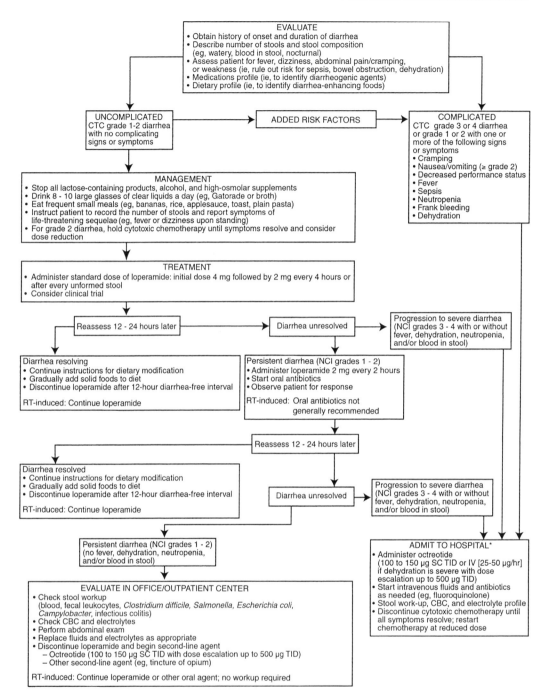

Fig. 1. Proposed algorithm for the assessment and management of treatment-induced diarrhea. For radiation-induced cases and select patients with CID, consider intensive outpatient management, unless the patient has sepsis, fever, or neutropenia. CTC, common toxicity criteria; NCI, National Cancer Institute; RT, radiotherapy, SC, subcutaneous; tid, three times per day; IV intravenous; CBC, complete blood count; CID, chemotherapy-induced diarrhea. Adapted with permission from Kornblau et al. *(11)*

Advantages/disadvantages: Not metabolized. Patients with Phenylketonuria should avoid the sugar-free preparation as this contains aspartame.

Prostaglandin Inhibitors

Preparations and doses: Aspirin, 300 mg 4hourly, up to 4 g per day; mesalazine, 1.2–2.4 g per day; bismuth subsalicylate, 525 mg tablets up to 5 mg per day.

Mechanism: Antiinflammatory, antioxidant properties.

Advantages/disadvantages: Both oral and rectal preparations are available. Careful monitoring for renal and liver impairment should be implemented. Risk of bleeding and bruising.

Opioid Agents

Codeine: 10–60 mg 4hourly, duration of action: 4–6 h.

Loperamide: 4 mg initial dose, then 2mg after each loose stool up to 16 mg per day, duration of action 8–16 h.

Mechanism: Opioid receptor agonist that acts peripherally on the μ-opioid receptors in the large intestines. Decreases activity of the intestinal myenteric plexus resulting in decreased gut motility allowing for increased water absorption.

Advantages/disadvantages: Always rule out infectious etiology prior to use.

Somatostatin Analogues

Octreotide: 300–600 mcg per 24 h by subcutaneous injection.

Mechanism of action: Somatostatin is produced in intestinal D cells and acts on gut epithelial receptors to inhibit secretion and peristalsis. It acts as an inhibitor of growth hormone, glucagon, and insulin. Extended release preparations are available which can be given once a month.

Advantages/disadvantages: In addition to treating refractory diarrhea from various causes, it is indicated for the treatment of diarrhea associated with carcinoid syndrome and vasoactive intestinal peptide-secreting tumors and also indicated for the treatment of bowel obstruction.

CONSTIPATION

Etiology of Constipation

Constipation is a common and underestimated symptom in patients with gastrointestinal and other malignancies. According to the Rome Criteria, constipation is defined as a specific pattern of bowel habits over a period of at least 12 weeks in the previous years *(14)*. The bowel characteristics include straining, lumpy or hard stool, sensation of incomplete evacuation, sensation of anorectal obstruction, and bowel movements limited to three or less per week.

Causes of constipation may be classified as either primary or secondary *(15)*. Primary causes of constipation include three primary categories: functional constipation, slow transit constipation, and anorectal dysfunction. There are numerous factors which result in secondary constipation. In addition to the tumor itself resulting in obstruction, complications of specific malignancy, side effects of drug therapy from tumor-directed therapy or pain management, organ failure, and depression can result in constipation. Medications are commonly associated with constipation. These include anatacids, anticholinergics, iron, narcotics, and antihistamines. Constipation is frequently the result of autonomic neuropathy caused by the alkylating agents, vinca alkaloids, taxanes, and thalidomide. Table 3 lists the common chemotherapeutic agents that are associated with constipation.

Prevalence of constipation is greater among the elderly and is compounded by changes in dietary and medicinal habits, inadequate fluid intake, immobility, and deconditioning. It can be a presenting symptom of cancer, but can occur throughout the treatment and supportive course. Table 4 lists the common causes of constipation.

Opiates and anticholinergics (antidepressants and antihistamines) may lead to constipation secondary to decreased sensitivity to the defecation reflexes, decreased gut motility, reduced production of secretions, and increased fluid absorption. Patients who are taking opiates will invariably develop constipation. The degree of constipation is dose related and tolerance to the constipating effects of the medication does not occur. Prophylaxis with laxatives often in combination with a stool softener is essential for all patients taking opiates. Patients are frequently prescribed a stool softener alone to prevent or treat constipation. This prescribing pattern is not sufficient to alleviate constipation. Patients should continue a bowel regimen throughout the duration of opiate use.

Other diseases, such as diabetes (with autonomic neuropathy) and hypothyroidism, may cause constipation. Metabolic disorders, such as hypokalemia and hypercalcemia, also predispose cancer patients to developing constipation. Electrolyte imbalances should be identified and treated with aggressive repletion.

Untreated constipation may lead to several complications. Effective management of constipation starts with a careful assessment of the patient, including the history of the frequency and difficulty of defecation, symptoms caused by constipation, and physical and rectal examinations. When the diagnosis of constipation is unclear, an abdominal X-ray may be required. The treatment of constipation includes general interventions,

Table 3
Chemotherapeutic agents associated with constipation

Cyclophosphamide
Mechlorethamine
Chlorambucil
Melphalan
Carmustine (BCNU)
Lomustine (CCNU)
Semustine (Methyl-CCNU)
Thiotepa
Triethylenemelamine
Busulfan
Procarbazine
Dacarbazine
Hexamethylmelamine
Cisplatin
Vinblastine
Vincristine
Vinorelbine

Table 4
Causes of constipation

Diet
Insufficient fiber or bulk in diet
Inadequate fluid intake
Medications
Chemotherapy
Opioids or sedatives
Anticholinergic medications
Phenothiazines
Calcium- and aluminum-based antacids
Diuretics
Vitamin supplements (iron, calcium)
Bowel disorders
Irritable bowel syndrome
Diverticulitis
Gastrointestinal malignancy
Metabolic disorders
Hypothyroidism and lead poisoning
Uremia
Dehydration
Hypercalcemia
Hypokalemia
Hyponatremia
Depression
Chronic illness
Anorexia
Immobility
Antidepressants
Inability to increase intra-abdominal pressure
Emphysema
Neuromuscular impairment
Massive abdominal hernias
Atony of muscles
Malnutrition and cachexia
Environmental factors
Inability to get to the bathroom
Unfamiliar environment
Change in bathroom habits (e.g., requiring bedpan, commode)
Lack of privacy
Narrowing of colon lumen
Radiation therapy
Adhesions
Obstructing mass
Neurologic causes
Multiple sclerosis
Parkinson's disease
Stroke
Spinal cord injuries

such as the availability of comfort and privacy or the elimination of medical factors that may contribute to constipation, and therapeutic interventions including oral or rectal laxatives and the use of prokinetic medications. A brief review of the pathophysiology and causes of constipation is provided below.

Assessment of Constipation

A normal bowel pattern is having at least three stools per week, but this is frequently not achieved in cancer patients. Constipation should be evaluated individually in patients who complain of decreased frequency with incomplete passage of dry, hard feces. A careful history should be taken to identify the pattern and etiology of constipation. Patients and caregivers should be encouraged to record frequency and consistency of bowel movements. A dietary and medication list should be obtained and reviewed. The evaluation should also include assessment of associated symptoms such as distention, flatus, cramping, or rectal fullness. A digital rectal examination should always be done, unless medically contraindicated, to rule out fecal impaction at the level of the rectum. A test for occult blood will be helpful in determining the presence of an obstructing intraluminal lesion. A thorough examination of the gastrointestinal tract via endoscopy is necessary if cancer is suspected.

Management of Constipation

The hallmark of constipation treatment is prophylaxis and prevention. Some patients can be instructed to increase dietary fiber (leafy vegetables, whole grains) in conjunction with increased fluid intake to one-half ounce per pound of body weight daily (if not contraindicated by co-morbid conditions). A pivotal study supporting the use of dietary fiber was conducted by Hull et al. *(16)*. Constipation was alleviated in 60% of geriatric nursing home bound patients with dietary fiber alone. The regimen included increasing the total fiber supplementation by 25–40%. In 1 year, the institution was able to essentially eliminate laxative use and reduce cost. The findings of the study were limited to a small sample size, but do highlight the use of dietary ingredients to help prevent constipation. In the past two decades, the cost of laxatives has dropped significantly and routine use is encouraged for prevention and treatment of constipation.

The use of herbal medication is frequently encountered in oncology practice. Patients will use herbs and other naturally occurring products in hopes of treating disease and sequelae of treatment. Patients are unaware of the side effects of herbal agents and will often purchase herbal medications without discussing it with their physician. The 2002 NHIS Alternative Medicine Supplement estimated that approximately 19% of Americans use herbal medications *(17)*. Despite its widespread use, results are not validated and no agent has been identified to treat constipation.

Patients should be allowed to have appropriate privacy and equipment to facilitate bowel movements. If a patient has not had a bowel movement after a period of 3 days, stimulant laxatives in combination with stool softeners should be started. If another 24 h has passed, patients should be encouraged to take a saline laxative, (i.e., Milk of magnesia, 30–45 ml) every few hours until a bowel movement results. A thorough list of medical agents used for the prevention and treatment of constipation are listed in Table 5.

Table 5
Medical agents for constipation

Bulk producers
Examples: Methycellulose, Psyllium
Drugs and dosages:
Methylcellulose: 5–20cc, three times per day with water
Psyllium: 1 TBSP 1–3 times a day
Mechanism of action: Increase water retention in the intestines which will result in increased peristalsis. Onset is typically within 24h
Advantages: Beneficial for patients with irritable bowel syndrome
Disadvantages: Must maintain adequate hydration. Bowel obstruction is a side effect if inadequate fluids are consumed
Saline laxatives
Examples: Magnesium sulfate, Milk of Magnesia, Magnesium citrate, Sodium phosphate, Monobasic sodium phosphate
Dosages:
Magnesium sulfate: 15 g in a glass of water
Milk of magnesia: 10–20cc if concentrated, 15–30cc if regular
Magnesium citrate: 240cc
Sodium phosphate: 4–8 g dissolved in water
Monobasic and dibasic sodium phosphate (Fleet Phospho-soda): 20–40 ml mixed with 4 oz cold water
Mechanism of action: These solutions are highly osmolar and will draw fluid into the lumen of the intestine. Increased water in stool will result in peristalsis
Disadvantages: Electrolyte imbalance. Exercise caution with patients who have underlying renal dysfunction of congestive heart failure
Advantages: Optimal for bowel evacuation prior to endoscopic procedure
Stimulant laxatives
Examples: Senokot (1–2 tablets daily – can take up to 8 tablets daily in divided doses – TID), Bisacodyl 10 mg oral tablet taken once a day or rectal suppository preparation
Mechanism of action: Increase peristalsis of intestines. Onset typically within 6–8 h
Disadvantages: May result in abdominal cramping
Lubricant laxatives
Mineral oil 10–30cc daily
Mechanism of action: Lubricates intestinal mucous membrane. Limits the amount of water reabsorption from the intestines
Disadvantage: Must be given on an empty stomach, preferably at bedtime. Will interfere with fat soluble vitamins. Do not give with docusate sodium as increased absorption of mineral oil may result
Fecal softeners
Example: Docusate sodium
Dosage: 100 mg, may be taken up to 800 mg daily in divided doses
Mechanism of action: Soften the stool by increasing water retention in the stool
Advantages/disadvantages: Beneficial when the stool is difficult to pass and hard. Slow onset of action. Should not be used alone

(continued)

Table 5
(continued)

Lactulose

Dosage: 10–20 g each time, (15–30 ml) can be given up to three times a day

Mechanism of action: Acts as a synthetic disaccharide that will pass through the small intestine without being digested. Once it reaches the colon, it is broken down to form lactic acid, acetic acid, formic acid, and carbon dioxide. These metabolites will increase the osmotic pressure and increase the amount of water in the stool

Onset: 24–48 h

Polyethylene glycol and electrolytes

Dosage: Five packets are mixed with 1gal. (3.785l) of tap water. Can be stored up to 48 h in the refrigerator

Mechanism of action: Evacuate bowel with minimal water and sodium imbalance

Disadvantages: Large volume of intake. Patients with nausea and significant gastrointestinal symptoms may not be able to tolerate

---

Rectal agents should be avoided in cancer patients who have thrombocytopenia and/ or neutropenia. In the immunocompromised patient, no manipulation of the anus or stoma should occur (rectal examinations, suppositories, or enemas). These actions can result in complications including anal fissures or abscesses, and can induce bacteremia and prolong acute illness.

Constipation is a common symptom of patients in the hospital and outpatient setting. Often the appropriate history and physical examination are not completed and patients may develop pain, abdominal distension, nausea, and vomiting. Randomized clinical trials between different laxatives and/or prokinetic agents in cancer patients are needed, and future studies should focus on the validation of different clinical assessment tools for constipation.

SUMMARY

Gastrointestinal cancers are common and treatments are widely varied. Tumors and treatment-related sequelae are leading causes of distressing gastrointestinal complications. Diarrhea and constipation are extremely prevalent and should not be overlooked. These symptoms require aggressive attention and palliation. The preceding sections offered helpful strategies to identifying and managing diarrhea and constipation in oncology patients.

REFERENCES

1. Guerrant RL, Gilder TV, et al. Practice guidelines for the management of infectious diarrhea. Clin Infect Dis 2001; 32:331
2. Hogan CM. The nurse's role in diarrhea management. Oncol Nurs Forum 1998; 25:879–886
3. DuPont HL. Guidelines on acute infectious diarrhea in adults. The Practice Parameters Committee of the American College of Gastroenterology. Am J Gastroenterol 1997; 92:1962–75
4. Benson AB, 3rd, Ajani JA, Catalano RB, et al. Recommended guidelines for the treatment of cancer treatment-induced diarrhea. J Clin Oncol 2004; 22:2918

5. Arbuckle RB, Huber SL, Zacker C. The consequences of diarrhea occurring during chemotherapy for colorectal cancer: A retrospective study. Oncologist 2000; 5:250–259

6. Milles SS, Muggia AL, Spiro HM. Colonic histological changes induced by 5-fluorouracil. Gastroenterology 1962; 43:391

7. Rothenberg ML, Meropol NJ, Poplin EA, et al. Mortality associated with irinotecan plus bolus fluorouracil/leucovorin: Summary findings of an independent panel. J Clin Oncol 2001; 19:3801–3807

8. Common Toxicity Criteria, version 2.0. Http://ctep.cancer.gov/forms/CTCv20_4–30–992.pdf

9. Kulke MH, Mayer RJ. Carcinoid tumors. N Engl J Med 1999; 340:858

10. Akerstrom G, Hellman P, et al. Management of midgut carcinoids. J Surg Oncol 2005; 89:161–169

11. Janson ET. Treatment of neuroendocrine tumors with somatostatin analogs. Pituitary 2006; 9:249–256

12. Bartlett JG. Antibiotic-associated diarrhea. N Engl J Med 2002; 346:334

13. Kelly CP, Pothoulakis CN, et al. Clostridium difficile colitis. N Engl J Med 1994; 330(4):257–262

14. Rao SS. Constipation: Evaluation and treatment. Gastroenterol Clin North Am 2003; 32(2):659–683

15. Hsieh C. Treatment of constipation in older adults. Am Fam Physician 2005; 72(11):2277–2284

16. Hull C, Greco RS, Brooks DL. Alleviation of constipation in the elderly by dietary fiber supplementation. J Am Geriatr Soc 1980; 28(9):410–414

17. Barnes PM, Powell-Griner E, McFann K, Nahin RL. Complementary and alternative medicine use among adults. Advance Data from Vital and Health Statistics, US Dept of Health and Human Services, Rockville, MD, 2004

13 Menopausal Symptoms

Debra L. Barton, Aditya Bardia, and Charles Loprinzi

ABSTRACT

Menopause is considered to be a major turning point in a women's life. It is accompanied by a variety of physical and psychological changes that can significantly impair one's quality of life. Menopausal symptoms among cancer survivors often occur at an earlier age, and can be more frequent, last longer, and be more severe than are seen in women experiencing natural menopause. A recent NIH state of the science report listed four symptoms as strongly associated with menopause: hot flashes with/without night sweats, osteoporosis, vaginal dryness, and insomnia. Other symptoms variably associated with menopause include urinary incontinence, mood swings, irritability, and cognitive impairment.

Traditionally, hormone replacement therapy (HRT) (estrogen and progesterone) has been the mainstay of therapy for menopausal symptoms. However, recent trials have raised concerns about risks of breast cancer, thrombosis, stroke, and cardiovascular mortality. Various novel nonhormonal therapeutic options have emerged for the management of menopausal symptoms. Newer antidepressants appear to be efficacious in reducing hot flashes. Bisphosphonates, along with calcium and vitamin D, remain the front line therapy for prevention and treatment of osteoporosis, but long-term efficacy has not been established. Vaginal dryness responds well to local estrogens and vaginal lubricants. There is evidence that new nonbenzodiazepines have efficacy in treating insomnia. However, despite progress in effective nonhormonal therapies, menopausal

From: *Cancer and Drug Discovery Development: Supportive Care in Cancer Therapy*
DOI: 10.1007/978-1-59745-291-5_13, Edited by: D. S. Ettinger © Humana Press, Totowa, NJ

symptoms remain a major cause of morbidity among cancer survivors and compassionate management of individual symptoms is crucial.

Key Words: Menopause, Cancer survivors, Hot flash, Osteoporosis, Vaginal dryness, Insomnia.

INTRODUCTION

Menopause is defined by the World Health Organization as the "permanent cessation of menstrual flow for more than 12 consecutive months, not associated with a physiological cause (such as lactation)" *(1)*. It generally occurs, naturally, as part of a woman's aging process but can occur prematurely secondary to surgery (oophorectomy), pelvic radiation, or drug therapy (usually chemotherapy) *(2–4)*.

About one-third of the female population is estimated to be postmenopausal worldwide. In the United States, it is estimated that there are currently over 30 million postmenopausal women. This is expected to rise further with the increase in the aging population as well as the increase in the number of cancer survivors *(4)*.

Most women in the United States experience menopause between the age of 40 and 58, with a median age of 52 years. Several factors, including higher parity, oral contraceptive use, higher body mass index (BMI), and high socioeconomic status, have been associated with a later onset of menopause, while smoking is associated with earlier menopause. The natural transition from menstrual cycles to menopause is usually associated with changes in menstrual cycle length; the change can span many years. On the other hand, treatment-induced menopause may be abrupt. It is estimated that up to 50% of premenopausal breast cancer survivors have chemotherapy-induced menopause within a year of receiving chemotherapy *(5)*.

Menopause is accompanied by a variety of physical and psychological changes that can significantly impair one's quality of life. A recent National Institute of Health (NIH) state of the science conference report listed four symptoms as strongly associated with menopause: hot flashes with/without night sweats, osteoporosis, vaginal dryness, and insomnia. These occur in more than one-third of women with menopause *(1)*. Other symptoms variably associated with menopause include urinary incontinence, mood swings, irritability, and cognitive impairment *(1)*. Generally, the first symptom of the menopause transition is hot flashes with or without night sweats. These can begin several years before the menstrual cycle ceases. Insomnia is another early symptom associated with hormone changes. Symptoms such as osteoporosis and vaginal dryness do not generally occur until after ovarian function has stopped.

There are some data to support that menopausal symptoms related to premature menopause due to cancer treatment or surgery result in more morbidity than natural menopause. The menopausal symptoms among cancer survivors and those experiencing surgical menopause can be more frequent, last longer, and be more severe, than those experiencing natural menopause *(5, 6)*.

The gold standard treatment for menopause has historically been HRT consisting of estrogen and progesterone. During the last decade, prospective trials by the Women's Health Initiative have demonstrated an unfavorable risk/benefit ratio for oral hormonal therapy with the suggestion that risks of breast cancer, thrombosis, and strokes may outweigh the benefits of hot flash management, vaginal dryness, and bone health; thus, other options to manage these symptoms are required *(7)*.

Given the prevalence of menopausal symptoms and the need for alternate treatment options, this chapter will review the four symptoms clearly delineated by the state of the science panel as being attributable to menopause, and the evidence base for various therapies, including complementary and alternative medicine (CAM) therapies, where appropriate.

HOT FLASHES AND NIGHT SWEATS

Definition and Natural Course

A hot flash can be defined as an intense episode of heat sensation, usually over the face and upper chest, often accompanied by sympathetic symptoms such as sweating, palpitations, and anxiety. A hot flash is generally transient, lasting for a few minutes, but can occur several times during a day. Hot flashes usually begin in the perimenopausal period (the menopausal transition phase), peak in the first year after the onset of menopause, and can variably continue for up to 15 or more years. Night sweats are episodes of profuse sweating that occur during sleep and can be a significant source of sleep disruption.

Prevalence

Hot flashes are one of the earliest and most distressing aspects of menopause. Bothersome hot flashes are known to occur in 75% of women and also in 80% of men with prostate cancer who receive androgen ablation therapy *(8)*. They can significantly impair one's ability to work, general functional ability, sleep, sexuality, self-image, and overall quality of life *(9–11)*. Cancer survivors can have more frequent and severe hot flashes, especially with the use of hormonal agents such as tamoxifen, raloxifene, and aromatase inhibitors.

Pathophysiology

The pathophysiology of hot flashes is complex. In simplistic terms, it involves the dysregulation of central nervous system (CNS) thermoregulatory centers, probably due to the withdrawal effects of estrogens and progesterones. The change is probably mediated by central neurotransmitters *(12)*. One of the leading hypotheses is that hot flashes are centrally mediated by serotonin *(13)*. Serotonin is also recognized as one of the major neurotransmitters involved in temperature regulation at the level of the hypothalamus *(14)*.

Management

HORMONAL THERAPIES

Estrogen Hot flashes are a major reason why women seek HRT, which has historically been the front line therapy for the relief of hot flashes. Comprising estrogens and/or progesterones, HRT is the most effective therapy to date in reducing hot flashes (by about 80–90%, with a dose–response relationship) *(15, 16)*. However, there have been recent concerns about using HRT in healthy women because of the increased risks of stroke, pulmonary embolism, and breast cancer *(17–19)*. Current recommendations include low-dose, short-term hormonal therapy for particularly distressing symptoms, such as hot flashes. The risk/benefit of this new approach, however, has not been fully explored.

Progestational Agents Progestational agents such as medroxyprogesterone acetate (MPA) and megestrol acetate are effective agents in reducing hot flashes (Table 1). A randomized, crossover, placebo-controlled clinical trial involving 163 patients found oral megestrol acetate (20 mg twice per day) to have similar efficacy as would be expected with estrogen therapy in reducing hot flashes, decreasing hot flashes by 85% over 4 weeks. The only side effect experienced in this trial was withdrawal vaginal bleeding. Similarly, intramuscular depot medroxyprogesterone acetate was evaluated against oral megesterol acetate in an Italian trial (20). Investigators reported that injections of 500 mg of MPA on days 1, 14, and 28 and daily oral megestrol acetate of 40 mg per day each resulted in an 86% reduction of hot flashes, with no difference of efficacy between groups. Similarly, a randomized trial comparing a single dose of intramuscular MPA (400 mg) with oral venlafaxine 75 mg (extended release) reported a 79% reduction in hot flashes with the single progesterone injection vs. a 55% reduction with venlafaxine (21).

NONHORMONAL TREATMENTS

Older Treatments Historic nonhormonal remedies for hot flashes included Bellergal (low-dose phenobarbitol, ergotamine tartrate, and levorotatory alkaloids of belladonna), methyldopa (an alpha adrenergic agonist), and clonidine (an alpha-2 adrenergic agonist). Little data exist for Bellergal and methyldopa, and significant toxicity of these agents is possible, making them a poor choice for hot flash treatment. Clonidine, both oral and transdermal, has been shown in randomized trials to be effective at reducing hot flashes by about 40–45% (22). Toxicities associated with clonidine include dry mouth, constipation, drowsiness, difficulty sleeping, and itchiness related to the patch. The modest efficacy coupled with the side effects make clonidine a less preferred choice for hot flash management.

Newer Antidepressants Various newer antidepressants, including paroxetine and venlafaxine, have been found to be efficacious in reducing hot flashes. Large, well-designed, randomized, controlled trials have been completed. One study involving 151 women,

Table 1
Evaluation and management of hot flashes

Evaluation	Clinical diagnosis (intense episode of heat sensation, usually over the face and upper chest, often accompanied by sympathetic symptoms such as sweating, palpitations, and anxiety)
	Determine frequency, severity and effect on quality of life, particular sleep
Management options	Paroxetine 10–20 mg per day
	Venlafaxine 37.5 mg titrating to 75 mg per day
	Gabapentin 300 mg titrating to 300 mg TID, and possibly to 2,400 mg per day
	MPA 400–500 mg IM for one dose

MPA medroxyprogesterone acetate

mostly breast cancer survivors, found that short-acting paroxetine reduced hot flashes by 41% with 10 mg per day and 52% in the 20 mg per day group, compared to 14% in the placebo arms (23). Long-acting paroxetine 12.5 mg and 25 mg was also studied in a placebo-controlled trial, demonstrating a 46% and 50% reduction for the 12.5-mg and 25-mg arms, respectively (24). Side effects were minimal, with nausea being the only side effect statistically significant different than placebo. However, more women in the 20 mg per day arm withdrew from the short-acting study, so investigators felt the 10 mg per day arm was the preferred treatment. Similarly, a randomized double-blind, controlled trial among 191 women with symptomatic hot flashes found 37.5 mg per day of venlafaxine (extended release) to reduce hot flashes by 40%, as compared to 27% with a placebo, and a higher dose of 75 mg per day venlafaxine resulted in a 60% reduction. Increasing the drug dosage to 150 mg per day did not add to efficacy (25). The main side effects of venlafaxine, different than placebo, included nausea, dry mouth, and a decrease in appetite. Constipation was only experienced at the 150 mg per day dose.

The efficacy of fluoxetine and sertraline appear to be slightly lower than venlafaxine and paroxetine. Both have been studied in placebo-controlled trials at a single dose. Fluoxetine 20 mg was evaluated and found to provide a 42% reduction in median hot flash frequency (26). Likewise, one sertraline trial demonstrated a 27% reduction in frequency over 6 weeks (27), while another reported a reduction of five fewer hot flashes per week over placebo (28). These reductions are very modest. Tolerance of these medications was good, with only nausea being significantly different from the placebo group with sertraline. Citalopram has mostly been studied in phase II trials, being associated with a 53–58% reduction in hot flash frequency (29). A recent randomized trial comparing citalopram and fluoxetine in 150 postmenopausal women found both of these agents to reduce hot flashes by about 70% but this was not significantly different from placebo which provided more than a 60% reduction in hot flashes (30). Due to the extremely large response rates for all arms, the long duration of the trial (9 months), and a high withdrawal rate, definitive conclusions regarding the true efficacy of citalopram and fluoxetine cannot be made from this study.

Many drugs, including antidepressants, are metabolized through cytochrome P450 pathways and interactions can occur that adversely affect the metabolism of one or more drugs. Studies have demonstrated that paroxetine effectively shuts down the CYP2D6 pathway that is necessary for the metabolism of tamoxifen to endoxifen (31). Studies are being done to clarify agents that have no or weak inhibitory effects on CYP2D6 vs. those that are potent inhibitors and should be avoided when tamoxifen is being used. Venlafaxine is believed to have no effect on CYP2D6 metabolism, while citalopram and sertraline are thought to be weak inhibitors; fluoxetine and paroxetine are potent inhibitors (32).

Gabapentin Gabapentin is another centrally acting agent that has been shown to be efficacious in reducing hot flashes. In two randomized, placebo-controlled trials involving postmenopausal women with a history of breast cancer as well as those naturally or surgically postmenopausal, gabapentin (300 mg three times per day) was found to reduce hot flashes by 46–54% (33, 34). Gabapentin at a lower dose (100 mg three times per day) was found to be less efficacious (30% reduction). A higher dose of gabapentin was also compared to estrogen therapy as well as a placebo for hot flash relief in a randomized trial involving 60 women (35). Gabapentin (2,400 mg per day) was reported to be equally as effective as conjugated estrogens (0.625 mg per day) for relieving hot flashes, with hot flash scores (frequency × severity) decreasing to just over 70% at 4 weeks and remaining there for the rest of the 12-week trial. The placebo effect in this trial was 54%. Ideally, this finding should be confirmed in a subsequent trial. Gabapentin also appears to be efficacious among women with inadequate relief from antidepressants and in such women the antidepressant should be weaned off slowly (while continuing gabapentin) to avoid potential antidepressant withdrawal effects *(36)*. Gabapentin is generally well tolerated with the major adverse effect being light-headedness and dizziness. Gabapentin has also been found to decrease serum albumin concentrations causing a fluid shift resulting in fluid retention and weight gain.

COMPLEMENTARY THERAPIES AND DIETARY SUPPLEMENTS

Complementary therapies, such as dietary supplements (including herbs) and acupuncture, are popular remedies for hot flashes. Vitamin E is one such dietary supplement that has been reported to have modest efficacy in a large placebo-controlled, randomized trial. Vitamin E reduced hot flashes, on average, by one hot flash per person per day over the placebo *(37)*. Considering its low cost, wide availability, safety profile (for those people who do not have diabetes or vascular disease), and nonhormonal mechanism, vitamin E alone might be a reasonable adjunctive therapy in women with mild to moderate hot flashes.

To date, none of the other interventions studied in randomized, placebo-controlled trials have demonstrated efficacy. These include soy, black cohosh, or acupuncture *(38, 39)*. There are a couple of dietary supplements (DHEA and flaxseed) that have been studied in phase II, nonrandomized trials that look promising and will go on to evaluation in phase III, placebo-controlled trials. Several popular herbs that are touted as hot flash remedies have estrogenic properties and should be avoided if estrogen supplementation is contraindicated. These products include red clover, licorice, chasteberry, hops, and dong quai *(40)*.

OSTEOPOROSIS

Definition and Natural Course

Osteoporosis literally means "porous bones." It refers to a skeletal process characterized by decreased bone mass and structural weakening of the bones, making them more vulnerable to fractures. The latter is often the first sign of ongoing osteoporosis. It is estimated that women lose 20–30% of cancellous bone and about 10% of cortical bone in the 10 years following menopause *(41)*. The rate of bone loss then slows down and declines to about 70% of its maximum value by the age of 80 *(42)*. Women with osteoporosis have a predilection for fractures of the vertebral body, hip, and distal forearm, in the order of decreasing frequency. However, osteoporosis can result in an increased risk of almost any fracture. Furthermore, people who have one fracture have a multifold risk of having another fracture.

While X-rays of the long bones or vertebral column can suggest the presence of significant osteoporosis, measuring bone density by Dual Isotope X-ray Absorption (DEXA) is the preferred method of diagnosing osteoporosis. According to World

Health Organization (WHO) criteria, a *T* score of less than −2.5 confirms the diagnosis of osteoporosis and a score of −1 to −2.5 is considered as osteopenia. Various osteoporosis calculators are now available that can estimate the risk of developing a fracture, based on the degree of osteoporosis (*T* score), as well as additional factors such as history of fracture, family history of fracture, smoking, alcohol use, steroid use, and body weight. Osteoporosis screening among postmenopausal women is recommended by the US Preventive Services Task Force, as well as other agencies. Other risk factors for bone loss include chemotherapy and aromatase inhibitors used to treat breast cancer *(43)*. Women experiencing chemotherapy-induced menopause have been shown to experience a 4% bone loss at their lumbar spine after 6 months *(44)*.

Prevalence

Osteoporosis is the most common bone disease among women. Currently, it is estimated that about 15–20% of postmenopausal women have osteoporosis, and about 40–50% have osteopenia *(45)*. Nearly 1.5 million fractures are attributed to osteoporosis each year and one in six Caucasian women over the age of 50 years are expected to develop a hip fracture over their lifetime (the risk is lower for other ethnic groups). This risk is expected to rise further with the increase in the aging population, and it is estimated that the number of hip fractures worldwide will rise to 6.3 million by the year 2050.

Pathophysiology

The pathophysiology of osteoporosis involves accelerated bone loss secondary to a deficiency of estrogen (either primary or secondary). Conceptually, osteoporosis can be thought of as an increase in the activity of osteoclasts (bone destroyers) over osteoblasts (bone builders), due to an increase in estrogen-regulated cytokines such as interleukin-1 (IL-1) and tumor necrosis factor (TNF), as well as a decrease in osteoclast inhibitors such as transforming growth factor β (TNF-β) and osteoprotegerin. The latter has received considerable recent interest due to its role in inhibiting the NFκB receptor (RANK) and its ligand (RANKL), which plays a key role in osteoclast differentiation, maturation, and functional activity.

Management

The pharmacologic agents that are approved by the Food and Drug Administration (FDA) for the treatment of osteoporosis include oral bisphosphonates (alendronate, risedronate, and ibandronate), raloxifene, nasal calcitonin, and teriparatide as summarized in Table 2. While *T* scores are helpful in deciding whom to treat, a risk-based assessment considering other factors is recommended. According to the National Osteoporosis Foundation, a pharmacologic intervention should be instituted in patients with a *T* score below −2.0, in patients with a *T* score below −1.5 if additional risk factors are present (previous fracture as an adult, history of fragility fracture in a first-degree relative, body weight <57 kg, current smoking, use of oral corticosteroid therapy for >3 months), and/or in any patient with a previous vertebral or hip fracture.

Table 2
Evaluation and management of osteoporosis

Evaluation	DEXA
	T score of less than −2·5 confirms diagnosis of osteoporosis
	T score of −1 to −2·5 confirms osteopenia
	Determine other risk factors
	Previous fracture as an adult
	History of fragility fracture in a first-degree relative
	Body weight <57 kg
	Current smoking
	Use of oral corticosteroid therapy for >3 months
	Medical illness, such as hyperparathyroidism
Management options	Bisphosphonates
	Alendronate 10 mg per day or 70 mg per week
	Risedronate 5 mg per day or 35 mg per day
	Ibandronate 2.5 mg per day or 150 mg per month
	Raloxifene 60 mg per day
	Calcitonin 200 IU per day
	Teriparatide 20 μg per day s/c
	Calcium 1,250–1,500 mg per day
	Vitamin D 400–800 IU per day
	Life Style changes, including exercise and fall prevention

DEXA dual isotope X-ray absorption

HORMONE REPLACEMENT THERAPY

HRT has been the "back bone" for osteoporosis prevention among postmenopausal women. Various clinical trials, including Women's Health Initiative trial, have shown the short-term and long-term efficacy of HRT in improving bone density and reducing the risk of postmenopausal fractures, particularly bone fractures *(46, 47)*. However, given the concern over possible deleterious effects of HRT, as outlined previously, there is a need for alternative treatments.

BISPHOSPHONATES

Bisphosphonates are the most effective, and frequently the first line therapy, for treatment of osteoporosis. Various randomized trials and a few meta-analyses have found these agents (alendronate, risedronate, and ibandronate) to increase bone density and reduce the incidence of fractures, especially vertebral fractures by as much 50% *(48–50)*. Alendronate and risedronate have also been found to be effective in reducing nonvertebral fractures in several meta-analyses *(51, 52)*. Bisphosphonates are recommended as first line therapy for the primary prevention of osteoporosis, especially among those on long-term glucocorticoid therapy *(53, 54)*. While intravenous bisphosphonates, such as pamidronate and zoledronate, are not routinely recommended for osteoporosis prevention or treatment, these agents are preferred for those with skeletal metastasis or those intolerant to oral preparations. The major side effects of bisphosphonates include upper gastrointestinal symptoms, particularly esophagitis. It is thus recommended that these agents be consumed with the patient fasting, and the person should remain upright for at least 30 min after administration. Oral bisphosphonates should be avoided (or used cautiously) in people with impaired renal function or esophageal diseases such as strictures or dysmotility. Finally, bisphosphonates have recently been associated with osteonecrosis of the jaw *(55, 56)*. Osteonecrosis of the jaw associated with bisphoshonates was first described in a letter to the editor in 2003 *(57)*. Since then, there have been a large number of articles related to this problem *(58–61)*. Osteonecrosis has been associated with frequent doses of intravenous bisphophonates; 5–10% of cases have been associated with oral bisphosphonates. Almost two-thirds of cases have been associated with dental procedures. Clinicians should be aware of the problem and the need for dental surgery should be evaluated before bisphosphonate therapy is initiated.

RALOXIFENE

Raloxifene has received considerable recent attention as it has been shown to have beneficial effects on the bone, but not to have unwanted effects on the breast and endometrium in terms of cell proliferation. In a large randomized trial involving 7,705 postmenopausal women, raloxifene (60 mg per day) significantly reduced vertebral fractures by 50% *(62)*. Similar results have been seen in other trials *(63, 64)* and raloxifene is FDA approved for both prevention and treatment of osteoporosis. However, the efficacy of raloxifene in reducing nonvertebral fractures has not yet been shown *(65)*. The major side effects include an increased frequency of venous thromboembolism and hot flashes.

CALCITONIN

Calcitonin is an endogenous hormone postulated to inhibit bone resorption by decreasing osteoclast formation. In a large multicenter clinical trial involving 1,255 postmenopausal women with established osteoporosis, a nasal spray of salmon calcitonin (200 IU per day, in alternating nostrils), was found to reduce the risk of vertebral fractures by 33%, as compared to placebo *(66)*. A higher (400 IU per day) or lower dose (100 IU per day) was found to be no more efficacious than placebo. The efficacy of calcitonin in reducing nonvertebral fractures and primary prevention of osteoporosis is less clear. The most common side effect includes rhinitis.

TERIPARATIDE

Teriparatide, a recombinant human parathyroid hormone analog that stimulates osteoblasts to increase bone formation, is an FDA-approved anabolic agent for prevention of bone loss among those at high risk for fracture. Parathyroid hormone can stimulate bone formation as well as resorption; therefore, attention to dose and administration is important if using this therapy. A randomized trial involving 1,637 postmenopausal women found teriparatide (20 µg per day subcutaneously) to be efficacious in increasing bone density as well as in reducing both vertebral (65% reduction) and nonvertebral (53% reduction) fractures *(67)*. Common adverse effects include dizziness, arthralgias, hypercalcemia, and gastrointestinal side effects. The safety of this agent in women with a history of breast cancer has not been established, as elevated levels of parathyroid hormone related peptide have been found in women with bone metastasis *(68)*. Teriparatide has been found to increase the incidence of osteosarcoma in rats but no cases of osteosarcoma among humans have been observed *(69)*. Furthermore, currently it is recommended that this treatment be used for a maximum of 2 years after which it should be followed by antiresorptive agents such as a bisphosphonate.

NEWER THERAPIES

Strontium ranelate, containing stable strontium, has been postulated to stimulate bone formation and decrease bone resorption. In one large clinical trial involving 1,649 postmenopausal women, strontium ranelate (2 g per day) was found to significantly increase bone density and reduce the incidence of vertebral fractures (41% reduction), as compared to placebo (70). Similar findings were observed in another large trial (71). The major side effects include gastrointestinal upset such as diarrhea.

Denosumab, a RankL inhibitor, is an upcoming novel therapy against osteoporosis. A phase II trial among 412 postmenopausal women found two injections of denosumab spaced 6 months apart increased lumbar spine bone density by 6.7%, compared to a 4.6% increase in patients receiving alendronate and 0.8% percent by placebo (72).

Other upcoming agents include cathepsin K and *SOST* gene inhibitors (sclerostin) (73). Both of these agents are involved in bone remodeling/resorption, and phase II trials assessing their efficacy are currently underway. Finally, observational studies have suggested that thiazides as well as statins are associated with decreased incidence of fractures, but this needs confirmation in large randomized trials (74–76).

BEHAVIORAL INTERVENTIONS

Physical exercise, particularly weight bearing exercise, has been postulated to play an important role in the primary prevention of osteoporosis. In early adulthood, physical exercise promotes bone density, and in postmenopausal individuals, exercise can slow the rate of bone loss. Physical exercise also improves muscle mass and body coordination which can reduce the incidence of falls by 25% and thus reduce the incidence of fractures (77). Other *life style modifications*, particularly fall prevention, are important for preventing fractures among postmenopausal women.

DIETARY SUPPLEMENTS, HERBS, AND COMPLEMENTARY THERAPIES

Adequate intake of *calcium and vitamin D* provides modest benefit for both primary prevention as well as secondary prevention of osteoporosis. Increased intake of calcium (1,500 mg per day) with vitamin D (400–800 IU per day) reduces the risk of fractures by 25% among postmenopausal women at high risk for fractures (78). However, the recent Women's Health Initiative, involving 36,282 general risk postmenopausal women, found that calcium (1,000 mg per day) and vitamin D (400 IU per day) increased bone density, but did not reduce the incidence of hip fractures. The lack of benefit has been attributed to many factors including a low incidence of hip fractures in the study and a high drop-out rate. A higher dose of vitamin D (800 IU per day) may be preferred among those at high risk for fractures and this dose appears to be more effective in reducing fractures as compared to 400 IU per day, as suggested by a recent meta-analysis involving 12 randomized trials (79). Thus, these agents are generally recommended for primary prevention of osteoporosis especially among those at high risk for fractures; for patients with osteoporosis, these should be used as adjunctive therapy rather than monotherapy.

There is limited evidence that DHEA, a prohormone created by the adrenal glands and available as a dietary supplement, may have bone protective effects.

DHEA supplementation in a dose of 50 mg per day over 12 months was shown to improve bone turnover in women over 70 years old *(80)*. Similarly, a small pilot study ($N = 14$) reported improvement in bone mineral density in the hip after 12 months of using a 10% DHEA cream *(81)*. Only postmenopausal women with systemic lupus erythematosus were found to benefit from 200 mg per day of DHEA in terms of increased BMD, while their premenopausal counterparts did not *(82)*. Prospective studies are needed to determine the risk/benefit ratio of DHEA.

VAGINAL DRYNESS AND DYSPAREUNIA

Definition and Natural Course

Atrophy refers to the wasting away, or decrease in size, of an organ or tissue. Vaginal atrophy refers to a loss of vaginal rugation and secretions resulting in the visual appearance of a thin, pale, and parched vaginal epithelium. The associated painful intercourse (dyspareunia) is a major cause of sexual decline during menopause. Other symptoms of vaginal atrophy include dryness, burning, itching, vaginitis, and increased risk of urinary tract infections. While the diagnosis of atrophic vaginitis is usually clinical, two simple tests (maturation index test, vaginal pH measurement) can confirm the diagnosis as outlined below.

Prevalence

Vaginal dryness affects up to half of menopausal women. It is estimated that vaginal dryness is bothersome in 3% of women of reproductive age, 4% of women in the early perimenopause, 21% of women in late menopausal transition, and 30–47% of women who are postmenopausal *(83)*. Smokers have a higher prevalence of vaginal dryness due to the toxic effects of smoking on the vaginal epithelium *(84)*.

Pathophysiology

Estrogen maintains the growth and integrity of the vaginal epithelium keeping it moist, smooth, and elastic. A decline in estrogen levels results in the loss of epithelial secretions, collagen, vascularity, and superficial squamous cells, resulting in increased epithelial atrophy. Vaginal smears reveal a paucity of glycogen laden and superficial squamous cells, with an increase in intermediate and parabasal cells. The change in ratio of the squamous, intermediate, and parabasal cells can be objectively used to confirm the diagnosis of atrophic vaginitis using the maturation index test.

Another simple test involves measuring the vaginal pH. The loss of glycogen laden cells results in decreased activity of vaginal lactobacilli and thus decreased lactic acid production. This results in increased vaginal pH among postmenopausal women (pH > 5.5), as compared to premenopausal women (pH < 4.5) *(85)*. The loss of pH also results in higher risk of vaginitis and urinary tract infections among menopausal women.

Management

The treatment of vaginal dryness usually involves the use of topical estrogen creams. Other therapies, such as oral estrogen-based therapy, have also been used but systemic treatment is less efficient if the target symptom is the vaginal epithelium. Finally, behaviors such as the maintenance of sexual activity can also be useful to keep maximal blood flow to the tissues. Management strategies are outlined in detail below and summarized in Table 3.

VAGINAL ESTROGEN

Multiple types of vaginal estrogen are available in the form of rings, vaginal tablets, and creams. Manufacturer recommendations for vaginal creams include the use of 0.5–4 g several times per week (even daily), which can significantly raise serum estradiol levels *(86)*. Products delivering lower doses of estrogen are becoming more popular. Noncream forms of vaginal estrogen tablets and rings result in lower, constant doses of estrogen and have been found to be effective in ameliorating vaginal symptoms. A vaginal tablet provides 25 mg of estrogen in 24 h and the ring can provide as low as 7.5 mg of estrogen in 24 h. The ring actively delivers estrogen for 90 days, while the tablet is active over a 24-h period.

Prospective, randomized trials, comparing both the tablet and ring with estrogen vaginal cream, provide efficacy data on the ring and tablet with less systemic estradiol absorption than 500–1,250 mg or more seen with estrogen cream *(87–89)*. However, one study comparing an estrogen cream (1 g) with a vaginal estrogen tablet (25 mg) reported that the cream was superior in terms of alleviating vaginal dryness and dyspareunia compared with the tablet *(90)*. Further, one advantage to the use of cream is that it can be targeted to areas of discomfort on the external genitalia and thus alleviate vulvar as well as vaginal symptoms. Thus estrogen containing cream provides a uniquely effective solution to the problem of vulvo-vaginal atrophy.

All forms of vaginal estrogen, including vaginal rings which are purported to have the lowest dose and thus the lowest systemic absorption, have been shown to be systemically absorbed *(91)*. Therefore, more studies are needed to find a dose that can be used effectively in the vagina that does not afford systemic absorption and would, therefore, be safe to use when estrogen should be totally avoided.

VAGINAL LUBRICANTS AND MOISTURIZERS

For women who wish to avoid estrogens, vaginal lubricants and moisturizers can provide temporary, symptomatic relief. Randomized trials involving a polycarbophil base

Table 3
Evaluation and management of vaginal dryness

Evaluation	Clinical diagnosis (visual appearance of a thin, pale and parched vaginal epithelium)
	Objective tests
	Maturation index test
	Vaginal pH
Management options	Local estrogen therapy
	Estrogen cream (various preparations)
	Estrogen tablet (such as Vagiderm)
	Estrogen ring (such as Estring)
	Vaginal lubricants (such as Replens)

lubricant, Replens, evaluated it against dienoestrol cream, and against a placebo water-based lubricant *(92, 93)*. In each study, all lubricants appeared to be effective in decreasing symptoms of dryness, dyspareunia, itching, and irritation. Replens was noted to be preferable and more effective than a pectin-based lubricant in a comparative study *(94)*. However, none of the nonhormonal lubricants appear to improve the overall health of the vaginal tissues as well as estrogen. A potential benefit of polycarbophil-based lubricants reported was the increase in local moisture and improved tissue elasticity.

Behavioral Imnterventions

Maintenance of sexual activity has been found to be helpful in preventing vaginal dryness. It increases vaginal blood flow and, therefore, can potentially reduce vaginal atrophy.

Complementary Therapies and Dietary Supplements

Vitamin E has been studied for its potential role in reducing vaginal atrophy. A phase II trial involving 100 postmenopausal women reported that a vaginal gel (containing hyaluronic acid, liposomes, phytoestrogens from Humulus lupulus extract, and vitamin E) was associated with a reduction in vaginal dryness after the first week of treatment throughout the duration of the 12-week study *(95)*. Further evaluation of this is needed in order to recommend to use.

INSOMNIA

Definition and Natural Course

Sleep disturbance, subjectively related to difficultly sleeping and dissatisfaction with sleep quality, is common in postmenopausal women *(96)*. Studies have suggested that with the onset of perimenopause, women start experiencing sleep difficulties as well as sleep-disordered breathing *(97–100)*. Troubles with sleep can include problems falling asleep, staying asleep, or waking up too early. Sleep disturbance can be associated with poor work performance, an increase in anxiety and depression, poor cognitive functioning, and impairment of overall quality of life *(101–103)*.

Prevalence

It is estimated that about 25–40% of women have sleep difficulties in their late forties and early fifties. The prevalence increases with age. However, the true prevalence due to menopause is less clear, given the relative effect of other factors such as hot flashes and mood symptoms and a lack of definitive research.

Pathophysiology

The etiology of sleep disturbance during menopause is probably multifactorial involving the aging process which includes changes in levels of hormones and neurotransmitters, as well as the presence of menopausal symptoms such as hot flashes *(104–106)*. A high density of estrogen receptors has been found in certain areas of the brain that regulate sleep cycle, and deficiency of estrogen is postulated to lead to a disruption in the sleep cycle patterns *(107)*. Other changes include less night time secretion of melatonin, an important regulator of sleep, by the pineal gland *(108)*. Polysomnographic studies evaluating sleep in perimenopausal and postmenopausal women have reported that women have long REM latency in menopause, compared to premenopausal women. The presence of vasomotor symptoms further decreases the polysomnographs sleep efficiency index *(109)*. However, the physiology is undoubtedly complex as studies with HRT do not uniformly demonstrate a resolution of sleep difficulties *(110)*.

Management

While there have been many studies assessing the effect of various pharmacologic agents, such as benzodiazepines, for the treatment of insomnia, there have been few trials evaluating the efficacy of therapies for insomnia specifically in postmenopausal women. Treatment for insomnia includes, behavioral therapy, specifically sleep hygiene, as well as pharmacologic therapy, particularly benzodiazepines and newer nonbenzodiazepine agents such as zolpidem and eszopiclone. These are discussed briefly below and listed in Table 4.

BEHAVIORAL INTERVENTIONS

Sleep hygiene incorporates life style changes to promote an effective sleep. It includes sleeping and waking up at a regular time, relaxing before going to bed, creating a comfortable sleep environment, avoiding watching television in the bedroom, getting sufficient daylight, avoiding napping, avoiding too much caffeine during the day, and exercising no closer than 3 h before bedtime *(111)*. Multiple trials and a few meta-analyses have shown sleep hygiene strategies to be effective in treating chronic insomnia and are comparable to conventional pharmacological therapies *(112)*.

BENZODIAZEPINES

Benzodiazepines, nonselective activators of the benzodiazepine receptors 1 and 2, have traditionally been the cornerstone of treatment of insomnia. The commonly used agents include flurazepam, triazolam, quazepam, estazolam, and temazepam. Although effective, long-acting benzodiazepine medications such as flurazepam can lead to daytime sedation and should be avoided *(113)*. Intermediate and short-acting agents such as temazepam (15–30 mg) are therefore preferred, and more widely used. These agents have the potential to cause tolerance, addiction, significant drug interactions, withdrawal effects, and thus have now been largely replaced by newer nonbenzodiazepine hypnotics.

NONBENZODIAZEPINE HYPNOTICS

There are several nonbenzodiazepine sleep aids which are selective benzodiazepine omega-1 receptor agonists, including zolpidem (5–10 mg per day) and zaleplon (5–10 mg per day). These agents help in sleep onset, improve sleep efficiency, decrease the number of awakenings, and increase total sleep duration *(114, 115)*. Unlike benzodiazepines, nonbenzodiazepines do not modify the normal sleep pattern, and do not carry the risk of tolerance or withdrawal, but they do have dependency potential *(116)*. There appears to be fewer major side effects as compared to benzodiazepines, and include nausea, dizziness, and drowsiness. Moreover, zaleplon appears to cause no psychomotor impairment or residual sedation *(117)*.

Table 4
Evaluation and management of insomnia

Evaluation	Clinical diagnosis (difficulty initiating or maintaining sleep)
	Assess for co existing illness particularly hot flashes and depression
Management options	Sleep hygiene
	Relaxation techniques (such as PMR, hypnosis, yoga)
	Nonbenzodiazepine hypnotics
	Zolpidem (10 mg per day)
	Zaleplon (10–20 mg per day)
	Eszopiclone (2–3 mg per day)
	Ramelteon (4–8 mg per day)
	Benzodiazepie (such as Temazepam)
	Treat co-existing symptoms

PMR progressive muscle relaxation

Eszopiclone (Lunesta) is a new nonbenzodiazepine hypnotic that mediates its hypnotic effects through interaction with the GABA (γ aminobutyric acid) receptor in the central nervous system *(118)*. A systematic review, based on five randomized double-blinded controlled studies, reported that eszopiclone (1–3 mg per day) was more efficacious than was placebo in reducing sleep latency, improving sleep efficiency, and increasing total sleep duration *(119)*. Unlike other hypnotics, it was found to be effective even after 6 months of use *(120)*, and is the only hypnotic approved for long-term use in insomnia. The major side effects include bitter taste, dry mouth, dizziness, hallucinations, edema, and viral infection. Eszopiclone does not have the risk of tolerance or withdrawal, there are no major contraindications, and usually no laboratory monitoring is needed. However, patients should be cautioned to avoid alcohol, other hynotics, and activities requiring high level of mental activity, such as operating machinery. Indiplon is a similar agent cited to help insomnia *(121)*, but has not been FDA approved to treat insomnia yet.

Ramelteon is another novel nonbenzodiazepine hypnotic that selectively targets melatonin receptors. Ramelteon has been reported to be more efficacious than placebo in reducing sleep latency, improving sleep efficiency, and increasing total sleep duration in three trials involving 829, 375, and 107 patients with chronic primary insomnia, respectively *(122–124)*. The major side effects included headache, somnolence, dizziness, and sore throat. Ramelteon does not alter sleep architecture, has no risk of tolerance or withdrawal, and appears to cause minimal (if any) residual sedation and/or memory impairment.

Complementary Therapies and Dietary Supplements

Herbal therapies such as valerian and melatonin have been reported to help insomnia *(125–130)*. In a large randomized, placebo-controlled trial involving 128 participants with sleep disorder, valerian (187-mg native extracts) was found to significantly improve subjective sleep parameters as compared to placebo *(131)*. Relaxation therapies such as progressive muscle relaxation (PMR), hypnosis, and yoga have also been shown to be effective with combination therapy being generally more beneficial than monotherapy *(132–134)*

REFERENCES

1. National Institutes of Health. National Institutes of Health State-of-the-Science Conference statement: Management of menopause-related symptoms. Ann Intern Med 2005; 142(12 Pt 1):1003–13

2. Loprinzi CL, Zahasky KM, Sloan JA, Novotny PJ, Quella SK. Tamoxifen-induced hot flashes. Clin Breast Cancer 2000; 1(1):52–6

3. Boekhout AH, Beijnen JH, Schellens JH. Symptoms and treatment in cancer therapy-induced early menopause. Oncologist 2006; 11(6):641–54

4. Carpenter J, Andrykowski M: Menopausal symptoms in breast cancer survivors. Oncol Nurs Forum 1999; 26(8):1311–17

5. Goodwin PJ, Ennis M, Pritchard KI, Trudeau M, Hood N. Risk of menopause during the first year after breast cancer diagnosis. J Clin Oncol 1999; 17:2365–70

6. Gallicchio L, Whiteman M, Tomic D, Miller K, Langenberg P, Flaws J. Type of menopause, patterns of hormone therapy use, and hot flashes. Fertil Steril 2006; 85(5):1432–40

7. Rossouw JE, Anderson GL, Prentice RL, LaCroix AZ, Kooperberg C, Stefanick ML, Jackson RD, Beresford SA, Howard BV, Johnson KC, Kotchen JM, Ockene J. Writing Group for the Women's Health Initiative Investigators. Risks and benefits of estrogen plus progestin in healthy postmeno-pausal women: Principal results from the Women's Health Initiative randomized controlled trial. J Am Med Assoc 2002; 288(3):321–33

8. Schow DA, Renfer LG, Rozanski TA, Thompson IM. Prevalence of hot flushes during and after neoadjuvant hormonal therapy for localized prostate cancer. South Med J 1998; 91(9):855–7

9. Carpenter J, Adrykowski M, Cordova M, et al. Hot flashes in postmenopausal women treated for breast carcinoma. Cancer 1998; 82:1682–91

10. Finck G, Barton DL, Loprinzi CL, et al. Definitions of hot flashes in breast cancer survivors. J Pain Symptom Manage 1998; 16(5):327–33

11. Greendale GA, Reboussin BA, Hogan P, et al. Symptom relief and side effects of postmenopausal hormones: Results from the postmenopausal estrogen/progestin interventions trial. Obstet Gynecol 1998; 92:982–8

12. Shanafelt TD, Barton DL, Adjei AA, Loprinzi CL. Pathophysiology and treatment of hot flashes. Mayo Clin Proc. 2002; 77(11):1207–18. Review

13. Berendsen HH. The role of serotonin in hot flushes. Maturitas 2000; 36(3):155–64. Review

14. Dalal S, Zhukovsky DS. Pathophysiology and management of hot flashes. J Support Oncol 2006; 4(7):315–20, 325

15. Loprinzi CL, Michalak JC, Quella SK, et al. Megesterol acetate for the prevention of hot flashes. N Engl J Med 1994; 331:347–52

16. Nand SL, Webster MA, Baber R, et al. Menopausal symptom control and side-effects on continuous estrone sulfate and three doses of medroxyprogesterone acetate. Climacteric 1998; 1:211–8

17. Lacey JV Jr, Mink PJ, Lubin JH, et al. Menopausal hormone replacement therapy and risk of ovarian cancer. J Am Med Assoc 2002; 288:334–41

18. Colditz GA, Hankinson SE, Hunter DJ, Willett WC, Manson JE, Stampfer MJ, Hennekens C, Rosner B, Speizer FE. The use of estrogens and progestins and the risk of breast cancer in postmenopausal women. N Engl J Med. 1995; 332(24):1589–93

19. Steinberg KK, Thacker SB, Smith SJ, Stroup DF, Zack MM, Flanders WD, et al. A meta-analysis of the effect of estrogen replacement therapy on the risk of breast cancer. J Am Med Assoc 1991; 265:1985–90

20. Bertelli G, Venturini M, Del Mastro L, Bergaglio M, Sismondi P, Biglia N, Venturini S, Porcile G, Pronzato P, Costantini M, Rosso R. Intramuscular depot medroxyprogesterone versus oral megestrol for the control of postmenopausal hot flashes in breast cancer patients: A randomized study. Ann Oncol 2002; 13(6):883–8

21. Loprinzi CL, Levitt R, Barton D, Sloan JA, Dakhil SR, Nikcevich DA, Bearden D 3rd, Mailliard JA, Tschetter LK, Fitch TR, Kugler JW. Phase III comparison of depomedroxyprogesterone acetate to venlafaxine for managing hot flashes: North Central Cancer Treatment Group Trial N99C7. J Clin Oncol 2006; 24(9):1409–14. Epub 2006 Feb 27

22. Pandya KJ, Raubertas RF, Flynn PJ, Hynes HE, Rosenbluth RJ, Kirshner JJ, Pierce HI, Dragalin V, Morrow GR. Oral clonidine in postmenopausal patients with breast cancer experiencing tamoxifen-induced

hot flashes: A University of Rochester Cancer Center Community Clinical Oncology Program study. Ann Intern Med 2000; 132(10):788–93

23. Stearns V, Slack R, Greep N, Henry-Tilman R, Osborne M, Bunnell C, Ullmer L, Gallagher A, Cullen J, Gehan E, Hayes DF, Isaacs C. Paroxetine is an effective treatment for hot flashes: Results from a prospective randomized clinical trial. J Clin Oncol 2005; 23(28):6919–30

24. Stearns V, Beebe KL, Iyengar M, Dube E. Paroxetine controlled release in the treatment of menopausal hot flashes: A randomized controlled trial. J Am Med Assoc 2003; 289(21):2827–34

25. Loprinzi CL, Kugler JW, Sloan JA, Mailliard JA, LaVasseur BI, Barton DL, Novotny PJ, Dakhil SR, Rodger K, Rummans TA, Christensen BJ. Venlafaxine in management of hot flashes in survivors of breast cancer: A randomised controlled trial. Lancet 2000; 356(9247):2059–63

26. Loprinzi CL, Sloan JA, Perez EA, Quella SK, Stella PJ, Mailliard JA, Halyard MY, Pruthi S, Novotny PJ, Rummans TA. Phase III evaluation of fluoxetine for treatment of hot flashes. J Clin Oncol 2002; 20(6):1578–83

27. Kimmick GG, Lovato J, McQuellon R, Robinson E, Muss HB. Randomized, double-blind, placebo-controlled, crossover study of sertraline (Zoloft) for the treatment of hot flashes in women with early stage breast cancer taking tamoxifen. Breast J 2006; 12(2):114–22

28. Gordon PR, Kerwin JP, Boesen KG, Senf J. Sertraline to treat hot flashes: A randomized controlled, double-blind, crossover trial in a general population. Menopause 2006; 13(4):568–75

29. Loprinzi CL, Flynn PJ, Carpenter LA, Atherton P, Barton DL, Shanafelt TD, Rummans TA, Sloan JA, Adjei AA, Mincey BA, Fitch TR, Collins M Pilot evaluation of citalopram for the treatment of hot flashes in women with inadequate benefit from venlafaxine. J Palliat Med 2005; 8(5):924–30

30. Suvanto-Luukkonen E, Koivunen R, Sundstrom H, Bloigu R, Karjalainen E, Haiva-Mallinen L, Tapanainen JS. Citalopram and fluoxetine in the treatment of postmenopausal symptoms: A prospective, randomized, 9-month, placebo-controlled, double-blind study. Menopause 2005; 12(1):18–26

31. Goetz MP, Rae JM, Suman VJ, Safgren SL, Ames MM, Visscher DW, Reynolds C, Couch FJ, Lingle WL, Flockhart DA, Desta Z, Perez EA, Ingle JN. Pharmacogenetics of tamoxifen biotransformation is associated with clinical outcomes of efficacy and hot flashes. J Clin Oncol 2005; 23(36):9312–8

32. Borges S, Desta Z, Li L, Skaar T, Ward B, Nguyen A, Jin Y, et al. Quantitative effect of CYP2D6 genotype and inhibitors on tamoxifen metabolism: Implication for optimization of breast cancer treatment. Clin Pharmacol Ther 2006; 80:61–74

33. Pandya KJ, Morrow GR, Roscoe JA, Zhao H, Hickok JT, Pajon E, Sweeney TJ, Banerjee TK, Flynn PJ. Gabapentin for hot flashes in 420 women with breast cancer: A randomised double-blind placebo-controlled trial. Lancet 2005; 366(9488):818–24

34. Guttuso T Jr, Kurlan R, McDermott MP, Kieburtz K. Gabapentin's effects on hot flashes in postmenopausal women: A randomized controlled trial. Obstet Gynecol 2003; 101(2):337–45

35. Reddy SY, Warner H, Guttuso T Jr, Messing S, DiGrazio W, Thornburg L, Guzick DS. Gabapentin, estrogen, and placebo for treating hot flushes: A randomized controlled trial. Obstet Gynecol 2006; 108(1):41–8

36. Loprinzi CL, Kugler RW, Barton DL, etal. A phase III randomized trial of gabapentin alone or in conjunction with an antidepressant in the management of hot flashes in women who have inadequate control with an antidepressant alone. J Clin Oncol 2007; 25:308–12

37. Barton DL, Loprinzi CL, Quella SK, Sloan JA, Veeder MH, Egner JR, Fidler P, Stella PJ, Swan DK, Vaught NL, Novotny P. Prospective evaluation of vitamin E for hot flashes in breast cancer survivors J Clin Oncol 1998; 16(2):495–500

38. Nelson HD, Vesco KK, Haney E, Fu R, Nedrow A, Miller J, Nicolaidis C, Walker M, Humphrey L. Nonhormonal therapies for menopausal hot flashes: Systematic review and meta-analysis. J Am Med Assoc 2006; 295(17):2057–71. Review

39. Vincent A, Barton DL, Mandrekar JN, Cha SS, Zais T, Wahner-Roedler DL, Keppler MA, Krcitzer MJ, Loprinzi C. Acupuncture for hot flashes: A randomizcd, sham-controlled clinical study. Menopause 2006; [Epub ahcad of print]

40. Liu J, Burdette J, Xu H, Gu C, van Breemen R, Bhat K, et al. Evaluation of estrogenic activity of plant extracts for the potential treatment of menopausal symptoms. J Agric Food Chem 2001; 49:2472–79

41. Shanafelt TD, Loprinzi CL. Improving quality of life for women at high risk for breast cancer: Symptom management without estrogen. In: Managing Breast Cancer Risk. Morrow M, Jordan VC (eds), BC Decker, Inc., Hamilton, Ontario, pp. 227–38, 2003

42. Mauck KF, Clarke BL. Diagnosis, screening, prevention, and treatment of osteoporosis. Mayo Clin Proc 2006; 81(5):662–72. Review

43. Lester J, Dodwell D, McCloskey E, Coleman R. The causes and treatment of bone loss associated with carcinoma of the breast. Cancer Treat Rev 2005; 31:115–42

44. Shapiro C, Maola J, Leboff M. Ovarian failure after adjuvant chemotherapy is associated with rapid bone loss in women with early stage breast cancer. J Clin Oncol 2001; 19:3306–11

45. Looker AC, Orwoll ES, Johnston CC Jr, et al. Prevalence of low femoral bone density in older U.S. adults from NHANES III. *J Bone Miner Res* 1997; 12:1761–8

46. Anderson GL, Limacher M, Assaf AR, et al. Women's Health Initiative Steering Committee. Effects of conjugated equine estrogen in postmenopausal women with hysterectomy: The Women's Health Initiative randomized controlled trial. *J Am Med Assoc* 2004; 291:1701–12

47. Cauley JA, Robbins J, Chen Z, et al. Women's Health Initiative Investigators. Effects of estrogen plus progestin on risk of fracture and bone mineral density: The Women's Health Initiative randomized controlled trial. *J Am Med Assoc* 2003; 290:1729–38

48. Cranney A, Tugwell P, Adachi J, Weaver B, Zytaruk N, Papaioannou A, Robinson V, Shea B, Wells G, Guyatt G; Osteoporosis Methodology Group and The Osteoporosis Research Advisory Group. Meta-analyses of therapies for postmenopausal osteoporosis. III. Meta-analysis of risedronate for the treatment of postmenopausal osteoporosis. Endocr Rev. 2002; 23(4):517–23. Review

49. Cranney A, Wells G, Willan A, Griffith L, Zytaruk N, Robinson V, Black D, Adachi J, Shea B, Tugwell P, Guyatt G; Osteoporosis Methodology Group and The Osteoporosis Research Advisory Group. Meta-analyses of therapies for postmenopausal osteoporosis. II. Meta-analysis of alendronate for the treatment of postmenopausal women. Endocr Rev 2002; 23(4):508–16. Review

50. Chesnut CH, Skag A, Christiansen C, et al. Effects of oral ibandronate administered daily or intermittently on fracture risk in postmenopausal osteoporosis, J Bone Miner Res 2004; **19**:1241–9

51. Nguyen ND, Eisman JA, Nguyen TV. Anti-hip fracture efficacy of biophosphonates: A Bayesian analysis of clinical trials. J Bone Miner Res 2006; 21(2):340–9

52. Karpf DB, Shapiro DR, Seeman E, Ensrud KE, Johnston CC Jr, Adami S, Harris ST, Santora AC 2nd, Hirsch LJ, Oppenheimer L, Thompson D. Prevention of nonvertebral fractures by alendronate. A meta-analysis. Alendronate Osteoporosis Treatment Study Groups. J Am Med Assoc 1997; 277(14):1159–64

53. Homik JE, Cranney A, Shea B, Tugwell P, Wells G, Adachi JD, Suarez-Almazor ME. A metaanalysis on the use of bisphosphonates in corticosteroid induced osteoporosis. J Rheumatol 1999; 26(5):1148–57

54. Homik J, Cranney A, Shea B, Tugwell P, Wells G, Adachi R, Suarez-Almazor M. Bisphosphonates for steroid induced osteoporosis. Cochrane Database Syst Rev 2000; (2):CD001347. Review

55. Ruggiero SL, Mehrotra B, Rosenberg TJ, Engroff SL, Osteonecrosis of the jaws associated with the use of bisphosphonates: A review of 63 cases, J Oral Maxillofac Surg (2004); 62:527–34

56. Migliorati CA, Siegel MA, Elting LS. Bisphosphonate-associated osteonecrosis: A long-term complication of bisphosphonate treatment. Lancet Oncol 2006; 7(6):508–14. Review

57. Marx RE. Pamidronate (Aredia) and zoledronate (Zometa) induced avascular necrosis of the jaws: A growing epidemic. J Oral Maxillofac Surg 2003; 61(9):1115–7

58. Marx RE, Sawatari Y, Fortin M, Broumand V. Bisphosphonate-induced exposed bone (osteonecrosis/osteopetrosis) of the jaws: Risk factors, recognition, prevention, and treatment. J Oral Maxillofac Surg 2005; 63(11):1567–75

59. Durie BG, Katz M, Crowley J. Osteonecrosis of the jaw and bisphosphonates. N Engl J Med. 2005; 353(1):99–102; discussion 99–102

60. Woo SB, Hellstein JW, Kalmar JR. Narrative [corrected] review: Bisphosphonates and osteonecrosis of the jaws. Ann Intern Med 2006; 144(10):753–61. Review

61. Badros A, Weikel D, Salama A, Goloubeva O, Schneider A, Rapoport A, et al. Osteonecrosis of the jaw in multiple myeloma patients: Clinical features and risk factors. J Clin Oncol 2006; 24:945–52

62. Ettinger B, Black DM, Mitlak BH et al. Reduction of vertebral fracture risk in postmenopausal women with osteoporosis treated with raloxifene: Results from a 3-year randomized clinical trial, J Am Med Assoc 1999; 282:637–45

63. Maricic M, Adachi JD, Sarkar S, Wu W, Wong M, Harper KD. Early effects of raloxifene on clinical vertebral fractures at 12 months in postmenopausal women with osteoporosis. Arch Intern Med 2002; 162(10):1140–3

64. Kanis JA, Johnell O, Black DM, Downs RW Jr, Sarkar S, Fuerst T, Secrest RJ, Pavo I. Effect of raloxifene on the risk of new vertebral fracture in postmenopausal women with osteopenia or osteoporosis: A reanalysis of the Multiple Outcomes of Raloxifene Evaluation trial. Bone 2003; 33(3):293–300

65. Siris ES, Harris ST, Eastell R, Zanchetta JR, Goemaere S, Diez-Perez A, Stock JL, Song J, Qu Y, Kulkarni PM, Siddhanti SR, Wong M, Cummings SR. Continuing Outcomes Relevant to Evista (CORE) Investigators. Skeletal effects of raloxifene after 8 years: Results from the continuing outcomes relevant to Evista (CORE) study. J Bone Miner Res 2005; 20(9):1514–24

66. Chesnut CH 3rd, Silverman S, Andriano K, Genant H, Gimona A, Harris S, Kiel D, LeBoff M, Maricic M, Miller P, Moniz C, Peacock M, Richardson P, Watts N, Baylink D. A randomized trial of nasal spray salmon calcitonin in postmenopausal women with established osteoporosis: The prevent recurrence of osteoporotic fractures study. PROOF Study Group. Am J Med 2000; 109(4):267–76

67. Neer RM, Arnaud CD, Zanchetta JR, et al. Effect of parathyroid hormone (1–34) on fractures and bone mineral density in postmenopausal women with osteoporosis. N Engl J Med 2001; 344:1434–41

68. Southby J, Kissin MW, Danks JA et al. Immunohistochemical localisation of parathyroid hormone-related protein in human breast cancer, Cancer Res 1990; **50:**7710–6

69. Gold DT, Pantos BS, Masica DN, Misurski DA, Marcus R. Initial experience with teriparatide in the United States. Curr Med Res Opin 2006; 22(4):703–8

70. Meunier PJ, Roux C, Seeman E, Ortolani S, Badurski JE, Spector TD, Cannata J, Balogh A, Lemmel EM, Pors-Nielsen S, Rizzoli R, Genant HK, Reginster JY. The effects of strontium ranelate on the risk of vertebral fracture in women with postmenopausal osteoporosis. N Engl J Med 2004; 350(5):459–68

71. Reginster JY, Seeman E, De Vernejoul MC, Adami S, Compston J, Phenekos C, Devogelaer JP, Curiel MD, Sawicki A, Goemaere S, Sorensen OH, Felsenberg D, Meunier PJ. Strontium ranelate reduces the risk of nonvertebral fractures in postmenopausal women with osteoporosis: Treatment of Peripheral Osteoporosis (TROPOS) study. J Clin Endocrinol Metab 2005; 90(5):2816–22

72. McClung MR, Lewiecki EM, Cohen SB, Bolognese MA, Woodson GC, Moffett AH, Peacock M, Miller PD, Lederman SN, Chesnut CH, Lain D, Kivitz AJ, Holloway DL, Zhang C, Peterson MC, Bekker PJ. AMG 162 Bone Loss Study Group. Denosumab in postmenopausal women with low bone mineral density. N Engl J Med 2006; 354(8):821–31

73. Sambrook P, Cooper C. Osteoporosis. Lancet 2006; 367(9527):2010–8. Review

74. Schoofs MW, van der Klift M, Hofman A, de Laet CE, Herings RM, Stijnen T, Pols HA, Stricker BH. Thiazide diuretics and the risk for hip fracture. Ann Intern Med 2003; 139(6):476–82

75. LaCroix AZ, Wienpahl J, White LR, Wallace RB, Scherr PA, George LK, Cornoni-Huntley J, Ostfeld AM. Thiazide diuretic agents and the incidence of hip fracture. N Engl J Med. 1990; 322(5):286–90

76. Bauer DC, Mundy GR, Jamal SA, Black DM, Cauley JA, Ensrud KE, van der Klift M, Pols HA. Use of statins and fracture: Results of 4 prospective studies and cumulative meta-analysis of observational studies and controlled trials. Arch Intern Med 2004; 164(2):146–52

77. Taaffe DR, Duret C, Wheeler S, Marcus R. Once-weekly resistance exercise improves muscle strength and neuromuscular performance in older adults. *J Am Geriatr Soc* 1999; 47:1208–14

78. NIH Consensus Development Panel on Osteoporosis Prevention, Diagnosis, and Therapy. Osteoporosis prevention, diagnosis, and therapy. J Am Med Assoc 2001; 285(6):785–95. Review

79. Bischoff-Ferrari HA, Willett WC, Wong JB, Giovannucci E, Dietrich T, Dawson-Hughes B. Fracture prevention with vitamin D supplementation: A meta-analysis of randomized controlled trials. *J Am Med Assoc* 2005; 293:2257–64

80. Baulieu E, Thomas G, Legrain S, Lahlou N, Roger M, Debuire B, et al. Dehydroepiandrosterone (DHEA), DHEA sulfate, and aging: Contribution of the DHEAge Study to a sociobiomedical issue. *Proc Natl Acad Sci USA* 2000; 97:4279–84

81. Labrie F, Diamond P, Cusan L, Gomez J, Belanger A, Candas B. Effect of 12-month dehydroepi-androsterone replacement therapy on bone, vagina, and endometrium in postmenopausal women *J Clin Endocrinol Metab 1997;* 82:3498–505

82. Hartkamp A, Geenen R, Godaert G, Bijl M, Bijlsma J, Derksen R. The effect of dehydroepiandrosterone on lumbar spine bone mineral density in patients with quiescent systemic lupus erythematosus. *Arthritis Rheum* 2004; 50:3591–5

83. Dennerstein L, Dudley EC, Hopper JL, Guthrie JR, Burger HG. A prospective population-based study of menopausal symptoms, Obstet Gynecol 2000; **96**:351–8

84. Kalogeraki A, Tamiolakis D. Cigarette smoking and vaginal atrophy in postmenopausal women. In Vivo 1996; **10**(6):597–600

85. Smith P. Estrogens and the urogenital tract: Studies on steroid hormone receptors and a clinical study on a new oestradiol-releasing vaginal ring, Acta Obstet Gynecol Scand Suppl 1993; **157**:1–26

86. Santen RJ, Pinkerton JV, Conaway M, Ropka M, Wisniewski L, Demers L, Klein KO. Treatment of urogenital atrophy with low-dose estradiol: Preliminary results. Menopause 2002; 9(3):179–87

87. Rioux JE, Devlin C, Gelfand MM, Steinberg WM, Hepburn DS. 17beta-estradiol vaginal tablet versus conjugated equine estrogen vaginal cream to relieve menopausal atrophic vaginitis. Menopause 2000; 7(3):156–61

88. Ayton RA, Darling GM, Murkies AL, Farrell EA, Weisberg E, Selinus I, Fraser ID. A comparative study of safety and efficacy of continuous low dose oestradiol released from a vaginal ring compared with conjugated equine oestrogen vaginal cream in the treatment of postmenopausal urogenital atrophy. Br J Obstet Gynaecol 1996; 103(4):351–8

89. Suckling J, Lethaby A, Kennedy R. Local oestrogen for vaginal atrophy in postmenopausal women. Cochrane Database Syst Rev 2003; (4):CD001500. Review

90. Manonai J, Theppisai U, Suthutvoravut S, Udomsubpayakul U, Chittacharoen A. The effect of estradiol vaginal tablet and conjugated estrogen cream on urogenital symptoms in postmenopausal women: A comparative study. J Obstet Gynaecol Res 2001; 27(5):255–60

91. Naessen T, Rodriguez-Macias K, Lithell H. Serum lipid profile improved by ultra-low doses of 17 B-estradiol in elderly women. J Clin Endocrinol Metab 2001; 86:2757–62

92. Loprinzi CL, Abu-Ghazaleh S, Sloan JA, vanHaelst-Pisani C, Hammer AM, Rowland KM Jr, Law M, Windschitl HE, Kaur JS, Ellison N. Phase III randomized double-blind study to evaluate the efficacy of a polycarbophil-based vaginal moisturizer in women with breast cancer. J Clin Oncol. 1997; 15(3):969–73

93. Bygdeman M, Swahn ML. Replens versus dienoestrol cream in the symptomatic treatment of vaginal atrophy in postmenopausal women. Maturitas 1996; 23(3):259–63

94. Caswell M, Kane M. Comparison of the moisturization efficacy of two vaginal moisturizers: Pectin versus polycarbophil technologies. J Cosmet Sci 2002; 53(2):81–7

95. Morali G, Polatti F, Metelitsa EN, Mascarucci P, Magnani P, Marre GB. Open, non-controlled clinical studies to assess the efficacy and safety of a medical device in form of gel topically and intravaginally used in postmenopausal women with genital atrophy. Arzneimittelforschung 2006; 56(3):230–8

96. Rosenthal MB. Epidemiology, sleep, and menopause. Menopause 2003; 10:4–5

97. Kalleinen N, Polo O, Himanen SL, Joutsen A, Urrila AS, Polo-Kantola P. Sleep deprivation and hormone therapy in postmenopausal women. Sleep Med 2006; 7(5);436–47

98. Krystal AD. Insomnia in women. Clin Cornerstone.2003; 5(3):41–50

99. Kravitz HM, Ganz PA, Brombergerj, et al. Sleep difficulty in women at midlife: A community survey of sleep and the menopausal transition. Menopause 2003;10:19–28

100. Young T, Finn L, Austin D, Peterson A. Menopausal status and sleep-disordered breathing in the Wisconsin Sleep Cohort Study. Am J Respir Crit Care Med 2003; 167(9):1181–5. Epub 2003 Feb 13

101. Roth T, Ancoli-Israel S. Daytime consequences and correlates of insomnia in the United States: Results of the 1991 National Sleep Foundation Survey. II. Sleep 1999; 22(Suppl 2):S354–8

102. Katz DA, McHorney CA. The relationship between insomnia and health-related quality of life in patients with chronic illness. J Fam Pract 2002; 51(3):229–35

103. Benca RM.Consequences of insomnia and its therapies. J Clin Psychiatry 2001; 62(Suppl 10):33–8. Review

104. Krystal AD, Edinger J, Wohlgemuth. Sleep in peri-menopausal and postmenopausal. Sleep Med Rev 1998; 2:243–53

105. Brugge KL, Kripke DE, Ancoli-Israel S, Gaffinkel L. The association of menopausal status and age with sleep disorders. Sleep Res 1989; 18:208

106. Ohayon MM. Severe hot flashes are associated with chronic insomnia. Arch Intern Med 2006; 166(12):1262–8

107. McEwen BS, Alves SE. Estrogen action in the central nervous system. Endocrinol Rev 1999; 20:279–307

108. Gorfine T, Assaf Y, Goshen-Gottstein Y, Yeshurun Y, Zisapel N. Sleep-anticipating effects of melatonin in the human brain. Neuroimage 2006; 31:410–8

109. Shaver J, Zenk S. Sleep disturbance in menopause. J Womens Health Gend Based Med. 2000; 9:109–18

110. Krystal AD, Edinger J, Wohlgemuth W, Marsh GR. Sleep in peri-menopausal and postmenopausal women. Sleep Med Rev 1998; 2(4):243–53

111. Becker P. Pharmacologic and nonpharmacologic treatments for insomnia. Neurol Clin 2005; 23:1149–63

112. Edinger JD, Wohlgemuth WK, Radtke RA, et al. Cognitive behavioral therapy for treatment of chronic primary insomnia: A randomized controlled trial. J Am Med Assoc 2001; 285:1856–64

113. Kamel NS, Gammack JK. Insomnia in the elderly: Cause, approach, and treatment. Am J Med 2006; 119(6):463–9. Review

114. Holm KJ, Goa KL. Zolpidem: An update of its pharmacology, therapeutic efficacy and tolerability in the treatment of insomnia. Drugs 2000; 59(4):865–89. Review

115. Dooley M, Plosker GL. Zaleplon: A review of its use in the treatment of insomnia. Drugs 2000; 60(2):413–45. Review

116. Ancoli-Israel S, Ayalon L. Diagnosis and treatment of sleep disorders in older adults. Am J Geriatr Psychiatry 2006; 14(2):95–103. Review

117. Troy SM, Lucki I, Unruh MA, Cevallos WH, Leister CA, Martin PT, Furlan PM, Mangano R. Comparison of the effects of zaleplon, zolpidem, and triazolam on memory, learning, and psychomotor performance. J Clin Psychopharmacol 2000; 20(3):328–37

118. Najib J. Eszopiclone, a nonbenzodiazepine sedative-hypnotic agent for the treatment of transient and chronic insomnia. Clin Ther 2006; 28(4):491–516. Review

119. Melton ST, Wood JM, Kirkwood CK. Eszopiclone for insomnia. Ann Pharmacother 2005; 39(10):1659–66. Epub 2005 Aug 30. Review

120. Krystal AD, Walsh JK, Laska E, Caron J, Amato DA, Wessel TC, Roth T. Sustained efficacy of eszopiclone over 6 months of nightly treatment: Results of a randomized, double-blind, placebo-controlled study in adults with chronic insomnia. Sleep 2003; 26(7):793–9

121. Petroski RE, Pomeroy JE, Das R, Bowman H, Yang W, Chen AP, Foster AC. Indiplon is a high-affinity positive allosteric modulator with selectivity for alpha1 subunit-containing GABAA receptors. J Pharmacol Exp Ther 2006; 317(1):369–77

122. Roth T, Seiden D, Sainati S, Wang-Weigand S, Zhang J, Zee P. Effects of ramelteon on patient-reported sleep latency in older adults with chronic insomnia. Sleep Med 2006; 7(4):312–8

123. Roth T, Stubbs C, Walsh JK. Ramelteon (TAK-375), a selective MT1/MT2-receptor agonist, reduces latency to persistent sleep in a model of transient insomnia related to a novel sleep environment. Sleep 2005; 28(3):303–7

124. Erman M, Seiden D, Zammit G, Sainati S, Zhang J. An efficacy, safety, and dose-response study of Ramelteon in patients with chronic primary insomnia. Sleep Med 2006; 7(1):17–24. Epub 2005 Nov 23

125. Donath F, Quispe S, Diefenbach K, Maurer A, Fietze I, Roots I. Critical evaluation of the effect of valerian extract on sleep structure and sleep quality. Pharmacopsychiatry 2000; 33(2):47–53

126. Andrade C, Srihari BS, Reddy KP, Chandramma L. Melatonin in medically ill patients with insomnia: A double-blind, placebo-controlled study. J Clin Psychiatry 2001; 62(1):41–5

127. Hallam KT, Olver JS, McGrath C, Norman TR. Comparative cognitive and psychomotor effects of single doses of Valeriana officianalis and triazolam in healthy volunteers. Hum Psychopharmacol 2003; 18(8):619–25

128. Morin CM, Culbert JP, Schwartz SM. Nonpharmacological interventions for insomnia: A meta-analysis of treatment efficacy. Am J Psychiatry 1994; 151:1172–80

129. Sack RL, Brandes RW, Kendall AR, Lewy AJ. Entrainment of free-running circadian rhythms by melatonin in blind people. N Engl J Med 2000; 343(15):1070–7

130. Zieglcr G, Ploch M, Miettinen-Baumann A, Collet W. Efficacy and tolerability of valerian extract LI 156 compared with oxazepam in the treatment of non-organic insomnia – a randomized, double-blind, comparative clinical study. Eur J Med Res 2002; 7(11):480–6

131. Morin CM, Koetter U, Bastien C, Ware JC, Wooten V. Valerian-hops combination and diphenhydramine for treating insomnia: A randomized placebo-controlled clinical trial. Sleep 2005; 28(11):1465–71

132. Cohen L, Warneke C, Fouladi RT, Rodriguez MA, Chaoul-Reich A. Psychological adjustment and sleep quality in a randomized trial of the effects of a Tibetan yoga intervention in patients with lymphoma. Cancer 2004; 100(10):2253–60

133. Khalsa SB. Treatment of chronic insomnia with yoga: A preliminary study with sleep-wake diaries. Appl Psychophysiol Biofeedback 2004; 29(4):269–78

134. Manjunath NK, Telles S. Influence of Yoga and Ayurveda on self-rated sleep in a geriatric population. Indian J Med Res 2005; 121(5):683–90

14 Supportive Care of the Older Cancer Patient

Lodovico Balducci

ABSTRACT

Cancer mainly affects individuals aged 65 and over, so that supportive care for cancer treatment concerns mostly elderly patients. Age is a risk factor for increased incidence and severity of chemotherapy-related toxicity and also for the emergence of different forms of toxicity including delirium and malnutrition; in addition age may modulate the perception of pain and the response to analgesics, and may indicate the need of a caregiver.

The National Cancer Center Network (NCCN) guidelines recommend that all cancer patients aged 70 and older undergo some form of geriatric assessment, receive dose modification to the renal function for the first dose of chemotherapy, receive prophylactic filgrastim or peg-filgrastim for moderately cytotoxic chemotherapy, have hemoglobin levels maintained around 12 g dl^{-1} and be treated with drugs with best toxicity profiles when that is feasible.

Though the perception of pain may decline with age, pain is endemic in the older population. Special problems include assessment, especially in cognitively impaired elderly, reduced tolerance to nonsteroidal medications, and increased susceptibility to the complications of opioids.

From: *Cancer and Drug Discovery Development: Supportive Care in Cancer Therapy*
DOI: 10.1007/978-1-59745-291-5_14, Edited by: D. S. Ettinger © Humana Press, Totowa, NJ

Delirium is a common complication of hospitalized elderly and is associated with increased risk of functional decline and of mortality. A comprehensive geriatric assessment is helpful in the prevention of delirium.

The caregiver may represent the best ally of the practitioner in the management of the older cancer patient, in allowing patients to receive timely treatment and support during emergency, and in being the spokesperson for the family. It behooves the practitioner to advise, train, and support the caregiver.

Cancer is a disease of aging. Currently, 50% of all malignances occur in 12% of the population aged 65 and older. In the year 2030, older individuals will represent 20% of the population and account for 70% of all cancer (Balducci L., Aapro M., Epidemiology of cancer and aging. Cancer Treat Res 2005, 1–16). Clearly, cancer in the older aged person is becoming the most common form of cancer. In general, older individuals may need more supportive care than the younger ones, due to increased vulnerability to stress and reduced personal and social resources. This chapter highlights the special supportive needs of older individuals with cancer after a brief overview of the biology and clinics of aging.

Key Words: Elderly, Supportive care, Neutropenia, Infection, Anemia, Delirium, Pain, Caregiver.

AGING, CLINICAL, AND BIOLOGICAL ASPECTS

Biology of Aging

Aging has been described as loss of entropy and fractality *(3)*. Loss of entropy means that the functional reserve of multiple organ-systems becomes progressively exhausted, which impair their ability to mount an adequate response to stress. Fractality is a repetitive, albeit unpredictable pattern of subdivision of a certain unit. For example, one can predict that the branches of a tree will subdivide into minor branches, whose number and length is unpredictable. Fractals in the human body include the bronchial and the vascular trees as well as the neurons. Loss of fractality in the nervous system may ultimately compromise the ability of the older person to perform complex activities, such as walking.

Underlying these losses is a chronic and progressive inflammation that represents the combination of chronic diseases, environmental interactions, and individual genomes *(4)*. The influence of chronic inflammation on aging is supported by a direct relationship between the concentration of inflammatory markers in the circulation, and the risk of death, disability, and geriatric syndromes *(4–7)*. Other important systemic changes of aging include endocrine senescence and immune senescence. Endocrine senescence is characterized by hypogonadism, decreased production of growth hormone, increased insulin resistance, and increased production of adrenal corticosteroids *(4, 8, 9)*. Low levels of testosterone have been associated with fatigue, anemia, depression, and catabolism both in men and women *(10)*. Immune senescence involves a decline in cell-mediated immunity that enhances the susceptibility of older individuals to infections by intracellular organisms and to some tumors *(11)*.

Of special interest to our discussion are the changes occurring in organs and systems involved in pharmacokinetics and pharmacodynamics of drugs. These include:

- Reduced glomerular filtration rate (GFR) that is almost universal with aging *(8, 12)* and prevents the excretion of drugs and their active metabolites
- Reduced hepatic mass and splanchnic circulation that reduces the ability of the liver to extract and metabolize drugs *(8)*
- Reduced intestinal absorption of drugs, due to a combination of reduced gastric motility and secretions, absorptive intestinal surface, and splanchnic circulation *(8)*
- Increased susceptibility of the hemopoietic system to hemopoietic stress, associated with increased risk of myelodepression from cytotoxic chemotherapy *(13)*
- Increased susceptibility of the digestive mucosas to cycle-active chemotherapy, due to a reduction of the number of mucosal stem cells and increased proliferation of the surface cells *(14)*
- Increased susceptibility of the heart and the nervous system to chemotherapy-related complications *(14–17)*

Though outside the scope of this chapter, it is worthy mentioning that aging may modulate tumor growth. For example hypogonadism and low growth hormone may hamper the growth of hormone-sensitive tumors, while the increased prevalence of metabolic syndrome may favor the growth of colorectal cancer *(18)*, and immune-senescence may enhance the susceptibility to highly immunogenic tumors *(19)*.

Clinical Evaluation of Aging

The management of cancer in the older aged person involves three basic questions:

- Is the patient going to die of cancer or with cancer?
- Is the patient going to live long enough to experience the complications of cancer?
- Is the patient able to tolerate the treatment complications?

The answer to these questions involves an individualized assessment of each patient, as aging is highly individualized and poorly reflected in chronologic age. While one can assume that most aged persons are 70 and older, it would be wrong to assume that all persons in that age ranged are aged. Figure 1 shows how the mortality rate of individuals

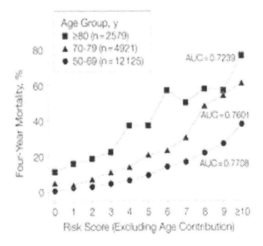

Fig. 1. Different risk of 4-year mortality for individuals of different ages and different degree of functional impairment and comorbidity. Adapted from (20), with kind permission from JAMA.

of the same age changes based on their function and presence of comorbidity *(20)*. Age 70 may be a landmark to start screening people for aging, the same way age 50 is a landmark to start screening women for breast cancer.

In the absence of direct measurements of entropy and fractality, one can use a multi-dimensional assessment for estimating the physiologic age of each individual.

The comprehensive geriatric assessment (CGA) is the time honored multidimensional assessment of the older person (Table1) *(8)*. As shown in Fig.1, the CGA may be utilized to estimate the risk of mortality and the life expectancy of different individuals *(20)*. Using 70 different pieces of information from the CGA, Mitnitsky et al. calculated a so-called "frailty index" that they used to estimate the physiologic, rather than the chronologic age of each person (Fig. 2) *(21)*. A practical example of how the CGA may be utilized for the management of older cancer patients is shown in Fig. 3 *(8)*.

The CGA is time consuming and sometimes exhausting for the patient. Then, a number of investigators have looked for simple and expedite instrument that may help screening older individuals and decide who may benefit from a full assessment. The cardiovascular health study (CHS) assessment has been validated on more than 8,500 independent individuals followed for more than 11 years and has gained almost universal acceptance *(3, 22)*. Based on whether these individuals had no abnormalities, one or two or more than two abnormalities in five simple parameters (Table 2), the investigators of the CHS have been able to identify three groups of patients, fit, pre-frail, and frail, with different risk of mortality, hospitalization, and functional decline over the following 11 years. The pre-frail and frail subgroups were more likely to benefit from the CGA than the fit one. Laboratory tests may also be used for screening purposes in the future. In a population of home dwelling individuals aged 70 and older, Cohen et al. demonstrated that increased levels of two markers of inflammation, Il6 and d-dimer, in the circulation, predicted risk of death and functional dependence over the next 2 years *(5)*.

A reasonable approach to patients 70 and older may include the CHS assessment with the first visit, followed by a more in depth CGA for those recognized as pre-frail or frail. The role of laboratory screenings remains to be determined. Given the high prevalence of functional dependence and comorbidity after aged 85, one may argue that all individuals 85 and older deserve a complete CGA.

Before leaving the clinical assessment of age, it is important to clarify a few terms that recur in the geriatric literature *(8)*. *Functional dependence* refer to inability to perform any of the activities of daily livings (ADLs) or instrumental activities of daily livings (IADLs) and implies the need of a caregiver that must reside with the patient in case of ADL dependence. Generally impairment, disability, and handicaps are associated with functional dependence. *Impairment* relates to the loss of a particular function (for example the movement of one leg); *disability* refers to the loss of a special activity, such as walking or climbing stairs; disability becomes a *handicap* when it is not compensated by environmental changes. For example, a paraplegic is not handicapped, and may be fully independent if provided with a motorized wheel chair, and if the bathroom and the bedroom have bars that allow that person to utilize the toilet and to get in and out of bed.

Another recurring term in the geriatric literature is frailty *(3, 21)*. For the majority of geriatricians today frailty includes a person who is at increased risk of suffering complications of an injury or of a disease. A disabled person, a dependent person, is definitely frail, but even an independent person may be frail if elective surgery requires

Table 1
The comprehensive geriatric assessment (CGA)

Domain	Assessment	Clinical implication
Functional status	Performance status (PS)	Dependence in ADL and IADLs:
	Activities of daily living (ADL):	Increased risk of mortality
	• Transferring	
	• Feeding	Increased vulnerability to stress
	• Grooming	
	• Dressing	
	• Use of the bathroom	
	Instrumental activities of daily living (IADL):	Dependence in ADLs: Need for a home caregiver
	• Use of transportations	
	• Use of telephone	Dependence in IADL: Need for a caregiver
	• Ability to take medications	
	• Financial management	
	• Shopping	Explore possibility of functional rehabilitation
	• Ability to provide to one's nutrition	
Comorbidity	Number of comorbid conditions	Risk of mortality and vulnerability to stress increases with the number and severity of comorbid conditions
	Comorbidity scales	Optimal management of diseases may improve patient health and prevent functional decline
Geriatric Syndromes	Dementia (screen)	Increased risk of mortality and functional dependence
	Depression (screen)	Increased vulnerability to stress
	Delirium	Medication may delay dementia, reverse depression, and ostoporosis
	Falls (screen for risk of falls)	
	Osteoporosis	Fall prevention
	Dizziness	
	Neglect and abuse	
	Failure to thrive	
Nutrition	Assessment of malnutrition and of risk of malnutrition	Malnutrition is associated with increased vulnerability to stress
Polypharmacy	Number of medications	Complications and cost
	Risk of drug interactions	
Social support	Personal resources	
	Social resources	

prolonged hospitalization and rehabilitation. A recent conference on frailty, described this condition as a syndrome of enhanced vulnerability characterized by sarcopenia, loss of mobility, force, resistance, and of neuromuscular coordination *(3)*. The identification

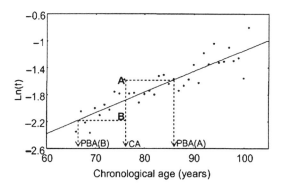

Fig. 2. Estimate of the physiologic age of a patient based on the Ln of the frailty index. Adapted from (21), with kind permission from Journal of Gerontology.

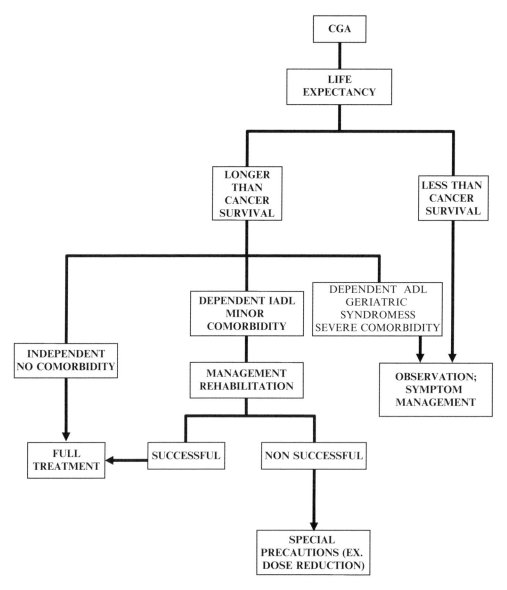

Fig. 3. Algorithm for the treatment of older cancer patients with cytotoxic chemotherapy.

Table 2
Parameters of the CHS study

1. Weight loss %10 lbs in 6 months)
2. Decreased energy level
3. Decreased grip strength
4. Decreased walk speed
5. Increased difficulty in initiating movements

of frailty is important not only because frail people are at increased risk of complications from cancer treatment (8), but also because frailty is at least in part reversible, as demonstrated by the ACOVE (advanced care of vulnerable elders) project (23). Thus, the CGA in cancer is helpful not only to estimate one person's life expectancy and functional reserve, but also to promote a series of interventions that may improve one's condition of frailty and make that person more suitable for treatment (24).

In discussing the supportive care of the older cancer patients, we will recognize problems that are common to all cancer patients but may be more serious in the elderly, and problems that are more typical of older individuals.

PROBLEMS RELATED TO CANCER AND CANCER MANAGEMENT THAT MAY HAVE PARTICULAR IMPORTANCE IN ELDERLY PATIENTS

In this section, the complications of chemotherapy, the complications of hormonal therapy, and pain will be examined.

Complications of Chemotherapy

Neutropenia, anemia, mucositis, cardiac and nervous complications become more serious and more common with age (8).

Neutropenia

The risk and severity of neutropenia and neutropenic infections increases with age. In a review of 500 patients treated in the community with CHOP and CNOP. Lyman et al. found the risk of neutropenic infections to be 38% among individuals, 65 and over, and 18% among the younger ones (25). The duration of hospitalization was more prolonged in older individuals by approximately 30% (26). This finding is worthy mentioning because hospitalization is associated with deconditioning and functional dependence in the elderly, in addition to increased cost. Similar results were reported by Morrison et al. also in older individuals treated for lymphoma (27). In addition, Kim et al. reported increased risk of myelotoxicity among patients managed in the South West Oncology Group (28) and Crivellari et al. among those managed in the International Breast Cancer Study Group (29). In a recent meta-analysis of 14 randomized controlled studies of myelopoietic growth factors, Kuderer et al. reported that the risk of infections and infection-related mortality increased with age (30).

The risk of neutropenia and neutropenic infection may compromise the outcome of older cancer patients, because these individuals are at increased risk of not receiving adequate dose or dose intensity of chemotherapy, in addition to the risk of mortality and functional dependence. In an analysis of patients receiving chemotherapy for lymphoma or for breast cancer in the adjuvant setting Lyman et al. reported that neutropenia accounted for more than 50% of dose delays and dose reductions, and more than 60% of older individuals receive less than 85% of the total planned dose of chemotherapy *(25, 31)*. This finding is extremely disturbing as the benefits of treatment are compromised when the total dose is reduced below 85%.

Three interventions have been proposed for limiting the incidence of neutropenia and neutropenic infections in older individuals: dose reduction, oral antibiotics, and prophylactic use of myelopoietic growth factors. Dose reduction is unacceptable when one try to administer curative treatment, as dose reduction may compromise tumor control. Prophylactic quinolones and trimetophrin/sulphametoxazole have reduced the risk of neutropenic infections in patients with acute myelogenous leukemia and bone marrow transplant, by favoring an overgrowth of anaerobic organisms in the gut that eliminates the more common Gram (−) organisms of the intestine *(32, 33)*. The value of prophylactic antibiotics in solid tumors has been reported in a randomized controlled study where the incidence of infections was determined not only by the presence of fever but also by the presence of so-called "signs of infections" *(34)*. At the same time, a randomized controlled study in lung cancer in the Netherlands reported that the combination of antibiotics and myeloid growth factors was superior to antibiotics alone in preventing infections *(35)*. A potentially serious complication of prolonged treatment with prophylactic antibiotics has been the emergence of antibiotic resistant bacteria *(33)*. At least five randomized controlled studies demonstrated that filgrastim or peg-filgrastim reduced the incidence of neutropenia and neutropenic infections in older individuals, and consequently this approach is the best documented *(36–40)*. The National Cancer Center Network (NCCN), the ASCO, and the EORTC all recommend that prophylactic growth factors be used with the first course of treatment in patients receiving CHOP or a CHOP-like chemotherapy regimens *(24, 41, 42)*

Anemia

The prevalence of anemia increases with age *(43, 44)* even in individuals without cancer. In cancer patients, anemia may be due to chronic inflammation, may represent an effect of chemotherapy, but may also be due to iron deficiency from occult bleeding or to B12 deficiency. The prevalence of B12 deficiency in persons over 60 may be as high as 15%, though only rarely this deficiency is manifested as anemia *(45)*. In the absence of simultaneous folate deficiency the most common manifestations of cobalamine deficiency in older individuals are neurological and include loss of vibratory sensations, peripheral neuropathy, and dementia. Both cancer and aging are chronic inflammations and these conditions may be synergistic in the pathogenesis of anemia. Inflammatory cytokines may blunt the response of erythropoietin to drops in hemoglobin and the response of erythropoietic progenitors in the marrow to erythropoietin *(46, 47)*. In addition, Il6 stimulates the hepatic production of hepcidin, a glycoprotein that inhibits the mobilization of iron from the stores and the absorption of iron from the duodenum, creating a condition of functional iron deficiency *(48)*. The age-related decline in GFR may also contribute to the pathogenesis of anemia, as GFR <60 min^{-1} may be associated to decreased production of epoietin *(12)*. The possible mechanism of anemia in the elderly is summarized in Fig. 4.

Anemia is detrimental to older patients for several reasons, including mortality of all causes, development, and worsening of congestive heart failure and kidney insufficiency, and increased risk of dementia and of delirium *(43)*. Five complications of anemia are germane to the management of older cancer patients. The risk of chemotherapy-related toxicity is increased in the presence of anemia, as the majority of antineoplastic agents are heavily bound to red blood cells *(49–53)*. A decline in hemoglobin is associated with increased concentration of free drug and enhanced risk of toxicity. The risk of functional dependence and falls increases inversely with the level of hemoglobin for levels below 13 dl^{-1} both in men and women *(54, 55)*. Functional dependence may represent a serious burden also for the caregiver of the older cancer patient, who often is compelled to limit the hours he/she can work *(56)*. Functional dependence may also limit the administration of more chemotherapy and compromise the treatment outcome. The response of tumors to chemotherapy and radiotherapy may be compromised in the presence of anemia, because the anoxia of the tumor tissue prevents the formation of free radicals necessary to the damage of the neoplastic DNA *(5)*. Symptomatic anemia requires management of blood transfusions that have been associated with poorer

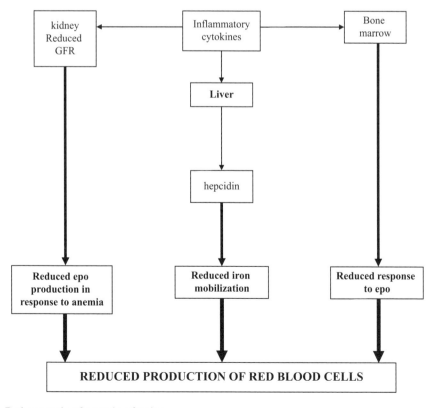

Fig. 4. Pathogenesis of anemia of aging.

cancer prognosis *(57)*. In addition, it is clear that in the presence of anemia cancer patients experience increased mortality *(58, 59)*.

In all patients with newly diagnosed anemia, a complete work up of potential causes is indicated, and specific causes such as iron or B12 deficiency should be corrected. In the absence of specific causes, the use of erythropoietic stimulating factors (ESF), such as epoetin α and β or darbepoetin α is indicated. These factors reduce the number of blood transfusions that a patient needs and improve the energy levels and quality of life *(58, 60)*. Unfortunately the use of these agents has not been associated so far with a reduction of chemotherapy-induced toxicity, improved response to chemotherapy, or improved survival. Paradoxically, according to at least two randomized controlled studies and a recent meta-analysis, they have been associated with a small shortening of the patients survival *(60 – 62)*. In patients with head and neck cancer, this phenomenon was ascribed to the presence of erythropoietin receptors in some of the tumors, for which ESF might have stimulated the growth *(63)*. Practical questions include:

* What hemoglobin levels should be the target? Current recommendations are to try to keep hemoglobin levels at 12 g dl^{-1}. The highest incremental change in energy is achieved when the hemoglobin levels rises from 11 to 13 dl^{-1}, and no risk of increased mortality were observed when hemoglobin was kept at 12 g dl^{-1} *(56, 58)*.
* When should ESF treatment be initiated? A recent study by Boccia et al. showed that lowest number of injections necessary to achieve target hemoglobin levels was employed when treatment was initiated for hemoglobin levels $\geq$10 g dl^{-1}. Thus, it appears to initiate the treatment for those hemoglobin levels *(64)*.
* Is administration of iron beneficial in combination of ESF? Intravenous administration of iron was associated with significantly higher response to ESF in a randomized controlled study. This strategy may be indicated in all patients and particularly in those with low serum iron *(65)*.
* Is there any difference between the available ESFs? No difference in terms of efficacy was demonstrated. The main advantage of darbepoetin α is that it can be utilized every 3 weeks, instead of weekly. Recent studies showed that also epoetin α may be administered at time intervals longer than weekly, when used in high doses.

Mucositis

According to the review of the North Central Cancer Treatment Group (NCCTG), the risk of muscositis from fluorinated pyrimidines was increased in individuals aged 65 and older. In these patients, mucositis occasionally led to death from volume depletion and renal failure *(66)*.

Two potential antidotes of mucositis have been proposed: a solution of glutamine and a keratinocyte growth factor (KGF). The clinical trials of glutamine so far have been inconclusive. KGF has proven effective in preventing mucositis for high doses of chemotherapy in patients undergoing allogeneic bone marrow transplantations, and in patients receiving hyperfractionated radiation therapy in combination with chemotherapy for cancer of the head and neck *(67)*. Problems related to this compound include high cost and cumbersome administrations.

Another simple measure to prevent mucositis includes the substitution of intravenous fluoropyrimidines with capecitabine. This prodrug is activated in the liver and the neoplastic tissues, so that normal tissues are spared from its toxic effects *(24)*.

Aggressive fluid resuscitation is recommended in all older individuals experiencing dysphagia and diarrhea. Given their limited water content, elderly are particularly susceptible to the risk of volume depletion.

Cardiotoxicity

The risk of anthracycline cardiomyopathy increases with age *(15–17)*. While the risk of overt congestive heart failure is relatively rare (around 1%) for total doses of doxorubicin up to 300 mg per m^{-2} of body surface area, approximately 20% of individuals aged 65 and older experience an asymptomatic decline in left ventricular ejection fraction after treatment with doxorubicin, detectable several years after discontinuance of the drug *(15–17)*. The natural history of this decline in cardiac function is unknown, but is of some concern as it affects individuals who have received potentially curative treatment for large cell lymphoma or for breast cancer in the adjuvant setting.

Anthracycline-related cardiotoxicity may be ameliorated in three ways: continuous infusion of doxorubicin in lieu of short-term infusion *(68)*, prophylactic treatment with dexrazoxane *(69)*, and substitution of doxorubicin with pegylated liposomal doxodubicin (PLD) *(70)*. Continuous infusions of doxorubicin may be somehow cumbersome to administer in older individuals and are associated with increased risk of mucositis. Dexarazoxane may enhance the risk of drug-related mucositis and myelosuppression. Furthermore, the drug may shelter the tumor from cytotoxicity, according to a study, PLD has many advantages, including minimal risk of myelodepression, alopecia, and nausea and vomiting. The elevated cost may be in part offset by the elimination of hemopoietic growth factors and antiemetics in the management of elderly patients. The indications for PLD are limited, however, and include metastatic breast cancer, multiple myeloma, and advanced ovarian cancer.

Neurotoxicity

The risk of peripheral neurotoxicity from vinca alkaloids, taxanes, and platinum congeners increases with age *(14)*. In older persons it may cause functional dependence by impeding the fine movement of the hands and causing uncertain gait. Seemingly, pre-existing neuropathy, such as the one due to diabetes, may predispose to more serious neurologic complications of cancer treatment Unfortunately, no antidotes to this complication are available. Current recommendations include avoidance of the combination of two neurotoxic agents such as cisplatin and paclitaxel, and discontinuance of the drug when weakness is detected or when movement impairment is a clear cause of functional dependence.

Cerebellar toxicity from high doses of cytarabin is also increased in older individuals due in part to decreased renal excretion of the toxic metabolite ara-uridine *(14)*. This treatment is generally avoided when the GFR is lower than 50 ml min^{-1}.

Treatment should be discontinued when physical signs of cerebellar dysfunction are apparent.

Based of the evidence reviewed so far, the NCCN has issued a number of guidelines for the management of older cancer patients with chemotherapy (Table 3).

Complications of Hormonal Therapy

Common form of hormonal therapy includes androgen deprivation for the management of prostate cancer and adjuvant treatment of breast cancer with aromatase inhibitors.

Table 3
NCCN guidelines for the management of the older cancer patient

1. A form of geriatric assessment is indicated in all individuals aged 70 and more to estimate life-expectancy, tolerance of treatment, and to recognize reversible conditions that may compromise the management of these individuals
2. The first dose of the drug should be adjusted to the GFR; subsequent doses should be increased if no toxicity has been observed
3. Prophylactic filgrastim or peg-filgrastim are indicated in persons aged 65 and older receiving treatment of dose-intensity comparable with CHOP, to prevent the risk of neutropenic infections, infectious deaths, and inadequate chemotherapy doses
4. Maintenance of hemoglobin around 12 g dl^{-1}
5. Preferential use, when feasible, of the following agents: capecitabine, PLD, vinorelbine, gemcitabine, premetrexed, weekly taxanes

Androgen Deprivation

This may be obtained with orchiectomy, LH–RH analogs, and high doses of ketoconazol and estrogens. Currently, orchiectomy and LH–RH analogs are the most common forms of treatment. Both of them may cause osteoporosis, anemia, fatigue, dementia, and diabetes, in addition to loss of libido *(71, 72)*. LH–RH treatment has also been associated with a 16% increase in coronary artery disease.

Osteoporosis is the most common complication of long-term androgen deprivation that has been associated with a 50% increase in bone fractures in older men. Current recommendation for the prevention of osteoporosis include monitoring the bone density of these patients and treatment with bisphosphonates in patients who already have severe osteopenia and osteoporosis and in those that experience a rapid bone loss *(73)*. More in general, however, it is time to revisit the role of long-term androgen deprivation in these patients. The main questions related to this treatment include:

- When should androgen deprivation begin?
- How long should it last?
- What alternative to androgen deprivation exists?

There is clear evidence that androgen deprivation prolongs the survival of prostate cancer patients when it is initiated prior to the development of symptoms in the presence of bone metastases or when it is used in the adjuvant setting in D1 diseases after surgery or in stage C disease with radiotherapy *(74)*. The benefit of the current practice to initiate hormonal treatment in patients with PSA recurrence after local treatment with surgery or radiation is unproven and should be discouraged, with the possible exception of patients at high risk (Gleason score of 8 or higher, PSA elevation within 2 years of local treatment, PSA doubling time of 10 months or less) *(74)*. Likewise, the primary treatment of prostate cancer with hormonal therapy in older patients who are considered unsuitable for surgery or radiation should be revisited, in view of the recent report of serious complications. In some of these patients, one should consider intermittent hormonal therapy that was found as effective as continuous treatment. Despite the risk of deep vein thrombosis and fluid retention, estrogens in low doses (1 daily mg of DES) may also be considered in these patients. Estrogens prevent ostoporosis and hot flashes and may be associated with lesser risk of fatigue, anemia, and loss of libido.

Adjuvant Treatment of Breast Cancer with Aromatase Inhibitors

This has become the most common adjuvant hormonal treatment of postmenopausal breast cancer in women with hormone receptor rich tumors. Bone fracture secondary to osteoporosis appears as the most common and consequential long-term complication of this treatment *(75)*. It has been common practice to treat these patients with bisphosphonates if they have severe osteopenia or overt osteoporosis.

Pain

The prevalence of pain increases with age and pain is underdiagnosed and under-treated in older people, especially in those hosted in assisted living *(76)*. Older individuals neglect pain until it becomes unbearable and may be reluctant to report pain for a number of reasons, including the misconception that pain is part of normal aging and that pain medication may cause addiction *(77)*.

Important characteristics of pain in the older aged person with cancer are described in Table 4.

Several studies indicate that the threshold of the stimulus for inducible somatic pain increases, and that the perception of visceral pain declines with age. The main consequence of these findings is that pain cannot be relied upon as a symptom of catastrophic events *(77)*. For example, more than 20% of myocardial infarctions are not associated with pain in individuals aged 70 and older. Likewise, visceral perforation may be asymptomatic in these patients.

In the same vein, the manifestations of pain may vary in older individuals. Instead of vocalizing her/his discomfort, the older person may react to pain with withdrawal and symptoms that are more typical of depression in the young *(77)*. The signs of pain may also vary: delirium is a common manifestation of underlying pain, whereas abdominal catastrophes, such as visceral perforation may not be accompanied by typical signs of peritonitis (guarding, rebound tenderness).

Comorbidity and polipharmacy may influence the perception of pain in different ways. Most important, they may mask new manifestations of cancer that are erroneously ascribed to pre-existing conditions. For example, the pain of new bony metastases may be mistakenly ascribed to pre-existing arthritis and osteoporosis, whereas the analgesics used for this condition may delay the recognition of new pain. Some diseases, including

Table 4
Features of pain in the older cancer patient

The perception of pain declines with age

The manifestations of pain may change with age

The assessment of pain may be problematic in older persons, especially those with cognitive impairment. Generally vertical pain scale are preferred to horizontal scales, as the visual field becomes progressively reduced with age

Comorbidity and polipharmacy may influence the perception of pain

The application of the WHO steps for pharmacological management of pain in older individuals is complicated by decreased tolerance of all classes of pain medication

Pain may cause deconditioning and functional dependence

depression, may enhance the perception of pain, and others, such as hypertension, may blunt it, though the mechanisms of these interactions are poorly understood.

The assessment of pain may be affected by decreased vision and hearing as well as by delirium and dementia. In general, vertical scales, such as the pain thermometer of the American Geriatric Society (AGS) are preferred to the horizontal ones, because aging is associated with a progressive restriction of the visual field (77, 78). Qualitative scales and pain maps may encourage patients to vocalize their discomfort and to identify their symptoms, but they may take time to administer. The absence of a quantitative assessment makes these instruments less suitable for clinical trials and for evaluating treatment outcome.

While it is true that the prevalence of dementia increases with age, seldom the dementia is so deep and disabling to prevent assessment of pain. Scales utilizing facial expressions "in lieu" of numbers have been proposed for cognitively impaired individuals, but these instruments may confuse some patients, as the expression of discomfort may be confused with an expression of sadness (77, 79). In individuals who cannot communicate, the observation of pain behaviors, such as groaning, grunting, and restlessness offer an adequate assessment of pain to the experienced observer (77, 79).

In addition to causing discomfort and compromising quality of life, pain, and the fear of pain usually limit the mobility of older individuals. They may cause deconditioning and functional dependence, which in turn may compromise the outcome of cancer treatment. Thus pain control is paramount to the management of older cancer patient.

Nonsteroidal anti-inflammatory drugs have limited use in the management of somatic pain in older individuals due to the risk of gastrointestinal and renal complications. Furthermore, recent studies have suggested that these agents may cause volume overload, congestive heart failure, and coronary artery diseases (77). Piroxicam, indomethacin, should always be avoided in older individuals. Acetaminophen appears safe, but it has no anti-inflammatory actions, and the risk of liver toxicity limits the doses of this drug. If tolerated, opioids are an effective management of pain in older individuals. General rules for the use of opioids include (77, 80):

• Mild opioids such as codein or tramadol are best avoided in the elderly, because they require activation by the P450 enzyme system in the liver. These reactions decline with age (14) and are a major site of drug interactions.
• Meperidine should be avoided, because its metabolite normeperidine, that is excreted from the kidneys, may cause seizures in presence of kidney insufficiency.
• The duration of action and the toxicity of morphine, hydromorphone, and oxycodone are unpredictable in older individuals. The 6 glucuronide and the 3 glucuronide of morphine are ten times as active and as toxic, respectively, than the parent compound and both of them are excreted though the kidneys. Furthermore, the ratio of δ and μ opioid receptors in the brain may increase with age, so that older individuals are more susceptible to the complications of opioids. It appears prudent to start opioid treatment in patients 65 and older with short acting medications, to establish "in vivo" the effects of the drugs, before administering long-lasting preparations.
• Whenever possible it appears prudent to avoid the systemic effects of opioids in older individuals. Radiation therapy to painful areas, radioactive isotopes for the management of bone metastases, local nervous block, intatecal administration of opioids, even cytotoxic chemotherapy should be tried before committing a patient to long-term opioid treatment. Prevention of constipation is mandatory in the management of older individuals with opioids.

- Neuropathic pain may represent a major problem in older cancer patients, and it may result from chemotherapy and radiation therapy, in addition to neurologic complications of cancer. As it is in younger patients, the mainstay of neurologic pain in the older ones involves the use of antiepileptic medications.

SUPPORTIVE ISSUES THAT ARE MORE COMMON IN OLDER CANCER PATIENTS

In this session we will describe delirium, malnutrition, and the need of a caregiver.

Delirium

Delirium is a disorder of attention that may include delusions and hallucinations and is associated with neurovegetative manifestations (fever, tachycardia) and an underlying systemic disease *(81, 82)*. Though it is generally the manifestation of an acute disease, delirium may sometimes be chronic or recurrent. Predisposing factors to delirium include dementia, anemia, infections, electrolyte and metabolic abnormalities, medications, and restrains *(81)*. When an older cancer patient presents with newly diagnosed delirium it is mandatory to review the list of the medications, especially the ones that have been instituted in the recent past, to rule out infections by chest radiography, urine analysis, urine and blood cultures, to check the serum electrolytes, including the magnesium, the glucose, and the BUN and creatinine, and to exclude stroke and brain metastases with an MRI of the brain. According to the clinical situation, one may also want to exclude a myocardial infarction with serum enzymes and troponin levels and with an electrocardiogram. Delirium is a common complication of acute changes in the living environment of the elder, including admission to a hospital or to assisted living facilities.

A multidimensional intervention based on CGA of older patients has proven effective in preventing "in hospital" delirium *(81)*. Management of polipharmacy aimed to avoid interactions and redundancy, correction of anemia, avoidance of restrains, provision of a familial caregiver during the hospital admission, may go a long way in preventing delirium. Treatment of delirium involves management of the underlying cause and prudent use of phenotiazines, such as haloperidol. Antipsychotic drugs such as zipradisone have also proven helpful in the management of delirium *(14, 81, 83)*. Delirium is a poor prognostic factor *(84, 85)* as it is associated with increased mortality, and incidence of functional dependence over the following year, and only half of the individuals who had experienced delirium have a complete cognitive recovery *(84)*. It is reasonable to consider delirium a geriatric syndrome and a manifestation of frailty *(3)*.

Malnutrition

Approximately 20% of individuals aged 70 and over are malnourished, and many more are at risk of malnutrition *(86–89)*. In addition to cancer, other risk factors in older people include loss of appetite, loneliness, depression, lack of access to regular meals, and increased concentration of inflammatory cytokines in the circulation that determine a condition of catabolism. Malnutrition is associated with functional dependence, and enhanced chemotherapy- and radiotherapy-related toxicity *(88)*. A mininutritional assessment should be included in the evaluation of all older cancer patients. It is important to make sure that patient at risk have access to at least three meals a day, and to motivate these individuals to pursue adequate nutrition. In patients with cancer of the esophagus and upper airways undergoing combined treatment with chemo and radiation a prophylactic gastrostomy may be indicated if they are at risk of obstruction.

Caregiver

Individuals dependent in ADLs do need a home caregiver; those dependent in IADLs need a reliable caregiver available to transport them to a care center on short notice in case of an emergency to monitor the patient's nutrition, medication, and general well being, and to support the patients during the ordeal of cancer and its treatment. The role of the caregiver in the management of older patients with cancer cannot be overemphasized *(90, 91)*. Under ideal circumstances, the caregiver is the best ally of the practitioner: In addition to providing a reliable presence in case of emergency, assuring timely medical attention to the older patient, the caregiver may act as the spokesperson for the family, and may be invaluable to mediate the conflicts that often occur within an extended family. It behooves the practitioner, therefore, to help in the selection of the caregiver, to counsel and to support the caregiver.

In the majority of cases, the caregiver of an older person is a spouse with health problem of his/her own, or an adult child, more often a daughter, who needs to reconcile the demands of her own family and of her job, with those of a sick parent.

Cancer treatment of the older person should include:

- Assessment of the pool of potential caregivers
- Choice of the person who appear better suited for the role
- Training and support of this person, to avoid burn out, depression and discouragement, that are common complications of caregiving

CONCLUSIONS

The management of cancer in the older aged person is becoming the most common condition faced by the practitioner of oncology, especially the medical oncologist. As a person's functional reserve declines progressively with age, timely and effective support treatment is essential to the well-being of this person, to the prevention of functional dependence, and to the administration of chemotherapy in adequate doses.

The NCCN guidelines (Table 3) recommend the most important provision for minimizing the complications of chemotherapy.

In addition, proper management of pain, prevention, and management of delirium and of malnutrition and provision of effective caregiving are essential to the management of older cancer patients.

REFERENCES

1. Balducci L, Aapro M: Epidemiology of cancer and aging. Cancer Treat Res 2005, 1–16
2. Lipsitz LA: Physiological complexity, aging, and the path to frailty. Sci Aging Knowledge Environ 2004, 2004(16):pe16
3. Walston A, Headley EC, Ferrucci L, et al: Research agenda for frailty in older adults: Toward a better understanding of physiology and etiology: Summary from the American Geriatrics Society/National Institute on Aging Research Conference on Frailty in Older Adults. J Am Geriatr Soc 2006, 54(6):991–1001
4. Ferrucci L, Corsi A, Lauretani F, Bandinelli S, Bartali B, Taub DD, Guralnik JM, Longo DL: The origin of age-related proinflammatory state. Blood 2005, 105(6):2294–2299
5. Cohen HJ, Harris T, Pieper CF: Coagulation and activation of inflammatory pathways in the development of functional decline and mortality in the elderly. Am J Med 2003, 114:180–187
6. Wilson CJ, Finch CE, Cohen HJ: Cytokines and cognition: The case for head to toe inflammatory paradigm. J Am Ger Soc 2002, 50:2041–2056
7. Hamerman D: Frailty, cancer cachexia and near death. In Balducci L,Lyman GH, Ershler WB, Extermann M: Comprehensive Geriatric Oncology, 2004, Taylor and Francis, London, pp. 236–249
8. Maggio, Cappola AR, Ceda GP, et al: The hormonal pathway to frailty in older men. J Endocrinol Invest 2005, 28(11 Suppl Proceedings):15–19
9. Duthie E: Physiology of aging: relevance to symptom perception and treatment tolerance. In: Balducci L, Lyman GH, Ershler WB, Extermann M: Comprehensive Geriatric Oncology, 2004, Taylor and Francis, London, pp. 207–222
10. Ferrucci L, Maggio M, Brandinelli S, et al: Low testosterone levels and risk of anemia in older men and women. Arch Intern Med 2006, 166:1380–1388
11. Effros R: Proliferative senescence of lymphoid cells and aging. In Balducci L, Ershler WB, DeGaetano G: Blood Disorders in the Elderly. Cambridge University Press, Cambridge, 84–94, 2008
12. Ble A, Fink J, Woodman R, et al: Renal function, erythropoietin and anemia of older persons: The In Chianti study. Arch Intern Med, 2005, 165, 2222–2227
13. Balducci L, Hardy CL: Hemopoietics tree and aging. In: Balducci L, Ershler WB, DeGaetano G: Blood Disorders in the Elderly. Cambridge University Press, 120–128, 2008
14. Carreca I, Balducci L, Extermann M: Cancer chemotherapy in the older patient. Cancer Treat Rev 2005, 31:380–402
15. Hoquet O, Le QH, Mollet I, et al: Subclinical late cardiomyopathy after doxorubicin therapy for lymphoma in adults. J Clin Oncol 2004, 22(10):1864–1871
16. Swain SM, Whaley FS, Ewer MS: Congestive heart failure in patients treated with doxorubicin: A retrospective analysis of three trials. Cancer 2003, 97(11):2869–2879
17. Doyle JJ, Neugut AI, Jacobson AS, et al: Chemotherapy and cardiotoxicity in older breast cancer patients: A population-based study. J Clin Oncol 2005, 23(34):8597–8605
18. Meyerhardt JA, Catalano PJ, Heller DG, et al: Impact of diabetes mellitus on outcomes in patients with colon cancer. J Clin Oncol 2003, 21(3):433–440
19. Ershler WB: Tumors and aging: The influence of age-associated immune changes upon tumor growth and spread. Adv Exp Med Biol 1993, 330:77–92
20. Lee SJ, Lindquist K, Segal MR, et al: Development and validation of a prognostic index for 4-year mortality in older adults. J Am Med Assoc 2006, 295(7):801–808. Erratum in: J Am Med Assoc 2006, 295(16):1900
21. Mitnitski AB, Song X, Rockwood K: The estimate of relative fitness and frailty in community dwelling older adults using self-report data. J Gerontol A Med Sci 2004, 59:M627–M632
22. Fried LP, Tangen CM, Walston J, et al: Frailty in older adults: Evidence for a phenotype. J Gerontol Med Sci 2001, 56A:M146–M156
23. Higashi T, Shekelle PJ, Adams JL, et al: Quality of care is associated with survival in vulnerable older patients. Ann Intern Med 2005, 143(4):274–281
24. Balducci L, Cohen HJ, Engstrom PF, et al: Senior adult oncology clinical practice guidelines in oncology. J Natl Compr Canc Netw 2005, 3(4):572–590
25. Lyman GH, Dale DC, Friedberg J, et al: Incidence and predictors of low chemotherapy dose-intensity in aggressive non-Hodgkin's lymphoma: A nationwide study. J Clin Oncol 2004, 22(21):4302–4311
26. Chrischilles E, Delgado DI, Stolshek BS, et al: Impact of age and colony stimulating factor use in hospital length of stay for febbrile neutropenia in CHOP treated non-Hodgkin's lymphoma patients. Cancer Control 2002, 9:203–211
27. Morrison VA, Picozzi V, Scotti S, et al: The impact of age on delivered dose-intensity and hospitalizations for febrile neutropenia in patients with intermediate – grade non-Hodgkin's Lymphoma receiving initial CHOP chemotherapy: A risk factor analysis. Clin Lymphoma, 2001, 2:47–56

28. Kim YJ, Rubenstein EB, Rolston KV, et al: Colony-stimulating factors (CSFs) may reduce complications and death in solid tumor patients with fever and neutropenia. Proc ASCO, 2000, 19:612a, abstr 2411

29. Crivellari D, Bonetti M, Castiglione-Gertsch M, et al: Burdens and benefits of adjuvant cyclophosphamide, methotrexate and fluorouracil and tamoxifen for elderly patients with breast cancer: The international Breast cancer Study Group Trial vii. J Clin Oncol 2000, 18(7):1412–1422

30. Kuderer NM, Dale DC, Crawford J, et al: Mortality, morbidity, and cost associated with febrile neutropenia in adult cancer patients. Cancer 2006, 106(10):2258–2266

31. Lyman GH, Dale DC, Crawford J: Incidence and predictors of low dose-intensity in adjuvant breast cancer chemotherapy: A nationwide study of community practices. J Clin Oncol 2003, 21(24):4524–4531

32. Gafter-Gvili A, Fraser A, Paul M, et al: Meta-analysis: Antibiotic prophylaxis reduces mortality in neutropenic patients. Ann Intern Med 2005, 142(12 Pt 1):979–995

33. Bucaneve G, Micozzi A, Menichetti F, et al, the Gruppo Italiano Malattie Ematologiche dell'Adulto (GIMEMA) Infection Program: Levofloxocin to prevent bacterial infections in patients with cancer and neutropenia. N Engl J Med 2005, 353:977–987

34. Cullen M, Steven N, Billingham L, et al., the Simple Investigation in Neutropenic Individuals of the Frequency of Infection after Chemotherapy +/– Antibiotic in a Number of Tumours (SIGNIFICANT) Trial Group: Antibiotic prophylaxis after chemotherapy for solid tumors and lymphoma. N Engl J Med 2005, 353:988–998

35. Timmer-Bonte JN, de Boo TM, Smit AJ, et al: Prevention of chemotherapy-induced febrile neutropenia by prophylactic antibiotics plus or minus granulocyte colony-stimulating factor in small-cell lung cancer: A Dutch Randomized Phase III Study J Clin Oncol 2005, 23(31):7974–7984

36. Zinzani PG, Storti S, Zaccaria A, et al: Elderly aggressive histology Non-Hodgkin's Lymphoma: First Line VNCOP-B Regimen: Experience on 350 patients. Blood 1999, 94:33–38

37. Sonneveld P, de Ridder M, van der Lelie H, et al: Comparison of doxorubicin and mitoxantrone in the treatment of elderly patients with advanced diffuse non-Hodgkin's lymphoma using CHOP vs CNOP chemotherapy. J Clin Oncol 1995, 13:2530–2539

38. Osby E, Hagberg H, Kvaloy S, et al: CHOP is superior to CNOP in elderly patients with aggressive lymphoma while outcome is unaffected by filgrastim treatment: Results of a Nordic Lymphoma Group randomized trial. Blood 2003, 101:3840–3848

39. Doorduijn JK, van derr Holt B, van der hem KG, et al: CHOP compared with CHOP plus granulocyte colony-stimulating factor in elderly patients with aggressive non-Hodgkin's lymphoma. J Clin Oncol 2003, 21(16):3041–3050

40. Balducci L, Tam J, Al-Halawani H, et al: A large study of the older cancer patient in the community setting: Initial report of a randomized controlled trial using pegfilgrastim to reduce neutropenic complications. ASCO Meeting Abstracts Jun 1 2005: 8111

41. Smith TJ, Katcheressian J, Liman GH, et al: 2006 Update of recommendations for the use of white blood cell growth factors: An evidence-based clinical practice guideline. J Clin Oncol 2006, 24(19):3187–3205

42. Repettol L, Biganzoli L, Koehne CH, et al: EORTC Cancer in the Elderly Task Force guidelines for the use of colony-stimulating factors in elderly patients with cancer. Eur J Cancer 2003, 39(16):2264–2272. Review

43. Balducci L: Anemia and aging or anemia of aging? Cancer Treat Res, In press

44. Balducci L: Anemia, cancer and aging. Oncology, In press

45. Stabler S: B 12 deficiency. In: Balducci L, Ershler WB, DeGaetano G: Blood Disorders in the Elderly. Cambridge University Press, 181–191, 2008 21–38

46. Ferrucci L, Guralnik L, Woodman RC, et al: Proinflammatory state and circulating erythropoietin in persons with and without anemia. Am J Med 2005, 118:1288–1296B

47. Ershler WB: The pathogenesis of late age anemia. In: Balducci L, Ershler WB, DeGaetano G: Blood Disorders in the Elderly. Cambridge University Press, 203–213, 2008

48. Ganz T: Regulation of iron metabolism. In: Balducci L, Ershler WB, DeGaetano G: Blood Disorders in the Elderly. Cambridge University Press, 2006, 171–180, 2008

49. Extermann M, Chen A, Cantor AB, Corcoran MB, Meyer J, Grendys E, Cavanaugh D, Antonek S, Camarata A, Haley WE, Balducci L: Predictors of tolerance from chemotherapy in older patients: A prospective pilot study. Eur J Cancer 2002, 38(11):1466–1473

50. Schrijvers D, Highley M, DeBruyn E, Van Oosterom AT, Vermorken JB: Role of red blood cell in pharma-cokinetics of chemotherapeutic agents. Anticancer Drugs 1999, 10:147–153

51. Ratain MJ, Schilsky RL, Choi KE, et al. Adaptive control of etoposide administration: Impact of interpatient pharmacodynamic variability. Clin Pharmacol Ther 1989, 45:226–233

52. Silber JH, Fridman M, Di Paola RS, et al. First-cycle blood counts and subsequent neutropenia, dose reduction or delay in early stage breast cancer therapy. J Clin Oncol 1998, 16:2392–2400

53. Wolff D, Culakova E, Poniewierski MS, et al: Predictors of chemotherapy-induced neutropenia and its complications: Results from a propsective nationwide Registry. J Support Oncol 2005, 3(6 supp 4):24–25

54. Penninx BW, Pahor M, Cesari M, et al: Anemia is associated with disability and decreased physical performance and muscle strength in the elderly. J Am Geriatr Soc 2004, 52:719–724
55. Penninx BW, Pluijm SM, Lips P, et al: Late life anemia is associated with increased risk of recurrent falls. J Am Geriatr Soc 2005, 53:2106–2111
56. Curt GA, Breitbart W, Cella D, et al: Impact of cancer-related fatigue on the lives of patients: New findings from the fatigue coalition. Oncologist 2000, 5(5):353–360
57. Heiss MM, Mempel W, Delanoff C, Jauch KW, Gabka C, Mempel M, Dieterich HJ, Eissner HJ, Schildberg FW. Blood transfusion-modulated tumor recurrence: First results of a randomized study of autologous versus allogeneic blood transfusion in colorectal cancer surgery. J Clin Oncol 1994, 12(9):1859–1867
58. Stasi R, Amadori S, Littlewood TJ, et al: Management of cancer-related anemia with erythropoietic agents: Doubts, certainties, and concerns. Oncologist, 2005, 10:539–554
59. Balducal Clinical consequences of anemia in the older person. In: Balducci L, Ershler WB, DeGaetano G: Blood Disorders in the Elderly. Cambridge University Press, 192–202, 2008
60. Bohlius J, Langersiepen S, Schwarzer G, et al: Recombinant human erythropoietins and cancer patients: Updated meta-analysis of 57 studies including 9353 patients. J Natl Cancer Inst 2006, 98(10):708–714
61. Henke M, Laszig R, Rube C, et al. Erythropoietin to treat head and neck cancer in patients with anaemia undergoing radiotherapy: Randomized, double-blind, placebo-controlled trial. Lancet 2003, 362:1255–1260
62. Leyland-Jones B. Breast cancer trial with erythropoietin terminated unexpectedly. Lancet Oncol 2003, 4:459–469
63. Henke M, Mattern D, Pepe M, et al: Do erythropoietin receptors on cancer cells explain unexpected clinical findings? J Clin Oncol 2006, 24(29):4708–4713
64. Boccia R, Malik AI, Raja V, et al: Darbepoetin alfa administered every three weeks is effective for the treatment of chemotherapy-induced anemia. Oncologist 2006, 11(4):409–417
65. Auerbach M, Ballard H, Trout JR, et al: Intravenous iron optimizes the response to recombinant human erythropoietin in cancer patients with chemotherapy-related anemia: A multicenter, open-label, randomized trial. J Clin Oncol 2004, 22:1301–1307
66. Jacobson SD, Cha S, Sargent DJ, et al: Tolerability, dose intensity and benefit of 5FU based chemotherapy for advanced colorectal cancer (CRC) in the elderly. A North Central Cancer Treatment Group Study. Proc Am Soc Clin Oncol 2001, 20:384a, abstr. 1534
67. Bijleven L, Sonis S: Palifermin (recombinant keratinocyte growth factor-1): A pleiotropic growth factor with multiple biological activities in preventing chemotherapy- and radiotherapy-induced mucositis. Ann Oncol 2006, 18(5):817–826
68. Hortobagy GN: Anthracyclines in the treatment of cancer. An overview. Drugs. 1997, 54(Suppl 4):1–7
69. Cvektovik RS, Scott LJ: Dexrazoxane: A review of its use for cardioprotection during anthracycline chemotherapy. Drugs 2005, 65(7):1005–1024
70. Ewer MS, Martin FJ, Henderson C, et al: Cardiac safety of liposomal anthracyclines. Semin Oncol 2004, 31(6 Suppl 13):161–181
71. Keating ML, O'malley AJ, Smith MR: Diabetes and cardiovascular disease during androgen deprivation therapy for prostate cancer. J Clin Oncol 2006, 24(27):4448–4456
72. Shainian VB, Kuo YF, Freeman JL, et al: Risk of fracture after androgen deprivation for prostate cancer. N Engl J Med 2005, 352(2):154–164
73. Smith MR: Bisphosphonates to prevent osteoporosis in men receiving androgen deprivation therapy for prostate cancer. Drugs Aging 2003, 20(3):175–183
74. Higano C: Androgen deprivation therapy: Monitoring and managing the complications. Hematol Oncol Clin North Am 2006, 20(4):909–923
75. Hirbe A, Morgan EA, Uluckan O: Skeletal complications of breast cancer therapies. Clin Cancer Res 2006, 12(20):6309s–6314s
76. Reiner A, Lacasse C: Symptom correlates in the gero-oncology population. Semin Oncol Nurs 2006, 22(1):20–30
77. Balducci L: Management of cancer pain in geriatric patients. J Support Oncol 2003, 1(3):175–191
78. Anonymous: Management of cancer pain in older patients. AGS Clinical Practice Committee. J Am Geriatr Soc 1997, 45(10):1273–1276
79. Stolee LM, Hillier: Instruments for the assessment of pain in older persons with cognitive impairment. J Am Geriatr Soc 2005, 53(2):319–326
80. Wilder-Smith OH: Opioid use in the elderly. Eur J Pain 2005, 9(2):137–140
81. Inouye SK: Delirium in older persons. N Engl J Med 2006, 354(11):1157–1165
82. McKusker J, Cole M, Dendukuri N, et al: The course of delirium in older medical inpatients: A prospective study. J Gen Intern Med 2003, 18(9):696–704
83. Lacasse H, Perrault MM, Willamson DR: Systematic review of antipsychotics for the treatment of hospital-associated delirium in medically or surgically ill patients. Ann Pharmacother 2006, 40(11): 1966–1973

84. Inouye SK, Zhang Y, Han L, et al: Recoverable cognitive dysfunction at hospital admission in older persons during acute illness. J Gen Intern Med 2006, 21(12): 1276–1281

85. McAway GJ, Van Ness TH, Bogardus PH, et al: Older adults discharged from the hospital with delirium: 1-year outcomes. J Am Geriatr Soc 2006, 54(8):1245–1250

86. Extermann M, Overcash J, Lyman GH, et al: Comorbidity and functional status are independent in older cancer patients. J Clin Oncol 1998, 16:1582–1587

87. Melton LJ, khosla S, Crowson CS, et al: Epidemiology of sarcopenia. J Am Ger Soc 2000, 48:625–630

88. Fisher A: Of worms and women. Sarcopenia and its role in disability and mortality. J Am Ger Soc 2004, 52:1185–1190

89. Guigoz Y, Vellas B, Garry PJ: Mininutritional assessment: A practical assessment tool for grading the nutritional state of elderly patients. In: Facts, Research, Interventions in Geriatrics, 1997, Serdi, New York, pp. 15–60

90. Weitzner MA, Haley WE, Chen H: The family caregiver of the older cancer patient. Hematol Oncol Clin 2000, 14:269–282

91. Haley WH, Burton AM, LaMonda LA: Family caregiving issues for older cancer patients. In Balducci L, Lyman GH, Ershler WB, Extermann M: Comprehensive Geriatric Oncology, 2004, Taylor and Francis, London, pp. 843–852

15 Integrative Oncology: Complementary Therapies in Cancer Care

Barrie Cassileth and Jyothirmai Gubili

CONTENTS

ABSTRACT

Many cancer patients experience both physical and emotional symptoms associated with cancer and cancer treatments. Complementary therapies are gentle, noninvasive techniques that alleviate symptoms. They are offered along with conventional care to improve quality of life. Alternative therapies, on the other hand, are unproved and potentially harmful. They are administered in lieu of mainstream treatment and should be avoided. Healthcare professionals and patients should be aware of this distinction.

Key Words: Cancer care, Complementary therapies, Acupuncture, Massage, Mind–body therapies.

INTRODUCTION

An increasing number of cancer patients seek treatments outside of conventional care to ease symptoms associated with cancer and cancer treatments. These modalities are generally defined under the heading, "Complementary and Alternative Medicine" (CAM) (Table 1). However, differences between complementary and alternative therapies are profound and essential to recognize. "Alternative" therapies include those offered in lieu of mainstream treatment. Typically these are invasive, expensive, and potentially harmful directly via physiologic effects or indirectly when patients delay or forego needed conventional treatment. Patients, who have lost hope or grown skeptical

From: *Cancer and Drug Discovery Development: Supportive Care in Cancer Therapy*
DOI: 10.1007/978-1-59745-291-5_15, Edited by: D. S. Ettinger © Humana Press, Totowa, NJ

Table 1
Reliable sources of information on complementary and alternative medicine

Medline Plus: http://www.nlm.nih.gov/medlineplus/druginformation.html
British Medical Journal: http://www.biomedcentral.com/bmccomplementalternmed/
Memorial Sloan-Kettering Cancer Center: http://www.mskcc.org/aboutherbs
National Center for Complementary and Alternative Medicine (NCCAM): http://nccam.nih.gov
American Cancer Society: http://www.cancer.org/docroot/ETO/ETO_5.asp
NIH Office of Dietary Supplements: http://dietary-supplements.info.nih.gov
US Pharmacopeia: http://www.usp.org/dietarySupplements

of mainstream medical care, are especially vulnerable to claims made for alternative therapies, when approaches are promoted as viable treatment options or even cures for advanced disease. Such "alternative" approaches, often associated with anecdotal reports, are not backed by scientific evidence and should be avoided.

Complementary therapies, conversely, are gentle, noninvasive, and used in conjunction with mainstream care. They control physical as well as emotional symptoms, and enhance patients' sense of physical and mental well-being. Complementary modalities include massage and other touch therapies, acupuncture, music therapy, relaxation and other mind–body approaches, fitness, nutritional guidance, and more. They are supported by evidence, although the strength of the evidence varies, and they have a favorable risk/benefit ratio. Their value lies not only in their effectiveness in providing symptom relief, but also in the fact that they are pleasant, noninvasive interventions among which patients can select according to their preference and use to help manage their own clinical care.

Although the origin of some complementary interventions predates the advent of modern biomedicine, most were incorporated into mainstream medical care only recently. They are important tools in the supportive care armamentarium.

PATIENTS' USE OF COMPLEMENTARY AND ALTERNATIVE THERAPIES

A survey of 604 cancer patients showed that 54% had initiated one or more forms of CAM, and a majority (86%) expressed satisfaction with the therapy they selected. Most patients cited the desire to improve general health as the reason for CAM use following cancer diagnosis and during treatment *(1)*. Across surveys, the most popular complementary therapies are herbs and other dietary supplements. Another consistent finding in virtually all patient surveys internationally is that users typically are young, better educated, and more affluent, a function of these patients' desire and ability to play an active role in their own care. Studies also show substantial use of herbs and other remedies self-sought by families of pediatric cancer patients *(2)*.

This chapter presents a review of complementary therapies, including acupuncture, massage, music, and mind–body approaches that are useful adjuncts in symptom management and that can contribute to pharmacologic and related technologies in the supportive care of cancer patients.

Acupuncture

Acupuncture is an intrinsic component of traditional Chinese medicine theory, which is based on the ancient theory of balance between yin and yang and the flow of Qi (energy) along hypothesized channels (meridians) in the body. Acupuncture points are located at specific points along the channels. The flow of Qi, and therefore health, was thought to be regulated by the needling of these points. Heat, pressure, and electrical stimulation are also used along with needling to achieve greater therapeutic effect.

Although the anatomic structures representing meridians remain elusive, some acupuncture points coincide with trigger points that are sensitive to pressure, indicating enriched enervation at the anatomic location. Stimulation of certain acupuncture points produces measurable physiologic change as demonstrated by functional magnetic resonance imaging (fMRI) as, for example, in a study of acupuncture for chronic pain *(3)*.

A 1997 NIH Consensus Conference concluded that acupuncture has a legitimate, useful role in the management of a number of symptoms, including nausea and vomiting. In the decade since that Conference, numerous methodologically sound studies have provided additional supporting data as well as efforts to understand the scientific mechanisms by which acupuncture achieves its results *(4)*.

In a randomized controlled study, 104 breast cancer patients receiving highly emetogenic chemotherapy received electroacupuncture at the PC6 acupuncture point, minimal needling at nonacupuncture points, or pharmacotherapy alone. Electroacupuncture significantly reduced the number of episodes of total emesis when compared with pharmacotherapy only *(5)*.

A systematic review of 11 clinical trials including 1,247 cancer patients revealed that acupuncture-point stimulation reduced the incidence of acute vomiting in the treatment group compared to the control group *(6)*. Preliminary results from another crossover study showed that when administered along with standard antiemetics, acupuncture reduced the need for additional antiemetic medication in pediatric cancer patients *(7)*.

Postchemotherapy fatigue has few reliable treatments in patients without a correctable cause such as anemia. It can be a major contributing factor in lowering the quality of life in palliative care patients. In an uncontrolled trial of fatigue after chemotherapy, acupuncture reduced fatigue 31% after 6 weeks of treatment. Among those with severe fatigue at baseline, 79% had nonsevere fatigue scores at follow-up *(8)*, whereas fatigue was reduced only in 24% of patients receiving usual care in another center *(9)*.

Acupuncture also appears to be effective in the treatment of xerostomia caused by salivary gland injury from head and neck radiotherapy. In a study involving 18 patients with head and neck cancer, acupuncture improved Xerostomia Inventory scores *(10)*. Larger, more definitive randomized trials are underway in North America and elsewhere.

Although the mechanism by which acupuncture controls emesis and other symptoms is not fully understood, research on acupuncture for pain has demonstrated the importance of serotonergic pathways. For example, serotonin antagonists and precursors, respectively, block and potentiate acupuncture analgesia in animal models *(11)*. In particular, the 5-HT3-receptor antagonist ICS 205–930 has been shown to block the analgesic effect of electroacupuncture in rabbits *(12)*.

Massage Therapy

Massage involves applying pressure to muscle and connective tissue to reduce pain, relieve tension, and anxiety, and to promote relaxation. Massage therapy may incorporate varying degrees of pressure, depending on the patient's clinical status. It has important emotional and psychological benefits and is used as a complementary adjunct in the treatment of many illnesses. Massage therapy is especially valued by cancer patients.

In a randomized crossover study, 230 cancer patients on chemotherapy received massage therapy, healing touch, or personal visit without therapy. Results showed that both massage therapy and healing touch reduced blood pressure, respiratory rate, and heart rate. Pain, mood disturbance, and fatigue were also decreased *(13)*.

In another study, 42 patients with advanced cancer were randomized to receive weekly massage with lavender oil, massage with inert oil, or no intervention for 4 weeks. Patients in both of the massage groups experienced improvement in sleep and significant reduction in depression scores compared to those in the control group *(14)*. A significant decrease in anxiety and pain following reflexology was observed in a crossover study involving 23 inpatients with breast or lung cancer *(15)*.

Massage has also been shown to be effective in control of nausea. In a randomized, crossover study conducted in Australia, nausea scores decreased by approximately one-third following a single massage, while little or no change occurred in control subjects *(16)*. A randomized trial of 33 patients undergoing autologous bone marrow transplant measured nausea before and after each of three massages or equivalent periods of "quiet time." Post treatment nausea scores were lower in the massage group at a statistically significant level *(17)*.

In the largest study of massage, 1,290 cancer patients were treated over a period of 3 years. Patients reported a 50% reduction in severity of symptoms following massage therapy. Symptoms included pain, fatigue, stress/anxiety, nausea, and depression *(8)*. Patients should be directed to massage therapists who have training or experience working with cancer patients.

Music Therapy

Music can evoke deep seated emotion and a particular type of music may hold special meaning to an individual depending on his/her life experience. Music therapy is provided by professional musicians who are also trained music therapists. They often hold professional degrees in music therapy, and are adept in dealing with the psychosocial as well as clinical issues faced by patients and family members.

Music therapy is particularly effective in the palliative care setting. Formal music therapy programs in palliative medicine exist in many major institutions. Although music therapy extends back to folklore and Greek mythology (Apollo was the god of both music and medicine), it has been studied scientifically only in recent years. Controlled trials indicate that music therapy produces emotional and physiologic benefits, reducing anxiety, stress, depression, and pain.

In the preoperative setting, randomized trials found that music reduced anxiety and its physiologic correlates such as blood pressure, and salivary cortisol, a biochemical marker of stress and anxiety. Music lowered blood pressure and anxiety scores during and after eye surgery *(18)*, and among women undergoing hysterectomies in a randomized, controlled trial *(19)*.

Music therapy was shown to be effective against pain among cancer patients *(20)*. Music also reduced intraoperative analgesic requirements when compared to controls, and patients randomized to a music intervention reported significantly less pain and required less pain medication. In a trial of 500 surgical patients, subjects were randomized to control, recorded music, jaw relaxation or a music/jaw relaxation combination. Music led to significant decreases in both pain intensity and pain-related distress *(21)*. Music also can help reduce depression *(22)*.

In a randomized trial of cancer patients undergoing autologous stem cell transplantation, anxiety, depression, and total mood disturbance scores were significantly lower in the music therapy group as compared with standard care controls *(23)*.

Mind–Body Therapies

Cognitive behavior therapy, biofeedback, guided imagery, hypnosis, meditation, and relaxation approaches comprise mind–body therapies, and all have a role in supportive cancer care.

Relaxation training involving progressive muscle relaxation has been studied in randomized controlled trials, which demonstrate that it significantly ameliorates anxiety and distress and is particularly effective when combined with imagery. A randomized study of relaxation therapy vs. alprazolam showed that both significantly decreased anxiety and depression, although the effect of alprazolam was slightly faster in anxiety and stronger on depressive symptoms.

A randomized trial of 82 radiation therapy patients found significant reduction in tension, depression, anger, and fatigue in those who received relaxation training or imagery *(24)*.

Hypnosis is a state of focused attention or altered consciousness in which distractions are blocked, allowing a person to concentrate intently on a particular subject, memory, sensation, or problem. It helps people relax and become receptive to suggestion. The suggestion, geared to affect the desired results, may come from the patient or the practitioner. Hypnosis has been studied extensively and found effective for a wide range of symptoms, including acute and chronic pain, panic, phobias, pediatric emergencies, surgery, burns, posttraumatic stress disorder (PTSD), irritable bowel syndrome (IBS), allergies, certain skin conditions, and unwanted habit control.

In a procedural study, 30 patients scheduled for interventional radiology procedure randomized to hypnosis or standard care. Subjects in the hypnosis group reported less pain and exhibited more stable oxygen saturation and hemodynamics *(25)*.

Recent perioperative trials demonstrate broad benefits from adjunctive hypnosis, including reduced presurgical and postsurgical anxiety and depression, fewer postsurgery complications, more stable vital signs perioperatively, faster healing, less postoperative pain medication use, and increased patient and surgeon satisfaction with the procedures.

Hypnosis also can control nausea and vomiting. A randomized controlled trial of 50 breast surgery patients assessed the ability of presurgical hypnosis to control nausea and vomiting. Results showed that patients in the hypnosis group experienced 29% less vomiting compared to the standard-care control group *(4)*. Hypnosis was also shown effective in children. Fifty-four pediatric cancer patients were randomly assigned to hypnosis, nonhypnotic distraction and relaxation, or attention control. Children in the hypnosis group reported the greatest reduction in anticipatory and postchemotherapy nausea and vomiting *(26)*.

Guided imagery may be considered a lighter form of hypnosis and is based on the reciprocal relationship between mind and body. It is another simple and powerful technique that directs imagination and attention in ways that produce symptom relief. Often termed "visualization" or "mental imagery," guided imagery lowers blood pressure and produces other physiologic benefits, including decreased heart rate. Imagery also can relieve pain and anxiety. A study of 96 women with locally advanced breast cancer compared standard treatment with relaxation training and imagery during chemotherapy. Women in the experimental group reported increased relaxation and better quality of life *(27)*. Similarly, guided imagery increased patient comfort in a randomized trial of 53 breast cancer patients receiving radiation therapy *(28)*. A review of 67 published studies indicates that relaxation, imagery, and suggestion impact cancer-related pain *(29)*.

Guided imagery also may be effective in controlling nausea, which is commonly experienced by cancer patients. In a study of 110 breast cancer patients undergoing autologous bone marrow transplantation, patients were randomized to standard care vs. education, cognitive restructuring, and relaxation with guided imagery. The experimental group experienced significantly reduced nausea and anxiety *(30)*.

The role of meditation in health care has been studied scientifically in the West throughout the last two decades. Its value in the management of physiologic symptoms such as chronic pain, hypertension, and symptoms associated with heart disease and cancer is well documented. Regular meditation also decreases generalized anxiety, wards off bouts of chronic depression, and enables patients to cope more effectively. A meta-analysis of 59 studies showed improved sleep induction and maintenance with psychological interventions, including meditation, biofeedback, and muscle relaxation *(31)*.

Yoga, a 5,000-year-old exercise regimen developed in India, also involves proper breathing, movement, and posture. Research documents its value in improving physical fitness and decreasing respiratory rate and blood pressure; yoga is often part of integrative management for heart disease, asthma, diabetes, drug addiction, acquired immunodeficiency syndrome (AIDS), migraine headaches, and arthritis, as well as cancer.

A randomized clinical trial of 39 lymphoma patients evaluated the effectiveness of Tibetan yoga, which incorporates controlled breathing, visualization, mindfulness, and low-impact postures. Patients under treatment or who had concluded treatment in the prior 12 months participated in seven weekly sessions. Researchers concluded that the yoga program significantly improved sleep-related outcomes, including better quality, longer duration, and decreased use of sleep medications *(32)*.

In another study, 59 breast cancer patients and 10 prostate cancer patients participated in an 8-week mindfulness-based stress reduction (MBSR) program that incorporated yoga as well as relaxation and meditation. Patients were assessed before and after the intervention. The MBSR program significantly enhanced patients' quality of life and decreased symptoms of stress *(33)*.

Herbal Supplements

Medicinal herbal agents, also termed phytomedicinals, are made from the whole plant or its leaves, stems, flowers, seeds, and/or roots. Herbal supplements may consist of a single herb or a combination of several, as used in traditional Chinese medicine and Ayurvedic medicine from India. Plants have been used as medicine since ancient times by all cultures worldwide. According to the World Health Organization, 80% of the world's population continues to use botanicals as the primary source of medicine today.

Many cancer patients use herbal supplements as an adjunct to chemotherapy or other cancer treatment to alleviate symptoms. They are typically considered to be "natural" and "safe" compared to invasive treatments with serious side effects. However, studies indicate that the misuse of herbs can be detrimental. For example, herbs such as ginger, ginseng, garlic, and ginkgo may cause postoperative hemorrhage because they have antiplatelet effects. Botanicals such as red clover and soy are known to have mild estrogenic effects *(34, 35)* and may stimulate the growth of hormone sensitive cancers.

Until more evidence is obtained from clinical trials, cancer patients should use caution before using herbal supplements. They should also be advised that herbal supplements are not viable substitutes for mainstream cancer treatment. Patients should consult their oncologists or pharmacists about potential supplement–drug interactions during cancer treatment.

CONCLUSION

Symptom control during and after cancer treatments remains a challenge for many physicians and their patients. Many cancer patients are interested in complementary and alternative therapies, which have variable benefit and risk ratios. Alternative therapies are unproved or disproved and potentially harmful.

Complementary therapies, on the other hand, are noninvasive, gentle techniques that help to manage symptoms and improve quality of life. Even though many of these therapies have been in use for centuries around the world, scientific examination of complementary therapies started only in the past few decades. Much of the data from research to date supports the use of acupuncture, music, massage, mind–body therapies for both physical and emotional symptoms. These are especially valuable for cancer patients and are being provided along with conventional care in many cancer hospitals and programs around the world.

REFERENCES

1. Vapiwala N, Mick R, Hampshire MK, Metz JM, DeNittis AS. Patient initiation of complementary and alternative medical therapies (CAM) following cancer diagnosis. Cancer J 2006;12(6):467–74
2. Kelly KM. Complementary and alternative medicines for use in supportive care in pediatric cancer. Support Care Cancer 2007; 15(4):457–60
3. Napadow V, Kettner N, Liu J, et al. Hypothalamus and amygdala response to acupuncture stimuli in carpal tunnel syndrome. Pain 2007; 130(3):254–266
4. Enqvist B, Bjorklund C, Engman M, Jakobsson J. Preoperative hypnosis reduces postoperative vomiting after surgery of the breasts. A prospective, randomized and blinded study. Acta Anaesthesiol Scand 1997; 41(8):1028–32
5. Shen J, Wenger N, Glaspy J, et al. Electroacupuncture for control of myeloablative chemotherapy-induced emesis: A randomized controlled trial. J Am Med Assoc 2000; 284(21):2755–61

6. Ezzo JM, Richardson MA, Vickers A, et al. Acupuncture-point stimulation for chemotherapy-induced nausea or vomiting. Cochrane Database Syst Rev 2006; (2):CD002285.

7. Reindl TK, Geilen W, Hartmann R, et al. Acupuncture against chemotherapy-induced nausea and vomiting in pediatric oncology. Interim results of a multicenter crossover study. Support Care Cancer 2006;14(2):172–6

8. Cassileth BR, Vickers AJ. Massage therapy for symptom control: Outcome study at a major cancer center. J Pain Symptom Manage 2004; 28(3):244–9

9. Escalante CP, Grover T, Johnson BA, et al. A fatigue clinic in a comprehensive cancer center: Design and experiences. Cancer 2001; 92(6 Suppl):1708–13

10. Johnstone PA, Peng YP, May BC, Inouye WS, Niemtzow RC. Acupuncture for pilocarpine-resistant xerostomia following radiotherapy for head and neck malignancies. Int J Radiat Oncol Biol Phys 2001; 50(2):353–7

11. Cheng RS, Pomeranz B. Monoaminergic mechanism of electroacupuncture analgesia. Brain Res 1981; 215(1–2):77–92

12. Yonehara N. Influence of serotonin receptor antagonists on substance P and serotonin release evoked by tooth pulp stimulation with electro-acupuncture in the trigeminal nucleus cudalis of the rabbit. Neurosci Res 2001; 40(1):45–51

13. Post-White J, Kinney ME, Savik K, Gau JB, Wilcox C, Lerner I. Therapeutic massage and healing touch improve symptoms in cancer. Integr Cancer Ther 2003; 2(4):332–44

14. Soden K, Vincent K, Craske S, Lucas C, Ashley S. A randomized controlled trial of aromatherapy massage in a hospice setting. Palliat Med 2004; 18(2):87–92

15. Stephenson NL, Weinrich SP, Tavakoli AS. The effects of foot reflexology on anxiety and pain in patients with breast and lung cancer. Oncol Nurs Forum 2000; 27(1):67–72

16. Grealish L, Lomasney A, Whiteman B. Foot massage. A nursing intervention to modify the distressing symptoms of pain and nausea in patients hospitalized with cancer. Cancer Nurs 2000; 23(3):237–43

17. Ahles TA, Tope DM, Pinkson B, et al. Massage therapy for patients undergoing autologous bone marrow transplantation. J Pain Symptom Manage 1999; 18(3):157–63

18. Allen K, Golden LH, Izzo JL Jr, et al. Normalization of hypertensive responses during ambulatory surgical stress by perioperative music. Psychosom Med 2001; 63(3):487–92

19. Mullooly VM, Levin RF, Feldman HR. Music for postoperative pain and anxiety. J N Y State Nurses Assoc 1988; 19(3):4–7

20. Beck SL. The therapeutic use of music for cancer-related pain. Oncol Nurs Forum 1991; 18(8):1327–37

21. Good M, Stanton-Hicks M, Grass JA, et al. Relaxation and music to reduce postsurgical pain. J Adv Nurs 2001; 33(2):208–15

22. Hanser SB, Thompson LW. Effects of a music therapy strategy on depressed older adults. J Gerontol 1994; 49(6):P265–9

23. Cassileth BR, Vickers AJ, Magill LA. Music therapy for mood disturbance during hospitalization for autologous stem cell transplantation: A randomized controlled trial. Cancer 2003; 98(12):2723–9

24. Decker TW, Cline-Elsen J, Gallagher M. Relaxation therapy as an adjunct in radiation oncology. J Clin Psychol 1992; 48(3):388–93

25. Lang EV, Joyce JS, Spiegel D, Hamilton D, Lee KK. Self-hypnotic relaxation during interventional radiological procedures: Effects on pain perception and intravenous drug use. Int J Clin Exp Hypn 1996; 44(2):106–19

26. Zeltzer LK, Dolgin MJ, LeBaron S, LeBaron C. A randomized, controlled study of behavioral intervention for chemotherapy distress in children with cancer. Pediatrics 1991; 88(1):34–42

27. Walker LG, Walker MB, Ogston K, et al. Psychological, clinical and pathological effects of relaxation training and guided imagery during primary chemotherapy. Br J Cancer 1999; 80(1–2):262–8

28. Kolcaba K, Fox C. The effects of guided imagery on comfort of women with early stage breast cancer undergoing radiation therapy. Oncol Nurs Forum 1999; 26(1):67–72

29. Mundy EA, DuHamel KN, Montgomery GH. The efficacy of behavioral interventions for cancer treatment-related side effects. Semin Clin Neuropsychiatry 2003; 8(4):253–75

30. Gaston-Johansson F, Fall-Dickson JM, Nanda J, et al. The effectiveness of the comprehensive coping strategy program on clinical outcomes in breast cancer autologous bone marrow transplantation. Cancer Nurs 2000; 23(4):277–85

31. Morin CM, Culbert JP, Schwartz SM. Nonpharmacological interventions for insomnia: A meta-analysis of treatment efficacy. Am J Psychiatry 1994; 151(8):1172–80

32. Cohen L, Warneke C, Fouladi RT, Rodriguez MA, Chaoul-Reich A. Psychological adjustment and sleep quality in a randomized trial of the effects of a Tibetan yoga intervention in patients with lymphoma. Cancer 2004; 100(10):2253–60

33. Carlson LE, Speca M, Patel KD, Goodey E. Mindfulness-based stress reduction in relation to quality of life, mood, symptoms of stress, and immune parameters in breast and prostate cancer outpatients. Psychosom Med 2003; 65(4):571–81

34. Beck V, Unterrieder E, Krenn L, Kubelka W, Jungbauer A. Comparison of hormonal activity (estrogen, androgen and progestin) of standardized plant extracts for large scale use in hormone replacement therapy. J Steroid Biochem Mol Biol 2003; 84(2–3):259–68
35. Hsieh CY, Santell RC, Haslam SZ, Helferich WG. Estrogenic effects of genistein on the growth of estrogen receptor-positive human breast cancer (MCF-7) cells in vitro and in vivo. Cancer Res 1998; 58(17):3833–8

16 End-of-Life Decisions

Sydney Morss Dy

ABSTRACT

Although end-of-life decision making is critical for good oncology care, physicians often do not initiate discussions until the last days of life and do not use good communication skills and evidence-based techniques. Research on deficits in decision making has found that patients often misunderstand information the first time it is provided or may not be ready to hear bad news, and that physicians often omit information about the terminal illness and options other than chemotherapy. Physicians also often fail to use basic communication techniques to elicit and improve understanding. Research supports the effectiveness of a variety of interventions to improve communication and decision making for outcomes such as reducing the use of interventions with a low likelihood of benefit, increasing hospice length of stay, and decreasing families' symptoms of bereavement. The widely used autonomy paradigm of presenting patients with options such as chemotherapy and allowing them to choose may not work well near the end of life. An evidence-based approach based on planning over time, a systematic approach to communication, and eliciting goals and values satisfactory to all involved in the decision-making process may be more appropriate. Using history-taking skills to explore patients' and families' emotion-laden statements about end of life care, and using a differential diagnosis approach when decision making does not occur smoothly or when conflict exists, can also be helpful in challenging situations.

From: *Cancer and Drug Discovery Development: Supportive Care in Cancer Therapy*
DOI: 10.1007/978-1-59745-291-5_16, Edited by: D. S. Ettinger © Humana Press, Totowa, NJ

Key Words: End of life decisions, Hospice, Palliative care, Communication, Autonomy.

To write prescriptions is easy, but to come to an understanding with people is hard.

– Franz Kafka

INTRODUCTION

Communication and decision making are critical to many aspects of quality care for patients with advanced cancer, including choosing between treatments, ensuring that care is consistent with patient preferences, and improving symptom management. However, studies have found that there are wide variations among physicians and hospitals in decision making and care at the end of life. In a national study of highly respected hospitals, the time hospitalized in the last 6 months of life ranged from 9 to 27 days and the percentage of patients dying in the hospital ranged from 16 to 56% *(1)*. In a nationwide survey of end-of-life care for critically ill patients, the proportion of patients who received aggressive treatments such as cardiopulmonary resuscitation and full life support ranged from 0 to 80% among intensive care units *(2)*.

The way that care is provided at the end of life changed somewhat during the 1990s. In one study of two intensive care units, the percentage of patients who had withdrawal of life support before they died increased from 51 to 90%, and resuscitation rates decreased from 49 to 10% *(3)*. Half of cancer patients currently receive hospice care before death, and hospice length of stay for cancer patients has decreased dramatically *(4)*. Although the likelihood of dying in a hospital has decreased somewhat, the proportion of patients who have an intensive care unit admission or undergo an invasive procedure at the end of life has increased *(5)*. Substantial numbers of patients receive chemotherapy near the end of life, with 31% of Medicare beneficiaries receiving treatment in the last 6 months and 23% in the last 3 months of life. Rates of use of chemotherapy for tumors generally responsive (e.g., breast) and unresponsive (e.g., pancreatic) to chemotherapy were the same in this study, suggesting that chemotherapy effectiveness may not have been well accounted for in many decisions *(6)*. The proportion of cancer patients receiving chemotherapy in the last few weeks or months of life also increased during the 1990s *(7)*.

These patterns of care all suggest that decisions about care near the end of life vary substantially and may often be suboptimal. Although many physicians are skilled at shared end-of-life decision making with patients, and many patients and families have excellent experiences, there remains much need for improvement in care and research into better methods of decision making and how best to train physicians and others in end-of-life discussions with patients and families. End-of-life conversations are often challenging due to professionals' and patients' reluctance to discuss painful issues; the difficulty of communicating in situations of strong emotion and deep grief; uncertainty of prognosis; and the time limitations, discontinuity, and complexity inherent in care for patients with serious illness.

The increasing availability of chemotherapy options and technological innovations that have the possibility of extending life only slightly, without necessarily improving function or quality of life, may also be significant barriers to conducting end-of-life discussions. Conflict between healthcare professionals, within families, and between professionals and patients is nearly universal, and often makes decision making difficult if it is not addressed *(8)*. Families often do not communicate about end-of-life issues among themselves, due to the desire to avoid difficult issues or distress and the complexity of the situations they face *(9)*. Avoiding decisions at the end of life may have adverse consequences, not only for patients and families, but also for nurses and other staff, whose morale may suffer from the inability to impact decisions and from providing interventions that they feel are unhelpful or increase patients' suffering. Other patients may also receive less attention because staff are working to provide aggressive care to patients who will not benefit.

Although advance directives are promoted through legislation and regulatory agencies, well-conducted studies have failed to show significant benefits *(10)*. Advance directives may be useful in some situations, but research has demonstrated marked deficiencies as they are used in clinical practice, including low rates of use, potentially incompatible requests for different treatments, terminology that severely limits the circumstances under which directives should apply, and lack of flexibility and real-world clinical relevance *(11)*. Decision making with patients and their families as the situation evolves is therefore critical, and there is much evidence and expert opinion on how to do it well.

This chapter will review both evidence and expert opinion on end-of-life decision making for patients with cancer, focusing on shared decision-making processes between physicians and patients and families. It includes reviews of research on potential deficits in decision-making processes and areas for improvement; the evidence for interventions to improve these decisions; and guidance on approaching these decisions based on the evidence and expert advice. The discussion focuses on general end-of-life decisions in cancer patients, with evidence from other populations where relevant, and includes more detailed information on specific areas, particularly artificial nutrition, the provision of palliative chemotherapy, and hospice.

RESEARCH ON DEFICITS IN END-OF-LIFE DECISION MAKING

Deficits in end-of-life decision making occur for a variety of reasons, including lack of communication and misunderstanding. One study of refractory and recurrent breast cancer patients who were told that chemotherapy was palliative and not curative found that 42% still believed they had a moderately high to high likelihood of cure. Whether differences in understanding of the limits of treatment are due to communication techniques or to patients hearing or believing what they wish to hear, decision making is often difficult when patients and physicians perceive the illness or treatments differently *(12)*.

Communication is often an issue; in one recent survey, 27% of families of patients who died in hospitals reported concerns about the communication that occurred (13). In a study which tape recorded chemotherapy decision making for patients with incurable cancer, a quarter of physicians did not discuss incurability, 43% did not address life expectancy, and more than half did not present an alternative to treatment. Physicians discussed quality of life issues associated with treatment in only a third of the tape recordings, and checked patients' understanding in only 10% *(14)*. In a study of patients who were transferred to intensive care and subsequently died, none had documentation that palliative care had been discussed as an option. In addition, in this as in other studies, most do-not-resuscitate decisions were made within a few days of death *(15)*.

The uncertainty of prognosis, and physicians' and patients' frequent discomfort with discussing it, are also barriers to end-of-life decisions and conversations. Prognosis is usually not a part of the history and physical and is often not considered in decisions about the approach to care and choice of aggressive interventions. There is insufficient science on determining prognosis, although evidence-based clinical recommendations now exist *(16)*, and even when there are good studies, tools for accurate calculation are not readily available. Prognostication includes significant uncertainty even when disease is very advanced or the dying process has begun, and physicians are frequently uncomfortable with the concept of prognostication, with addressing this uncertainty, and with addressing end-of-life issues when prognosis is unclear *(17)*. When physicians do estimate prognosis, they are frequently overoptimistic: A systematic review found overestimation of survival by at least 1 month in 25% of terminally ill cancer patients *(18)*.

Communication about prognosis is also sometimes lacking, which can be a barrier to shared decision making. Patients who do not know about their prognosis cannot participate fully in decision making; the choice for aggressive care is logical if a patient does not know that he likely has only weeks to live. Physicians are sometimes reluctant to share information about prognosis with patients, and may be overoptimistic in their communication about prognosis *(19)*. Patients may also be unwilling to hear about prognosis, although often they also do not ask because they are waiting for the physician to bring up the subject. Research suggests that readiness to hear prognosis may change over time, and current expert opinion advises asking patients and families their opinion on how much information they wish to hear *(17)*.

Physicians are often reluctant to bring up end-of-life issues, but research has found that patients and families often would like and appreciate discussions about difficult issues if done well. A discussion that is upsetting and emotional to professionals and family members, for example, may, if done appropriately and in the right situation, be very valued by a patient because of its honesty, usefulness, and compassion *(20)*. Physicians may avoid these discussions more than patients would wish: in one study, the idea for hospice care was brought up in 49% of situations by the patient or family rather than healthcare providers. Triggers for bringing up hospice were less often concerns about the end of life and more often worries about family needs; 42% were brought on by an increase in home care needs, and 16% by escalating pain and other symptoms *(21)*. In another study, the top-rated items that patients wanted to know about hospice were practical issues, such as payment, frequency of visits, and continuity of care, rather than end-of-life issues such as spirituality and life closure *(22)*. Physicians and patients may have different perceptions of the relative importance of elements of decision making; in another study, patients and families rated coordination of care and provision of information as most important in clinical encounters, while healthcare professionals were more focused on quality of life issues *(23)*.

Research has found that issues related to the provision of artificial nutrition are similar to general end-of -life decision making. Health professionals vary in their attitudes about artificial nutrition, and the benefit–risk ratios that they perceive for patients are often greater than the medical evidence supports. A study using scenarios found that the proportion of seriously ill patients for whom physicians recommended artificial nutrition varied with physicians' experience and beliefs about artificial nutrition *(24)*. Studies have also shown deficits in physician–patient decision making about gastrostomy feeding tube placement, including nurse reports of insufficient time for decision making and care planning, provision of inaccurate information, overuse of jargon, and lack of discussion about prognosis and complications (25, 26). In a study of patients (including those with cancer) or their surrogates, only about half reported receiving the information they wanted about the gastrostomy tube. In open-ended questions, respondents felt that there was not usually much of a decision-making process; the decision to place the feeding tube was made in the setting of emotional distress, was eclipsed by more difficult decisions, and was often seen as the only alternative (26).

INTERVENTIONS TO IMPROVE END-OF-LIFE DECISIONS

Improving end-of-life decision making can lead to improvement in a variety of areas, including the quality of decisions made, use of services, and family bereavement. Studies have addressed decision making and related communication issues, as well as structural changes and interventions to enhance decision making. Relatively simple interventions, such as providing a brochure to families of critically ill patients (27) or providing families with tape recordings of oncology consultations (28), can improve both comprehension of difficult issues and satisfaction. Routine provision of information relevant to decision making to physicians has also improved outcomes in some studies. For example, a randomized clinical trial (RCT) of screening nursing home patients for goals of care and needs for palliative care services and providing this information to the physician found a 30-day hospice referral rate of 20% in the intervention group compared to 1% in the control group. The intervention group also had decreased hospitalizations and improved ratings of end-of-life care (29).

Studies have also shown benefits of providing direct assistance with decision making. A multicenter randomized trial of ethics consultations for patients with value-related treatment conflicts found a significant reduction in intensive care unit length of stay (1.4 fewer days) with consultation compared to usual care, mainly due to less time on ventilators, with no significant increase in in-hospital mortality (30). Restructuring the way care is provided can also be effective. A multicenter RCT in dying intensive care unit patients compared usual care family conferences to conferences structured according to specific, evidence-based guidelines, combined with a brochure about bereavement. The conferences in the intervention group were significantly longer with greater family participation; the intervention patients received fewer nonbeneficial treatments; and at 90 days the intervention families had fewer symptoms of bereavement (e.g, symptoms of anxiety) than the families of patients receiving the usual practice at each center (31).

Increasing the timeliness of decision making can also be effective. A study requiring a multidisciplinary care meeting within 72 h of intensive care admission for all patients with a clinical probability of 50% of surviving the ICU stay, to discuss goals and expectations, clinical milestones, and palliative care options when appropriate, found that the meetings occurred in almost all cases. Median length of stay was reduced by 1 day with no increase in mortality, and the intervention and benefit was maintained for 4 years (32). Improving support to patients may also be effective. A study of interdisciplinary palliative care provided by a hospice team, including support and family conferences, for advanced lung cancer patients from the time of diagnosis demonstrated both increased hospice enrollment and longer hospice length of stay *(33)*. Other types of interventions may also be useful, including more standardization of chemotherapy decisions, do-not-resuscitate protocols, and professional and trainee education, although further research is needed in these areas.

Studies have also shown that interventions can decrease specific treatments sometimes used inappropriately at the end of life, such as artificial nutrition. Successful interventions regarding parenteral nutrition in general hospital populations have included an educational program about criteria for appropriate use, metabolic support service consults, requiring a formal approval process, and implementing a guideline or algorithm *(26)*. A trial of a decision aid for long-term enteral feeding in dementia patients found that surrogates felt that it was helpful by improving knowledge and decreasing uncertainty *(26)*.

DRAWBACKS OF THE CURRENT AUTONOMY PARADIGM

Much decision-making research in patients with life-limiting illness has focused on methods based on the autonomy paradigm, such as advance directives, that do not clearly impact outcomes and do not account for the complexity of palliative care. Focusing on advance care planning creates an illusion that we can make choices about death. In reality, it is often difficult to plan for the specifics of end-of-life care due to uncertainty about prognosis, clinical circumstances, and caregiving. In addition, asking patients and families to participate in end-of-life decision making requires that they accept the terminal prognosis, and promotes the view that this is necessary for good end-of-life care and that those who cannot make this transition, or accept responsibility for end-of-life decisions, are problematic.

The timing of death is often uncertain, and it is often unclear what terminal illness means, or patients are unwilling to accept physicians' views of the situation. The concept of decision making may not make sense when death is inevitable, and assumes that patients and families can accept and consider the possibility of death and make rational choices about relevant care in the setting of profound grief. In addition, the advance directive/do-not-resuscitate literature presupposes that patients and families can understand and make appropriate decisions about specific and complex medical procedures *(34, 35)*. Physicians, patients, and families often simply avoid issues related to death, and end-of-life decision making often does not occur: what happens is the result of a lack of decisions, and patients receive aggressive care because issues are not addressed. When end-of-life decision-making does occur, it may be suboptimal because options related to the concept of death, such as not providing further chemotherapy or opting for hospice care, are avoided by the physician or patient. Current research also has shown that many patients and families would prefer healthcare professionals to provide recommendations, help with decision making, or make the decisions themselves, rather than simply providing options *(36)*.

Following the autonomy paradigm, that patients have the right to whatever chemotherapy they choose, may be flawed because patients often are not told, do not understand, or are not willing to accept their prognosis, the odds of treatment success and the details of what it will entail, or the fact that treatment being offered is palliative. Chemotherapy may be the only option offered to patients, and they may choose it based on emotions or for reasons such as not wanting to give up, not wanting to disappoint the physician or family, uncertainty about another approach, or a (often justified) fear of being abandoned. The physician may find it easier to simply offer chemotherapy than to spend the time discussing why it would not be beneficial.

The complex issues in decision making in life-limiting illness may benefit from an approach different from traditional autonomy-based shared decision making. Rather than focusing on issues of death or dying or making decisions around issues of prognosis or terminal illness, addressing more concrete and easily addressable issues, such as goals of care and values, may both be more effective and be preferred by patients and families *(37)*. Research has found that what many patients with advanced illness value most is not autonomy, but excellent communication and medical care.

EVIDENCE-BASED APPROACH TO DECISION MAKING BASED ON GOALS OF CARE

An approach to decision making based on research and expert opinion involves four key elements: planning over time, a systematic approach, focus on values and goals of care, and using history-taking skills and differential diagnosis to determine how best to address difficult situations. Starting early is critical: When the possibility of bad outcomes has never been addressed, or news has been presented in a positive manner throughout an illness, it is not surprising when families balk at accepting a comfort care approach when this is brought up suddenly a few days before death. Gently talking about planning for the possibility of bad outcomes, in the setting of hoping for the best, and starting discussions early when bad outcomes start to become likely, can be helpful as multiple discussions over time are often necessary. If a family is unaware of the prognosis, or even of the extent of the disease, it may take several discussions before appropriate goals can be addressed.

Planning over time may be helped by identifying potential decision points in advance and directing communication accordingly; for example, if a patient is aware that decisions may be needed after a scan is done, or if they are asked to bring family at that time, they may be more ready for the needed discussions. Patients can also be educated about what signs to look for that may necessitate decisions, such as difficulty tolerating chemotherapy or more trouble with daily activities. Setting expectations appropriately, allowing for or redirecting hope but not encouraging unrealistic beliefs, is also important. It is also helpful to ensure that all staff are communicating consistently, as patients who hear different messages may focus on whatever they hear that is most positive.

The systematic approach includes having a plan and an agenda for each time that important issues are discussed with patients. Ensuring that all information is available, and discussing with other team members if needed, can help make discussions go more smoothly. It also includes using good skills for eliciting information and communication. It is often helpful to start with open-ended questions, such as, "What have you been told about your illness?" and, "How is treatment going for you?" to ensure patients' understanding and allow them to express concerns *(38)*. Allowing patients and families to start gives them control, which is important when they have so little control over their illness, and ensures that physician communication is properly targeted.

When patients share emotions, it is important to respond with validating statements, rather than to change the topic or retreat into technical discussions. Information should be provided simply and clearly, and prefaced when needed by statements making the meaning clear, such as, "I'm afraid I have some bad news." Communication should address what is known, as well as the range of possible outcomes, and acknowledge uncertainty. Assessing for understanding and gentle repetition (often in the next session or by other staff) is important as patients may not hear or understand the first time. Allowing for individual preferences for communication, and individual style, may be very important, as may multidisciplinary involvement to ensure that issues such as caregiving, family relationships and stress, and the care needs of the patient are included in decisions that otherwise may focus on the risks and benefits of technology. It is helpful to encourage talk about difficult topics, by asking questions like, "Do you have any concerns?," as well as to address nonmedical issues, such as caregiving needs.

Rather than focusing on specific treatment options, this approach focuses on eliciting patients' goals, hopes, and values. The goals of current or potential treatments must be clear to the medical team; when things are not going well, or there are concerns about the future, assessing patients' goals may help to align care. Patients' goals may range from trying all possible treatments and clinical trials, to living until a certain event, to staying out of pain and being at home with family. If the patient's goals are oriented toward quality of life, the appropriate treatment options may be clearer. These goals frequently change over time and with the availability of treatment options, and so should be addressed periodically, particularly when the situation changes.

Approaching complex decision-making situations using history-taking skills, by addressing challenging issues as though they were symptoms needing further investigation rather than directly as the patient frames them, may be effective in improving the decision-making process. This is a useful approach for clarifying difficult questions or statements; rather than answering the question, "How long do I have?," with an estimate of prognosis, it may be helpful to ask, "Can you tell me what you mean by that question?" Although some patients may want precise estimates, many others may be asking the question as a way to bring up fears about the future or concerns about their current situation. This may also help with other challenging statements. When a family says, "We believe there will be a miracle," or "He's a fighter," it may help to explore what that means and why they are focusing on that aspect of the situation.

When communication and decision making are not going well, or there is conflict between or among parties, considering a differential diagnosis for difficult discussions may help to resolve the situation, or at least help the staff understand and accept why there is conflict or differing perspectives (39). Misunderstanding or lack of information is common, and it may be helpful to ask again what patients or families have been told. Asking about the underlying reasoning or beliefs behind a decision may allow for specific issues, such as misperceptions about care, to be addressed, or at least for it to make sense to the staff. Patients or families may be in denial, which is often part of the grieving process; listening to and validating emotions may be the best approach in this situation. Finally, families may act out of guilt and grief; this can be addressed by focusing on positive goals oriented toward comfort, or addressing positive issues such as the value of the patient's life or the dedication of the family. Staff should also consider possible reasons for difficult decision making from their perspective, such as difficulties with communication or discussing death, giving conflicting information, or not taking enough time. Other potential issues include viewing the patient's decline as a failure or overemphasis on technology.

CONCLUSION

Decision making at the end of life is an essential part of the continuum of cancer care. Although many professionals have not been trained well in communication, or may avoid decision making at the end of life because of the difficult issues and emotions, good decision making is critical for good outcomes and can be improved by an evidence-based approach including planning over time and communication based on guidelines. Eliciting and clarifying goals should use open-ended questions, such as "What do you think will happen in the future? What are your concerns?" Responses to such questions should be summarized, and appropriate recommendations framed in the context of these goals: "You've said you now want to get as much help for your family as possible. I think hospice may be a good way to help achieve that goal." Finally, discussions should emphasize the positive aspects of what medical care can provide: "I understand that you want to be at home, and with the help of hospice, I believe we'll be able to support you well there." Using this approach may help to make these end-of-life decisions easier and more productive for medical professionals, patients, and families, and increasing the quantity and quality of end-of-life decision making may improve outcomes such as patient and family satisfaction, family bereavement symptoms, appropriate use of interventions, and hospice length of stay.

REFERENCES

1. Wennberg JE, Fisher ES, Stukel TA, Skinner JS, Sharp SM, Bronner KK. Use of hospitals, physician visits, and hospice care during last six months of life among cohorts loyal to highly respected hospitals in the United States. Br Med J 2004; 328:607
2. Prendergast TJ, Claessens MT, Luce JM. A national survey of end-of-life care for critically ill patients. Am J Respir Crit Care Med 1998; 158:1163–7
3. Prendergast TJ, Luce JM. Increasing incidence of withholding and withdrawal of life support from the critically ill. Am J Respir Crit Care Med 1997; 155:15–20
4. Han B, Remsburg RE, McAuley WJ, et al. National trends in adult hospice use: 1991–1992 to 1999–2000. Health Aff 2006; 25:792–9
5. Barnato AE, McClellan MB, Kagay CR, et al. Trends in inpatient treatment intensity among medicare beneficiaries at the end of life. Health Serv Res 2004; 39:363–75
6. Emanuel EJ, Young-Xu Y, Levinsky NG, Gazelle G, Saynina O, Ash AS. Chemotherapy use among medicare beneficiaries at the end of life. Ann Intern Med 2003; 138:639–43
7. Earle CC, Neville BA, Landrum MB, et al. Trends in the aggressiveness of cancer care near the end of life. J Clin Oncol 2004; 22:315–21
8. Breen CM, Abernethy AP, Abbott KH, Tulsky JA. Conflict associated with decisions to limit life-sustaining treatment in intensive care units. J Gen Intern Med 2001; 16:283–9
9. Zhang AY, Siminoff LA. Silence and cancer: Why do families and patients fail to communicate? Health Commun 2003; 15:415–29
10. Lorenz K, Lynn J, Morton S, et al. End-of-Life Care and Outcomes. Agency for Healthcare Research and Quality, Rockville, MD, 2004. Available at www.ahrq.gov
11. Nolan MT. Could lack of clarity in written advance directives contribute to their ineffectiveness? A study of the content of written advance directives. Appl Nurs Res 2003; 16:65–9
12. Doyle C, Crump M, Pintilie M, Oza AM. Does palliative chemotherapy palliate? Evaluation of expectations, outcomes, and costs in women receiving chemotherapy for advanced ovarian cancer. J Clin Oncol 2001; 19:1266–74

13. Teno JM, Clarridge BR, Casey V, et al. Family perspectives on end-of-life care at the last place of care. J Am Med Assoc 2004; 291:88–93

14. Gattellari M, Voigt KJ, Butow PN, Tattersall MH. When the treatment goal is not cure: Are cancer patients equipped to make informed decisions? J Clin Oncol 2002; 20:503–13

15. Rady MY, Johnson DJ. Admission to intensive care unit at the end-of-life: Is it an informed decision? Palliative Med 2004; 18:705–11

16. Maltoni M, Caraceni A, Brunelli C, et al. Prognostic factors in advanced cancer patients: Evidence-based clinical recommendations – a study by the Steering Committee of the European Association for Palliative Care. J Clin Oncol 2005; 23:6240–8

17. Christakis NA. Death Foretold: Prophecy and Prognosis in Medical Care. University of Chicago Press, Chicago, 1999

18. Glare P, Virik K, Jones M, et al. A systematic review of physicians' survival predictions in terminally ill cancer patients. Br Med J 2003; 327:195

19. Lamont EB, Christakis NA. Prognostic disclosure to patients with cancer near the end of life. Ann Intern Med 2001; 134:1096–105

20. Emanuel EJ, Fairclough DL, Wolfe P, Emanuel LL. Talking with terminally ill patients and their caregivers about death, dying, and bereavement: Is it stressful? Is it helpful? Arch Intern Med 2004; 164:1999–2004

21. Casarett D, Crowley R, Stevenson C, Xie S, Teno J. Making difficult decisions about hospice enrollment: What do patients and families want to know? J Am Geriatr Soc 2005; 53:249–54

22. Casarett D, Crowley RL, Hirschman KB. How should clinicians describe hospice to patients and families? J Am Geriatr Soc 2004; 52:1923–28

23. Snyder CF, Dy SM, Hendricks DE, et al. Asking the right questions: Investigating needs assessments and health-related quality-of-life questionnaires for use in oncology clinical practice. Support Care Cancer 2007; 15(9):1075–85

24. Smith DG, Wigton RS. Modeling decisions to use tube feeding in seriously ill patients. Arch Intern Med 1987; 147:1242–5

25. Elasy T, Carey T, Hanson L, et al. Gastrostomy use in the seriously ill. Perspectives of patients, families, physicians, and nurses. J Gen Int Med 1998;13(Suppl):108

26. Dy SM. Enteral and parenteral nutrition in terminally ill cancer patients: A review of the literature. Am J Hosp Palliat Care 2006; 23:369–77

27. Azoulay E, Pochard F, Chevret S, et al. Impact of a family information leaflet on effectiveness of information provided to family members of intensive care unit patients: A multicenter, prospective, randomized, controlled trial. Am J Respir Crit Care Med 2002; 165(4):438–42

28. Scott JT, Harmsen M, Prictor MJ, Entwistle VA, Sowden AJ, Watt I. Recordings or summaries of consultations for people with cancer. Cochrane Database Syst Rev 2003; 2:CD001539

29. Casarett D, Karlawish J, Morales K, Crowley R, Mirsch T, Asch DA. Improving the use of hospice services in nursing homes: a randomized controlled trial. J Am Med Assoc 2005; 294:211–7

30. Schneiderman LJ, Gilmer T, Teetzel HD, et al. Effect of ethics consultations on nonbeneficial life-sustaining treatments in the intensive care setting: A randomized controlled trial. J Am Med Assoc 2003; 290:1166–72

31. Lautrette A, Darmon M, Megarbane B, et al. A communication strategy and brochure for relatives of patients dying in the ICU. N Engl J Med 2007; 356:469–78

32. Lilly CM, De Meo DL, Sonna LA, et al. An intensive communication intervention for the critically ill. Am J Med 2000; 109:469–75

33. Ford Pitorak E, Beckham Armour M, Sivec HD. Project safe conduct integrates palliative goals into comprehensive cancer care. J Palliat Med 2003; 6:645–55

34. Drought TS, Koenig BA. "Choice" in end-of-life decision making: Researching fact or fiction? Gerontologist 2002; 42:114–28

35. Schneider CE. The Practice of Autonomy: Patients, Doctors, and Medical Decisions. Oxford University Press, New York, 1998

36. Nolan MT, Hughes M, Narendra DP, Sood JR, Terry PB, Astrow AB, Kub J, Thompson RE, Sulmasy DP. When patients lack capacity: the roles that patients with terminal diagnoses would choose for their physicians and loved ones in making medical decisions. J Pain Symptom Manage 2005; 30:342–53

37. Hawkins NA, Ditto PH, Danks JH, Smucker WD. Micromanaging death: Process preferences, values, and goals in end-of-life medical decision making. Gerontologist 2005; 45:107–17

38. Lo B, Quill T, Tulsky J. Discussing palliative care with patients. ACP-ASIM End-of-Life Care Consensus Panel. American College of Physicians-American Society of Internal Medicine. Ann Intern Med 1999; 130:744–9

39. Goold SD, Williams B, Arnold RM. Conflicts regarding decisions to limit treatment: a differential diagnosis. J Am Med Assoc 2000; 283:909–14

Index

Printed in the United States of America